Textbook of

OTOLARYNGOLOGY

Textbook of
OTOLARYNGOLOGY

COLLIN S. KARMODY, M.D.,
F.R.C.S.E., F.A.C.S.
Department of Otolaryngology
New England Medical Center
Tufts University, School of Medicine
Boston, Massachusetts

Lea & Febiger   1983   *Philadelphia*

Lea & Febiger
600 Washington Square
Philadelphia, PA 19106
U.S.A.

Library of Congress Cataloging in Publication Data

Karmody, Collin S.
    Textbook of otolaryngology.

    Bibliography: p.
    Includes index.
    1. Otolaryngology. I. Title. [DNLM: 1. Otorhinolaryn-
gologic diseases. WV 100 K18t]
RF46.K28 1983   617'.51   83-14868
ISBN 0-8121-0887-6

PRINTED IN THE UNITED STATES OF AMERICA

Print No. 3   2   1

To my family,

my teachers,

and my students.

PREFACE

The objective of this text is to provide a logical, rational, and easily comprehensible basis for the practice of modern otolaryngology with emphasis on diagnosis and management rather than on surgical techniques. I hope the content will be of substantial assistance to students of medicine at both the undergraduate and postgraduate levels and to the primary care physician. I have tried to detail fundamental and practical information on the diagnosis and treatment of disorders of the head and neck and to introduce the most recent thoughts in this specialty. Only the practical points on anatomy and physiology are emphasized except for a more detailed discussion of the anatomy and physiology of the ear, which is almost universally neglected in the curriculum of the modern medical school.

In the past three decades, the practice of otolaryngology has undergone significant changes in thought and scope, particularly in otology, the management of cancer of the head and neck, and in plastic surgery. The regional plastic surgery, although well within the province of the practicing otolaryngologist, is, however, not discussed in depth because it requires details of surgical technique that are beyond the scope of this text.

Single authorship, although currently out of vogue, is lovingly tedious, but has the advantage of consistency and balance in the presentation of the material. I hope this text combines these characteristics in a single volume that is manageable in both size and content.

Boston, MA   Collin S. Karmody

ACKNOWLEDGEMENTS

I am deeply indebted to Ms. Ruth Sigel for her painstaking typing of this manuscript, to Dr. Barbara Carter for her generous contribution of radiologic material and to Drs. Gerald Healy, Charles Vaughan, and Chris Doku for their clinical photographs. My colleagues Drs. Werner D. Chasin, Arnold E. Katz, and Victor E. Calcaterra have been most helpful, patient, and supportive. Finally, my thanks to the many medical students and residents who have read the manuscript and offered their suggestions.

CONTENTS

Chapter 1

HISTORY AND PHYSICAL EXAMINATION

HISTORY

Accurate medical diagnosis is based on the history, physical examination, and ancillary tests. Obtaining a detailed pertinent history is therefore absolutely essential and might even suggest the diagnosis. It is comparatively easy to attain if the examiner adheres to a set plan. First, obtain the details of the present illness and the past history of local and general problems. Follow this up by obtaining the pertinent family history. In the following pages the points regarding history-taking that are relevant to the individual areas of the head and neck are discussed.

Ear

SYMPTOMS. The symptoms to inquire about are pain, discharge, hearing loss, dizziness, and pain in the surrounding area, pharynx, and larynx.

PAIN. Pain (otalgia) might be caused by intrinsic otopathology or might be referred from elsewhere. The most common cause of otalgia and otorrhea is infection. Does the pain radiate? Severe otalgia frequently radiates to the jaw and neck. Furunculosis of the external ear canal may cause severe otalgia, which is accentuated by moving the jaw. Is there associated pain in the mouth or throat? Oral and pharyngeal symptoms might be referred to the ear (referred otalgia). Is fever present?

OTORRHEA. Inquire about the quantity, consistency, color, and odor of the discharge. Is it bloodstained? In acute otitis media profuse, bloodstained, mucoid discharge might occur suddenly. In external otitis the ear itches and usually weeps a small quantity of yellow material. In chronic otitis media drainage might be yellow and mucoid; it could be a small quantity and foul smelling, which is characteristic of a cholesteatoma.

HEARING LOSS. Question the patient regarding which side the hearing loss affects, its rapidity of onset, and its progression. Inquire about fluctuations in hearing; abnormal, constant or pulsatile painful responses to loud noises, and tinnitus (is it constant or pulsatile?). Does the patient's hearing ability change with position of the head (which indicates the presence of fluid in the middle ear)? Is there a previous history of exposure to loud noises, aminoglycoside antibiotics, ear infections, or to infectious diseases such as measles, mumps, meningitis, or syphilis? Is there a family history of hearing loss, renal disease, or pigmentary abnormalities?

DIZZINESS. "Dizziness" is a common

1

complaint, and it is surprising how patients describe widely diverse symptoms as dizziness. The examiner, therefore, must clarify this complaint by taking a careful and detailed history. Is the patient describing a sense of imbalance, light-headedness, or spinning (vertigo)? Vertigo is the subjective sensation of rotation of the patient or of his surroundings. Disorders of the labyrinth cause a sense of imbalance and vertigo. Is the sensation constant, intermittent, or related to posture? Does the patient lose consciousness or fall during an attack? Labyrinthine problems never cause a loss of consciousness. If the vertigo is episodic, what is the pattern of attacks? Are changes in hearing, tinnitus, or other aural symptoms associated with the attack?

OTHER FACTORS. Is there a history of recent or chronic ear infection? Acute and chronic otitis media may affect the vestibular labyrinth. Is there a history of recent or past injury to the head or neck, facial paralysis, cardiac problems, diabetes, or vascular disease? Is there a recent or past history of systemic infection such as syphilis, meningitis, or herpes? Does the patient have a history of allergies?

Nose, Sinuses, and Face

SYMPTOMS. The symptoms to inquire about are facial pain, nasal obstruction, nasal discharge, bleeding from the nose, sneezing, and loss of the sense of smell. There are two sides to the nose—always find out which side is the source of the problems.

FACIAL PAIN. Identify the exact location of the patient's facial pain. Pain in the lower third of the face is usually not caused by sinusitis. Does the pain begin in one area and then radiate? Does touching a specific point trigger pain (as in trigeminal neuralgia)?

NASAL OBSTRUCTION. Is nasal obstruction intermittent or constant? Is it unilateral or bilateral? Deviation of the nasal septum usually causes unilateral obstruc-

tion. Is obstruction triggered by a particular circumstance (e.g., exposure to pollens or animals, which is characteristic of allergic rhinitis)?

NASAL DISCHARGE. Nasal discharge (rhinorrhea) is an abnormal volume and consistency of nasal secretions. Are the secretions unilateral, yellow (purulent), malodorous, bloodstained, or frankly bloody? Purulent, even blood-streaked, secretions are common in suppurative sinusitis.

SNEEZING. Inquire about the pattern of sneezing. Sneezing is an important symptom of allergic rhinitis. Does the patient have swelling of the cheeks, forehead, or eyelids? Is there ophthalmia or diplopia?

OLFACTION. Is the sense of smell normal? Allergic polyps may cause total anosmia. Has the patient been exposed to specific allergens such as aspirin or detergents? Most patients complain about anosmia rather than hyperosmia. Is the anosmia constant or intermittent? Was there an antecedent viral upper respiratory infection? Chronic malodor might be caused by suppurative sinusitis, whereas a distortion of odors is associated with certain medications and intracranial lesions.

OTHER FACTORS. Is there a past history of recurrent sinusitis? "Sinusitis" is a much-abused term that is usually used as a diagnosis for all types of headaches and facial pain. A careful history of present and past episodes will usually clarify the problem. Does the patient have a recent or past history of allergy or clinical expression of allergy (e.g., hay fever or bronchospasm)?

Throat

SYMPTOMS. The symptoms to inquire about are local and referred pain, pain on swallowing (odynophagia), difficulty in swallowing (dysphagia), lump in the throat, and changes in vocal quality.

PAIN. Soreness of the throat is one of the most common human complaints. Are the symptoms acute, chronic, or recurrent?

How severe are the symptoms? Is the pain localized to one side, one area, or referred to the ear? Long-standing localized pain suggests a neoplasm.

SWALLOWING AND VOICE CHANGES. Can the patient swallow? Is swallowing difficult because of pain (odynophagia) or mechanical obstruction (dysphagia)? Has the patient noticed a change in his voice? Is fever present? All these symptoms may be present with a peritonsillar abscess.

OTHER FACTORS. Is there heartburn or a recent loss of weight? Does the patient have a past history of sore throat? If so, how frequent? Inquire about the treatment of these episodes. Tonsillitis tends to be recurrent. Has the patient had a tonsillectomy? Does he smoke or drink alcohol? Malignant neoplasms are more frequent in heavy smokers and heavy drinkers. Does the patient have specific allergies to dust, pollens, or foods? Inquire about a family history of tonsillitis, tonsillectomy, and neoplasms.

Larynx

SYMPTOMS. The symptoms to inquire about are hoarseness, local and referred pain, odynophagia, difficulty with breathing (stridor), and cough.

HOARSENESS. The usual symptom of a laryngeal disorder is hoarseness. The pertinent questions to ask about hoarseness are those regarding its duration, progression, episodes of aphonia, and associated pain and cough.

PAIN. Infection or extensive neoplasms of the larynx may cause local pain or odynophagia. Pain from the larynx and hypopharynx is frequently referred to the ear. Acute infection, as in epiglottitis, is accompanied by high fever.

STRIDOR. Obstruction of the airway at the laryngeal level causes difficulty with breathing, which may first be manifested by harsh, noisy breathing and dyspnea on exertion and may later progress to stridor. Stridor is a characteristic type of noisy breathing caused by significant compromise of the airway. The sound is that of air being sucked through a small opening with vibrating walls. Obstruction at the laryngeal level causes stridor on inspiration, while obstruction in the trachea or mainstem bronchi may cause expiratory stridor.

COUGH. Laryngeal disorders cause cough in two ways. Intrinsic irritation of the larynx, such as occurs with laryngitis or respiratory infections, is accompanied by a dry, annoying, nonproductive cough. Alternatively, if there is paralysis of a vocal cord, food might be aspirated on swallowing; the patient then experiences episodes of coughing whenever he eats or drinks.

OTHER FACTORS. Malignant neoplasms of the larynx are more common in the heavy smoker and drinker. Therefore, the examiner must ask about the use of cigarettes and alcohol. Is there a past history of injury or surgery to the patient's neck (e.g., thyroidectomy) or chest? Inquire about the recent or past history of systemic diseases, such as pulmonary tuberculosis or sarcoidosis. Inquire about a family history of malignancies and the smoking and drinking habits of the immediate family. Does a close relative of the patient have tuberculosis?

Esophagus

SYMPTOMS. The symptoms to inquire about are dysphagia, heartburn, pain in the midline of the back of the thorax, and soreness of the throat.

DYSPHAGIA. The most common esophageal symptom is difficulty with swallowing. Dysphagia can be either acute or chronic. Acute obstruction is caused by impacted foreign bodies, infections, or muscle spasm. Chronic obstructive dysphagia is frequently caused by neoplasms or long-standing strictures.

HEARTBURN. Reflux esophagitis causes heartburn but can also cause pain referred to the pharynx.

The questions listed in this section are only guidelines. The region of the head and neck, although anatomically complex, is comparatively small, and it is not uncommon for many areas to be symptomatically involved by the same pathologic process. Furthermore, the examiner should remember that disorders in this area may only be local expressions of systemic disease.

PHYSICAL EXAMINATION

The head and neck region is an area of crowded anatomy with close relationships among component structures. Therefore, examination of many structures is usually performed simultaneously. For purposes of descriptive clarity, however, the areas will be discussed individually.

General Points

Good lighting is a basic necessity of otolaryngologic examination, whether it be with a head mirror or headlight. The patient is comfortably seated, and the examiner stands or sits in front of him. Few instruments are needed to perform a thorough examination of the head and neck. These instruments are shown in Figure 1.1.

USE OF THE HEAD MIRROR. Most otolaryngologists prefer to use a head mirror or head light because they focus to a bright light and free both hands. With a head mirror, the light source should be easily adjustable directionally (e.g., on a "goose neck," angle poise, or ball-and-socket joint) and must be of about 100 watts in intensity. The light is positioned behind and just to one side of the patient's head on the same side as the head mirror (Figure 1.2). The most useful head mirror is 3.5 in. in diameter with a central aperture diameter of 0.5 to 0.75 in. The head mirror is positioned in front of the examiner's eye, to the right or left depending on personal preference and close to but not against the examiner's face. The mirror is adjusted so that the light focuses on the patient.

The Ear

The ear should be examined methodically so that nothing is missed. First, the pinna is examined and carefully palpated. Next, the mastoid process is examined and palpated. Finally, the periauricular area is palpated.

INSTRUMENTS. The following is a list of the instruments that are used to examine the ear.
1. Light source (head mirror, headlight, electric otoscope)
2. Aural speculum
3. Cerumen loop or curette
4. Suction apparatus

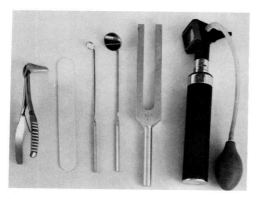

Fig. 1.1. The basic instruments required for examination of the ear, nose, and throat. From left to right: nasal speculum, tongue depressor, small- and large-angled mirrors, tuning fork, and electric otoscope. The otoscope is sealed with a magnifying lens and has a rubber bulb for pneumatic otoscopy.

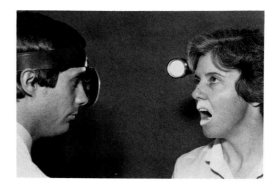

Fig. 1.2. Use of the head mirror. A light source is placed close to the patient's head. Light is reflected from the concave mirror and focuses on the patient. Note the position of the mirror close to the examiner's face.

5. Cotton-tipped applicators
6. Tuning forks

The external ear canal and tympanic membrane are examined through an aural speculum. An aural speculum is essentially a funnel that concentrates light at its narrower end. There are many designs of specula (Figure 1.3). Those with oval-shaped, smaller ends are easier to use. Siegle's speculum is a special type used

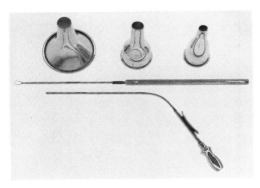

Fig. 1.3. Three types of aural specula, a wire loop for removing cerumen, and a cannula for suction. A different type of speculum is used for pneumatic otoscopy.

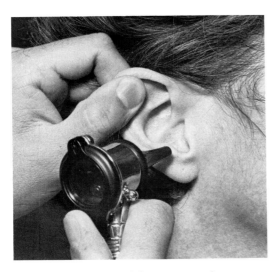

Fig. 1.4. Examination of the ear using a battery-powered otoscope. Note that the fingers of one hand are pulling the top of the pinna upward and backward. The instrument has been turned on and the beak of the speculum is about to be gently introduced into the meatus.

for pneumatic otoscopy, which is a procedure for determining mobility of the tympanic membrane. This speculum is rounded, with a thickened, narrower end. A glass-faced chamber fits snugly into the wider end, and a bulb is attached to this chamber. Squeezing the bulb alters pressure in the system and moves the tympanic membrane in and out.

TECHNIQUE. There are three essential steps to be taken in the examination of the external ear canal and tympanic membrane:

1. It is always necessary throughout the examination to straighten the canal by pulling the pinna upward and backward (Figure 1.4). This aligns the cartilaginous and bony canals.
2. The meatus of the canal should be inspected before a speculum is introduced. This determines whether a furuncle, cerumen, discharge, neoplasm, or other condition exists that might prevent a more thorough examination. Large amounts of cerumen should first be removed with a loop or curette under direct vision (see Chapter 5). Secretions are first sampled for bacteriologic study and then cleared by suctioning or with cotton-tipped applicators.
3. The external canal and tympanic membrane are inspected directly through a speculum. The speculum is introduced under direct vision and is passed to just a few millimeters beyond the hair-bearing areas but no further.

If an electric otoscope (Figure 1.1) is used, the light should be turned on before the speculum is introduced into the meatus. The examiner should keep his eye constantly applied to the instrument so that the end of the speculum is not introduced too far into the canal, in which case examination will become painful and, particularly in children, will no longer be tolerated.

The cartilaginous external canal is lined

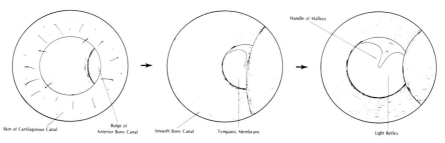

Handle of Malleus

Skin of Cartilaginous Canal   Bulge of Anterior Bony Canal   Smooth Bony Canal   Tympanic Membrane   Light Reflex

Fig. 1.5. Sequential views on examination of the external auditory canal. In the first frame the hair-bearing cartilaginous canal is seen (the tympanic membrane is not visualized). In the second frame, as the instrument is passed slightly deeper, the smooth nonhair-bearing walls of the bony canal are seen; the skin here is usually pink. At the deep end of the external auditory canal the posterior edge of the gray tympanic membrane is just visible. The third frame shows the view that is obtained with the instrument at its deepest position. The tympanic membrane is seen in its entirety. A small segment anteriorly may be obscured by the anterior wall of the canal.

with soft, thick skin that contains hair and ceruminous glands. The bony canal is lined with thin, smooth, pink skin (Figure 1.5).

The tympanic membrane is concave, pearl-gray, and smooth. It slopes downward, forward, and medially. The handle of the malleus is embedded in the middle of the upper half of the tympanic membrane. At the upper end of the handle is the white lateral process, which is the most prominent visible structure on the tympanic membrane. At the lower end of the handle of the malleus is the umbo, which is at the center of the membrane and at the fundus of its concavity. The direction of the membrane relative to the incidence of light causes a triangular-shaped area of brightness, the light reflex, which spreads anteroinferiorly from the umbo (Figure 1.5). The mobility of the membrane is assessed by altering the pressure in the ear canal with a Siegle's speculum. For further details of the tympanic membrane see Chapter 3.

After the physical examination is completed, the level of hearing is evaluated (see Chapter 4). Following this, the vestibular system is assessed (see Chapter 9).

Nose and Sinuses

INSTRUMENTS. The following is a list of the instruments that are used to examine the nose and sinuses.

1. Light source
2. Nasal speculum
3. Tongue depressor
4. Small-angled mirror
5. Mirror warmer
6. Suction apparatus
7. Vasoconstrictor spray (phenylephrine hydrochloride, 0.25%)

TECHNIQUE. The nose should be examined systematically by external examination, anterior rhinoscopy, posterior rhinoscopy, and testing of olfaction (see Chapter 13).

EXTERNAL EXAMINATION. Observe first and carefully for asymmetry, signs of inflammation or trauma, tumors, or anomalies. If injury or inflammation is present, palpate gently. Feel the nasal bones and

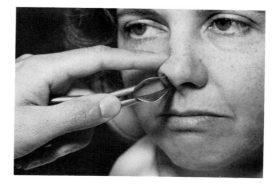

Fig. 1.6. The use of the Vienna model nasal speculum. The closed blades are introduced in an upward and downward position and do not reach the nasal mucosa. The blades are then gently opened.

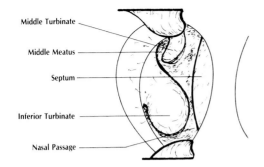

Fig. 1.7. The structures that are visible by anterior rhinoscopy. Greater detail can be obtained by gently rotating the patient's head.

then the cartilaginous nose. Test for patency of the airway one side at a time. Palpate by gentle pressure over the sinuses, over the cheeks for maxillary sinuses, over the forehead and on the roof of the orbit for the frontal sinuses, and on the medial wall of the orbit for the anterior ethmoid sinuses.

ANTERIOR RHINOSCOPY. Examination of the nasal passages requires a spreading speculum to displace the ala. The most popular speculum in use is the spring-loaded Vienna model (Figure 1.1). The light is first directed at the nose, and the blades of the speculum are gently introduced under direct vision to spread the nares upward and downward and not laterally (Figure 1.6). The tips of the blades should not touch the sensitive nasal mucosa. When the internal structures can be seen clearly, they should be examined carefully. Moving the patient and the examiner's head slightly in different directions will bring most of the available structures into view (Figure 1.7). Note the size of the turbinates and the condition of the mucosa. Look carefully for evidence of infection (velvety mucosa and a yellow or watery discharge). Look for polyps in the middle meatus. Are there any signs of neoplasm, such as a bloodstained discharge and obstructing masses? Examine the nasal septum. Is it in the midline or to one side? Are there ridges and spurs? Does the sep-

tum compromise the airway? If the mucosa is too swollen, it can be shrunk by spraying with phenylephrine hydrochloride, 0.25%; wait for 10 minutes and then reexamine.

POSTERIOR RHINOSCOPY. Posterior rhinoscopy is really an examination of the nasopharynx. It is achieved by the use of a small-angled mirror that is placed just posterior to the uvula. Depress the tongue with a spatula, and introduce the mirror gently and manipulate it to a position just behind and to one side of the uvula (Figure 1.8). Position the angle of the mirror so that the choana and the posterior edge of the septum can be seen. Systematically examine the choana, posterior ends of the turbinates, orifices of the eustachian tubes, median adenoid mass and the lateral walls of the nasopharynx, and the posterior surface of the soft palate (Figure 1.9). If a pu-

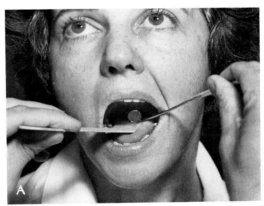

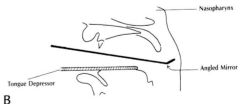

Fig. 1.8. *A.* Posterior rhinoscopy. The tongue is depressed by a spatula, and a small-angled mirror is introduced from the side. The mirror is passed farther posteriorly than is shown here. *B.* Diagram showing the principle of posterior rhinoscopy. The small-angled mirror has been passed just posterior to the soft palate.

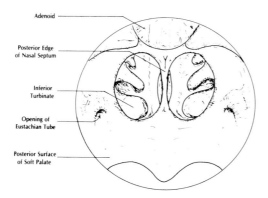

Adenoid

Posterior Edge
of Nasal Septum

Inferior
Turbinate

Opening of
Eustachian Tube

Posterior Surface
of Soft Palate

Fig. 1.9. The structures that are seen on posterior rhinoscopy. The small size of the mirror does not allow a panoramic view, such as is depicted in this diagram. The mirror must be rotated from side to side to view the entire nasopharynx.

rulent exudate is present, try to identify its source; that is, whether it is from the inferior, middle, or superior meatus. The maxillary and ethmoid sinuses drain into the middle meatus. A view of the choana can be prevented by poor technique, by the adenoid mass in children, or by neoplasms in adults.

Oral Cavity

INSTRUMENTS. The following is a list of the instruments that are used to examine the oral cavity.

1. Bright light source
2. Tongue depressor
3. Angled mirror
4. Gauze sponge
5. Finger cot

TECHNIQUE. The oral cavity is a deceptively large space with many expandible crevices that would be missed unless they were deliberately opened. Therefore, this cavity should be approached systematically, using the tongue depressor as the main instrument.

Examine sequentially the vestibule of the mouth, buccal mucosa, teeth and gums, tongue, floor of the mouth, salivary glands, and hard and soft palates.

VESTIBULE OF THE MOUTH. The vestibule of the mouth is the space between the lips

and gums. Open this with a tongue depressor or finger by everting the lips, and palpate the area carefully. The vestibule is followed posteriorly into the posterior buccogingival sulcus. At this stage examine the buccal mucosa, which is the inner surface of the cheek, paying particular attention to the ductal papillae of the parotid glands that are opposite the second upper molar teeth.

TEETH AND GUMS. Examine the teeth and gums. Use a warm, angled mirror to see the posterior surfaces of the teeth. Check for sensitivity by tapping gently on the teeth with a small metallic instrument. Look carefully at the gums—are they inflamed? Are the interdental papillae red and swollen?

TONGUE. Examine the tongue. Look at its dorsal surface. The surface is normally pink and rough because of numerous papillae. There are usually no deep furrows. If the papillae are absent, the surface becomes smooth, shiny, and reddened. Papillae are lost in many disorders such as vitamin B deficiency and anemia. Check the mobility and relative size of the two sides of the tongue. If one hypoglossal nerve is damaged, the ipsilateral tongue is paralyzed and atrophies. The tongue can-

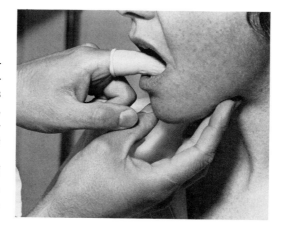

Fig. 1.10. Palpating the floor of the mouth and submandibular salivary glands and adjacent lymph nodes.

not then be voluntarily pushed to the opposite side.

FLOOR OF THE MOUTH AND SALIVARY GLANDS. Examine the undersurface of the tongue, the floor of the mouth, and submandibular salivary glands by the bidigital maneuver shown in Figure 1.10. Note the papillae of the salivary glands.

HARD AND SOFT PALATES. Examine the hard and soft palates (velum). Note the integrity of the hard palate and the shape of its arch (i.e., whether it is high or low). Next, examine the soft palate. Check its integrity. Complete clefting is obvious, but submucosal clefting is more subtle and is frequently missed. It is identified as a bluish line down the midline of the soft palate in association with a bifid uvula. Palpate the posterior edge of the hard palate. A notch in its posterior edge is usually associated with submucosal clefting of the soft palate. Check for the mobility of the soft palate by asking the patient to say "ah." The palate should move upward and posteriorly and should make contact with the midline of the posterior pharyngeal wall. With an incompetent velopharyngeal isthmus, the voice is hypernasal, air is emitted from the nostril during phonation, and food might be regurgitated through the nose on swallowing.

Oropharynx, Hypopharynx, and Larynx

INSTRUMENTS. The following is a list of the instruments that are used to examine the oropharynx, hypopharynx, and larynx.
1. Light source (head mirror or headlight)
2. Tongue depressors
3. Angled mirrors (small, medium, and large)
4. Gauze sponges
5. Mirror warmer (alcohol lamp)
6. Finger cots
7. Topical anesthetic

TECHNIQUE. In the following section the techniques of examining the oropharynx, hypopharynx, and larynx will be dis-

cussed separately. See the section on posterior rhinoscopy in this chapter for the technique of examining the nasopharynx.

OROPHARYNX. The oropharynx is an integral part of the examination of the oral cavity. Both are visible during the same examination. Direct bright light into the mouth and center it just below the uvula. The tongue stays in the mouth and does not protrude. Gently depress the tongue with a wooden or metal depressor. The palatine arch, palatine tonsils, and posterior pharyngeal walls are usually easily visible. If not, ask the patient to say "ah"; this makes the palate move upward, the tongue move downward, and exposes more of the tonsils and posterior pharynx. Note the symmetry and mobility of the soft palate. Unilateral paralysis of the soft palate is caused by neoplasms or by lesions of the fifth or tenth cranial nerves. Carefully assess the tonsils. Note whether they are symmetric, inflamed, or ulcerated. If a neoplasm is present, palpate with a gloved finger or with a soft-tipped, blunt instrument.

HYPOPHARYNX AND LARYNX. Examine the hypopharynx and larynx together by indirect laryngoscopy using a large-angled

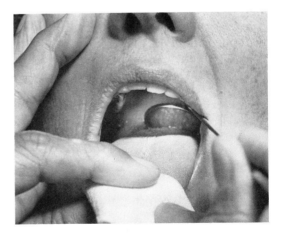

Fig. 1.11. The technique of indirect laryngoscopy. The tongue is pulled forward and held with a gauze sponge. The warm, angled mirror is passed gently superior to the tongue to a position that is more posterior than is shown here.

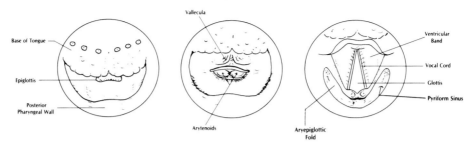

Fig. 1.12. Sequential views during indirect laryngoscopy. The following structures are seen in order: the dorsum of the tongue, the base of the tongue, the epiglottis, arytenoid eminences, aryepiglottic folds, pyriform sinuses, ventricular bands, vocal cords, and upper trachea.

mirror (Figure 1.1). A mirror gives an image that is turned around to 180° in all directions. The patient should be sitting upright with the neck straight and the head slightly thrust forward, but not extended. Encourage the patient to relax and breathe deeply and rhythmically. Have him open his mouth, and focus the light on the base of the uvula. Next, warm the mirror, testing it on the back of the examiner's hand. Have the patient stick out his tongue and gently but firmly grasp it with a gauze sponge, using the left hand. Introduce the mirror gently and carefully on the left side of the patient's mouth with the glass surface parallel to the tongue (Figure 1.11). When the mirror reaches the soft palate, rotate it so that the glass surface is 45° to the vertical. At this point, focus the light on the mirror. The position of the mirror and light should bring the structure of the hypopharynx and larynx into view. If not, rotate the mirror slowly and gently and displace the uvula upward and backward. For a better view and to assess the mobility of the structures, ask the patient to say "eh" and/or "ee." The following structures should come into view in sequence (Figure 1.12) (for greater detail see Chapter 19):

 Base of the tongue—anterior, irregular, pink.

 Epiglottis—anterior, flat, curved, freestanding, yellow to pink with a few delicate vessels on its surface.

Vallecula—anterior between the base of the tongue and the epiglottis. These are shallow depressions divided in the midline by a delicate fold of mucosa.

Arytenoid eminences—posterior, deep to the epiglottis. These are rounded, mucosa-covered masses of cartilage that are separated by a central depression. The arytenoids move with respiration and phonation.

Aryepiglottic folds—two delicate folds of mucosa, one on each side, which extend from the arytenoid eminences to the lateral borders of the epiglottis.

Ventricular bands (false cords)—two mucosa-covered, smooth, comparatively thick bands disposed in an anteroposterior direction, just inferomedial to the aryepiglottic folds and superior to the true vocal cords.

Vocal cords—normal vocal cords are white. There are two, one on each side, which meet in the midline anteriorly at the base of the epiglottis and diverge posteriorly as they join the arytenoids. The visible part of the vocal cords in adults is about 5 mm wide. Vocal cords move with breathing and phonation. They come together with high-pitched sounds, such as "ee," and are then more easily visible.

They abduct (spread apart) with deep inspiration.

Subglottic area and upper trachea—with a cooperative patient it is possible to see the anterior half of the subglottic area and three to four rings of the upper trachea. The mucosa is thin, and the white cartilaginous rings can be identified easily.

Salivary Glands

The major salivary glands are comparatively superficial and easy to examine. The sublingual and submandibular glands are best palpated with a finger in the floor of the mouth and two or three fingers externally (Figure 1.10). The parotid glands are posterior to the ramus of the mandible and inferior to the external auditory canal. They slip into the retromolar area when the mouth is open and, therefore, are best examined with the mouth closed. Feel both glands between thumb and index finger and with the flat of the fingers. Examine the floor of the cartilaginous ear canal for displacement or for salivary fistulas. Examine the ductal papillae of all the salivary glands. Milk the ducts to assess the quality and quantity of salivary flow and, if necessary, use a sialagogue (lemon juice).

Neck

The neck is examined by observation, palpation, and auscultation. Place the patient in a sitting position with both shoulders horizontally at rest. The chin and sternum should be in a straight vertical line. Look for obvious swelling, redness of the skin, and other signs of inflammation. Note any asymmetry from muscular wasting or spasm. View the neck from the front and side, noting whether the larynx and trachea are displaced. Palpation of the neck is done preferably with the examiner standing behind the patient. Use both hands, one on each side, and palpate with the pads of the fingers (Figure 1.13).

Palpation must be done systematically.

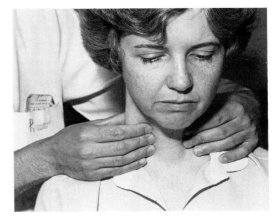

Fig. 1.13. Palpating the neck. The neck is slightly flexed. The examiner stands behind the patient and palpates with the flat of the hand and pads of the fingers. Deeper palpation is possible by curving the fingers around the sternocleidomastoid muscles as shown on the left.

All structures in the neck are palpable, and some are easily visible. The examiner's own neck provides a readily available model for practice. Begin superiorly at the chin and move inferiorly in the midline. Successively palpate the following: the submental area, containing a few salivary glands and lymph nodes; the hyoid bone; the thyrohyoid membrane; and the keel-like V-shaped thyroid cartilage with a lamina on each side joined in the midline. Next, feel a dimple inferior to the thyroid cartilage; this is the area of the cricothyroid membrane. Inferior to the cricothyroid membrane is the rounded eminence of the cricoid cartilage. Below the cricoid cartilage are the cartilaginous rings of the trachea. The isthmus of the thyroid glands can be felt as a soft structure anterior to the trachea. Deep palpation in the paratracheal groove gives some idea of the condition of the periesophageal area. Next, palpate the lobes of the thyroid gland. Ask the patient to swallow; the trachea and thyroid gland move upward and are momentarily more easily palpated.

The examiner then moves his fingers laterally, with the tips of the fingers curving deep to the inferior sternocleidomastoid muscles. Identify the carotid pulsations.

This determines the position of the jugular vein and the chain of the jugular lymph nodes. Palpate firmly, moving superiorly along the jugular vein and paying attention to the carotid pulsations, while simultaneously examining for lymphadenopathy. Continue the examination to the tips of the mastoids. Next, move both hands across the occipital region, feeling for lymph nodes. Then, with the flat of the fingers sweep the hands inferiorly over the posterior triangles to the clavicles. Palpate the supraclavicular fossa carefully. If a mass is identified in the neck, additional information can be obtained by standing in front of the patient and using the thumb and index fingers for assessment. Examine each mass for consistency and fluctuation; identify as far as possible its point of origin (e.g., thyroid gland, lymph node). Auscultate all neck masses; some vascular masses have audible bruits.

Examining Children

Children are inherently afraid of medical instruments. It is, therefore, wise to spend a few minutes with a child and allow him to play with the instruments, so that he loses some of his fear. At the same time, the examiner tickles the child's ear to acquaint him with the feel of the otoscope. (Remember that the normal tympanic membrane of the crying child quickly becomes hyperemic, which is easily misdiagnosed as infection.) If it is impossible to examine the child, he must be wrapped in a sheet and "mummified." He is then held in a sitting position on a nurse's lap. The nurse's right hand anchors the child's head across the forehead, the nurse's left arm holds him firmly across the chest, and the child's legs are locked between the nurse's crossed knees.

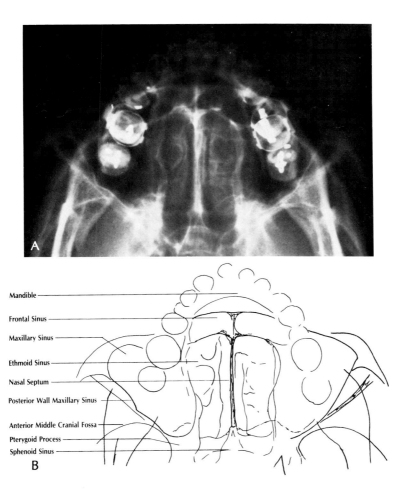

Mandible
Frontal Sinus
Maxillary Sinus
Ethmoid Sinus
Nasal Septum
Posterior Wall Maxillary Sinus
Anterior Middle Cranial Fossa
Pterygoid Process
Sphenoid Sinus
B

Fig. 2.4. Submental vertex position. The plane of the image is roughly horizontal. This position demonstrates the maxillary, sphenoid, and, sometimes, the frontal sinuses. The ethmoid labyrinths are overshadowed by the inferior turbinates.

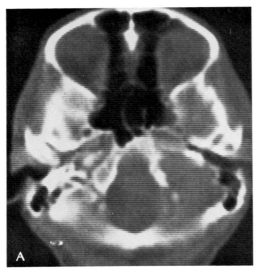

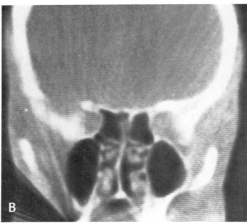

Fig. 2.5. Computed tomography of the paranasal sinuses. (Courtesy of Barbara Carter, M.D.)
A. Axial (transverse) plane through the ethmoid, frontal, and sphenoid sinuses and the orbits. The air-containing spaces are black.
B. Coronal plane through the maxillary and ethmoid sinuses. The detail of the bony walls of the sinuses and of the contained soft tissue that is revealed makes computed tomography a most useful technique.

ethmoid sinuses, and the nasal turbinates are also well demonstrated. This is the only position in which the foramen rotundum can be seen.

LATERAL. This position is good for the frontal and sphenoid sinuses and, to a lesser extent, the maxillary and ethmoid sinuses. This position is also useful for

showing the thickness of the skull and demonstrating the sella turcica. Lateral roentgenograms usually include the nasopharynx (Figure 2.3A and B). A true lateral roentgenogram is not easy to obtain because some degree of tilt usually exists that produces double lines (e.g., two "mandibles," two "zygomas," etc.).

SUBMENTAL VERTEX. This position is useful for the sphenoid and maxillary sinuses but is less so for the frontal sinuses. The nasopharynx and the foramina in the base of the skull are well shown in this position (Figure 2.4A and B). The plate is horizontal above the head and the roentgen tube is directed from below the lower jaw. The posterior walls of the maxillary and frontal sinuses and the pterygopalatine spaces, which are directly posterior to the maxillary sinuses, are seen only on lateral and submental vertex roentgenograms.

OBLIQUE LATERAL. The standard roentgenograms of the optic canals are oblique laterals of the sinuses, which show the posterior ethmoid sinuses very clearly. In England and Europe the oblique lateral position is included as one of the standard positions of the paranasal sinuses.

Multidirectional Tomography

Multidirectional tomography is a most useful technique for delineating the bony walls of the sinuses and for defining intracavitary soft tissues. Tomographic cuts can be obtained in the coronal, lateral, and horizontal (submental vertex) planes. Multidirectional tomography, however, is time-consuming and expensive.

Computed Tomography

Computed tomography (CT) shows the paranasal sinuses very clearly and is particularly valuable for defining the parameters of neoplasms (Figure 2.5A and B). Computed tomography provides excellent horizontal cuts through the sinuses. Coronal and lateral cuts, however, are not as sharply defined because they are recon-

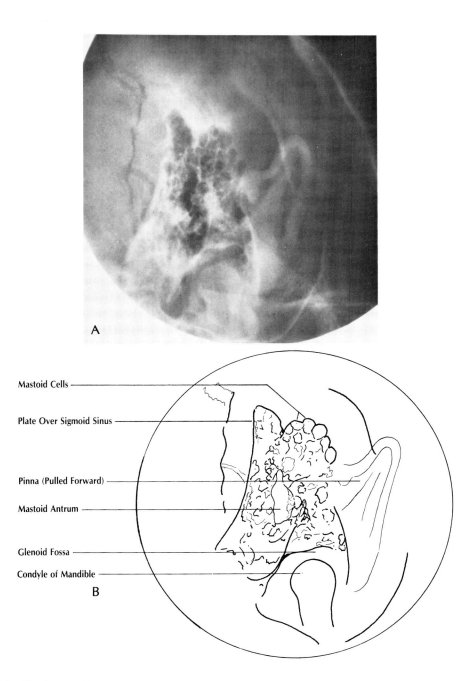

Fig. 2.6. The Law position.

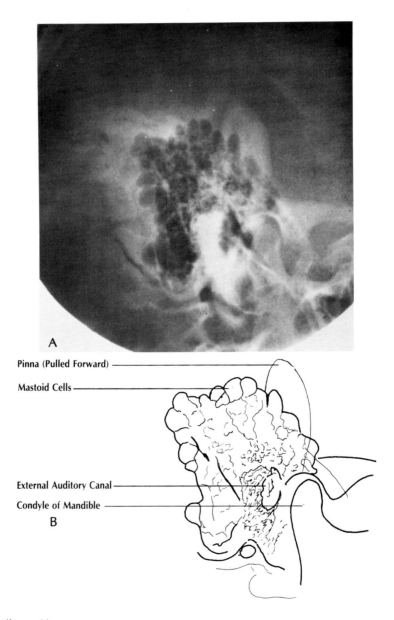

A

Pinna (Pulled Forward) ——————

Mastoid Cells ——————

External Auditory Canal ——————

Condyle of Mandible ——————

B

Fig. 2.7.   Schuller position

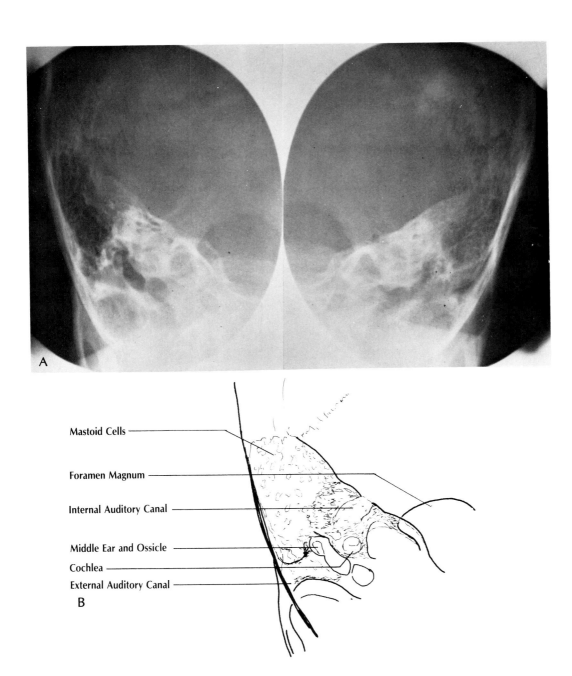

Fig. 2.8.   Towne position

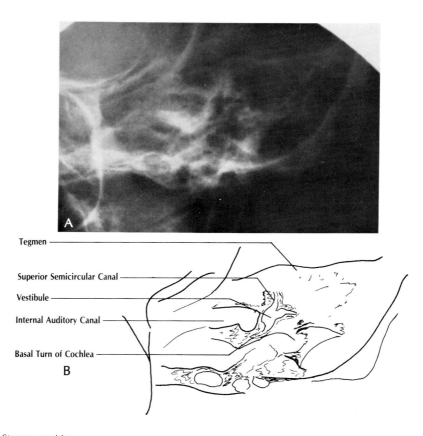

Fig. 2.9.   Stenver position

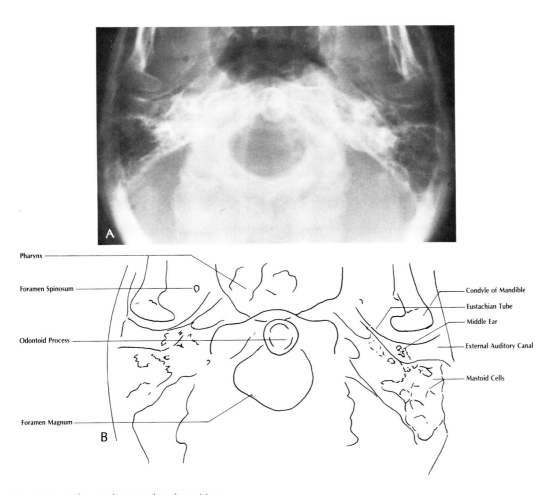

Fig. 2.10. Submental vertex (basal) position

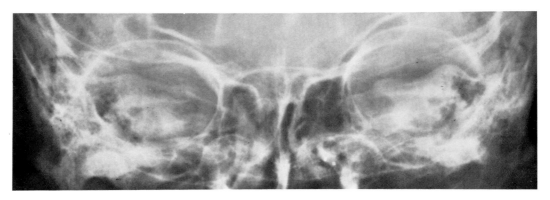

Fig. 2.11. Transorbital position. Both internal auditory canals are seen simultaneously through the orbits. The vestibules of the inner ears present as round lucencies, while there are faint outlines of the horizontal and superior semicircular canals.

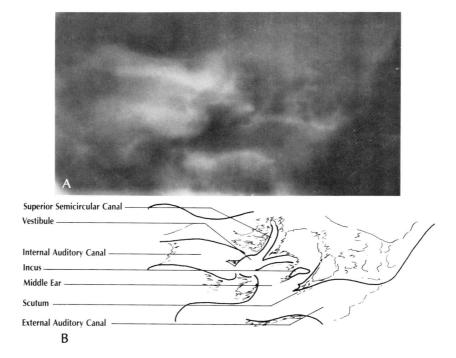

A

Superior Semicircular Canal

Vestibule

Internal Auditory Canal

Incus

Middle Ear

Scutum

External Auditory Canal

B

Fig. 2.12. Multidirectional tomography. This is a frame in an anteroposterior plane. The external auditory canal, middle ear, semicircular canals, and internal auditory canals are seen in detail. (Courtesy of Barbara Carter, M.D.)

structions by the computer rather than direct views.

THE EAR

Three types of mastoid bones are seen on roentgenograms: cellular, sclerotic, and diploic. A cellular mastoid represents normal development and has a large number of air-containing cells with very thin walls. A cellular mastoid looks like a blackened honeycomb on a roentgenogram. Diseased, fluid-filled cells are hazy and gray on a roentgenogram. A sclerotic mastoid contains only a few cells with thick walls. A diploic mastoid, which is the rarest type, contains virtually no cells, being a solid block of bone.

Standard Positions

Four standard positions are used to evaluate the mastoid cells, antrum, and epitympanum. These are: (1) the Law position (Figure 2.6); (2) Schuller's position (Figure 2.7); (3) Towne's position (Figure 2.8); and (4) Stenver's position (Figure 2.9). The fifth position, the submental vertex (basal) (Figure 2.10), is an optional view.

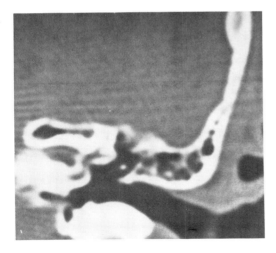

Fig. 2.13. Computed tomography of the temporal bones in the coronal plane. There is a faint outline of the ossicles. The superior and horizontal semicircular canals, the basal turn of the cochlea, and the internal auditory canal are well demonstrated. (Courtesy of Barbara Carter, M.D.)

In the first three positions the photographic plate is placed beneath the patient's head. The roentgen tube is angled to prevent superimposing the mastoids on each other.

LAW. This position gives a nearly true lateral view. The tube is angled a little superiorly, projecting the mastoid cells above the condyle of the mandible (Figure 2.6). The cell system is well demonstrated, and intercellular septa are sharply defined. The middle ear, however, is not visible. The smooth plate of bone that covers the sigmoid sinus can be seen clearly.

SCHULLER. As the angle of the tube is elevated, the dense petrous part of the temporal bone is more depressed away from the rest of the temporal bone. The mastoid cells are well demonstrated, and the intercellular septa are sharply defined. The bony part of the external canal and the middle ear are seen as a common space posterior to the glenoid fossa. The ossicles are usually visible.

TOWNE. In this position the temporal bones are raised above the facial skeleton. The entire vertical dimension of the mastoid bone and the tegmen mastoidea can be assessed. The internal auditory canal can be seen, as well as the cavity of the middle ear and the malleus (Figure 2.8). The cochlea is sometimes comparatively well defined.

STENVER. This position gives a view along the long axis of the temporal bone and shows the vestibule, and the horizontal and superior semicircular canals (Figure 2.9). The internal auditory canal is clearly demonstrated and can even be measured. The cavity of the middle ear and the scutum are not seen adequately, but are best defined in a Chausse III position, which is a slight modification of Stenver's position.

SUBMENTAL VERTEX (BASAL). The view obtained from this position is parallel to the base of the skull. The external auditory canal, middle ear, and mastoid bones are well demonstrated (Figure 2.10).

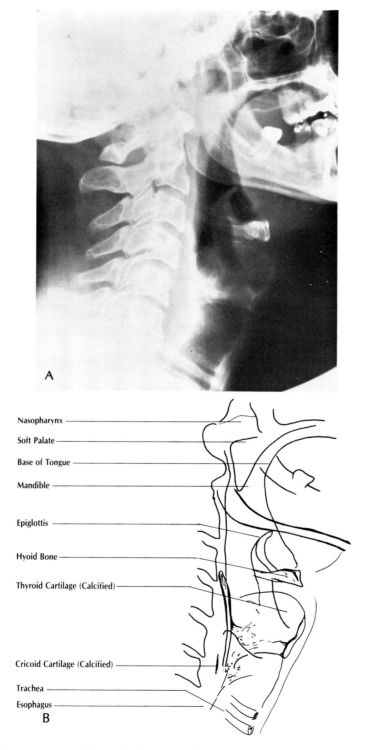

Nasopharynx

Soft Palate

Base of Tongue

Mandible

Epiglottis

Hyoid Bone

Thyroid Cartilage (Calcified)

Cricoid Cartilage (Calcified)

Trachea

Esophagus

Fig. 2.14. Lateral roentgenogram of the neck of a 60-year-old male. The laryngeal cartilages have calcified, which is a normal process of aging. The posterior lamina of the cricoid cartilage looks deceptively like a foreign body. The air-containing ventricle immediately above the vocal cord is seen as a faint horizontal line.

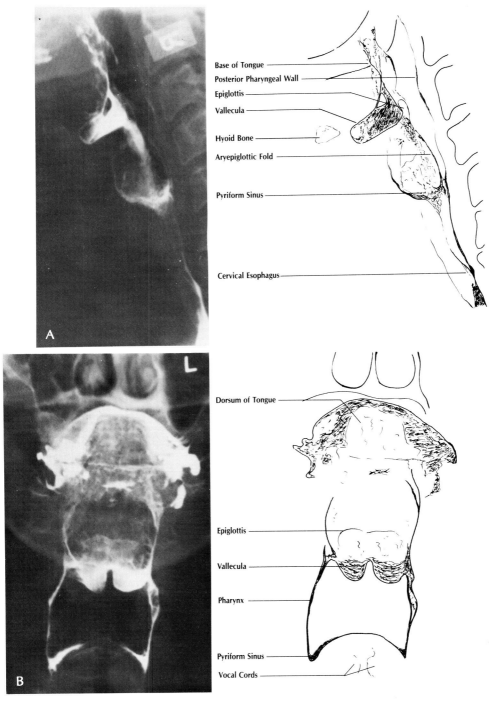

Fig. 2.15. Barium swallow. Barium sulfate is used to outline the pharynx and upper esophagus. The technique is popular and most useful.

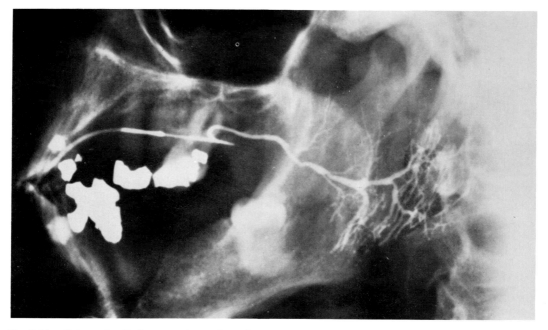

Fig. 2.16. Sialography. Radiopaque dye outlines the ductal system of the parotid gland, seen here on a lateral view. (Courtesy of Barbara Carter, M.D.)

Even the ossicles can be identified, and the line of the eustachian tube is visible. The stylomastoid foramen, through which the facial nerve exits, is sometimes seen easily.

TRANSORBITAL POSITION. The head and roentgen tube are aligned so that the apices of the petrous temporal bones are seen within the framework of the orbits. If this technique is successful, it provides the best undistorted view of the internal auditory canals. Both internal canals are visible on the same film and can be compared with some degree of accuracy.

The vestibule, cochlea, and internal auditory canals are demonstrated by Towne's (Figure 2.8), Stenver's (Figure 2.9), and transorbital (Figure 2.11) positions.

Multidirectional Tomography

Multidirectional tomography provides finer detail, particularly for the study of the external auditory canal, middle ear, inner ear, and internal auditory canal (Figure 2.12).

Contrast Radiography

Contrast radiography is used to define the contents of the posterior cranial fossa and the internal auditory canal. The contrast medium can be air, isophendylate (Pantopaque), or water-soluble metrizamide.

Computed Tomography

Computed tomography has become an important technique in evaluation of the ear and temporal bone and might soon replace multidirectional tomography (Figure 2.13). CT scans are particularly useful for studying the posterior cranial fossa and for demonstrating tumors of the cerebellopontine angle. CT scanning, combined with air as a contrast medium, can identify very small masses in the internal auditory canal.

THE THROAT

Radiologic evaluation of the pharynx is limited. The nasopharynx, oropharynx, and hypopharynx can all be seen on a standard lateral roentgenogram of the neck (Figure 2.14). Soft tissues show clearly, and their anatomic limits can be assessed. Better delineations can be obtained, using fluoroscopic techniques, with barium as a contrast medium. Computed tomography does show the pharynx in horizontal section and demonstrates soft tissues more clearly, and is, therefore, useful for assessing neoplasms and infections.

THE LARYNX

The larynx is seen reasonably well on the lateral roentgenogram of the neck. In infants and children most of the larynx is comparatively clearly outlined. The laryngeal cartilages begin to calcify in early adulthood and are clearly seen in middle-aged and elderly patients. Calcification is patchy and might be misinterpreted as a radiopaque foreign body or an invasion by a neoplasm (Figure 2.14). Contrast laryngography outlines the mucosal surfaces of the hypopharynx and larynx and clearly defines the supraglottic areas. Multidirectional tomography is also very useful for studying the larynx. Even the motion of the vocal cords can be determined. CT scanning is becoming an increasingly popular method of evaluating the larynx and is particularly useful for assessing the extent of soft-tissue neoplasms, the pre-epiglottic space, and adjacent structures.

Barium Swallow

This radiographic technique shows the base of the tongue, oropharynx, hypopharynx, and esophagus (Figure 2.15A and B). The technique also demonstrates competence of the glottis because barium will pass into the larynx and trachea if the glottis is incompetent.

Angiography

Radiographic examination of the major blood vessels in the neck is sometimes necessary. This can be achieved either by arteriography or venography.

Sialography

Sialography is the technique of contrast radiography of the salivary glands (Figure 2.16). Only the parotid and submandibular glands are amenable to this radiographic technique. Contrast material is injected to fill the ductal systems of the glands, and filling defects are easily demonstrated. Sialography is now combined with CT scanning for better definition.

Radioisotope Scans

Radioisotope scans are useful in the area of the head and neck. Technetium is concentrated in the salivary glands, particularly the parotids. [131]I delineates the thyroid gland. Gallium scans are useful for detecting lymphomatous disease because gallium is readily taken up by dividing leukocytes.

BIBLIOGRAPHY

Carter, B.L., and Karmody, C.S.: Computed tomography of the face and neck. Sem. Roentgenol., 22(No. 3):257–266, 1978.
Compere, W.C.: Radiographic Atlas of the Temporal Bone. Rochester, Minn., American Academy of Ophthalmology and Otolaryngology, 1964.
Dodd, G.D., and Jing, B.S.: Radiology of the nose, paranasal sinuses, and nasopharynx. Section 2. Golden's Diagnostic Radiology Series. Baltimore, The Williams and Wilkins Company, 1977.
Fletcher, G., and Jing, B.S.: An Atlas of Tumor Radiology—The Head and Neck. Chicago, Yearbook Medical Publishers, 1968.
Merrel, R.A., and Yanagisawa, E.: Radiographic anatomy of the paranasal sinuses. Arch. Otolaryngol., 87: 1968.
Valvassori, G.E., Mafee, M.T., and Dobben, G.D.: Computed tomography of the temporal bone. Laryngoscope, 92:562–565, 1982.
Valvassori, G.E.: Radiology in otolaryngology. Otol. Clin. North Am., 6(No. 2): 1973.

Chapter *3*

ANATOMY AND PHYSIOLOGY OF THE EAR

ANATOMY OF THE EAR

In the human there are three parts to the ear: the external, middle, and inner ears, plus the internal auditory canal. The middle and inner ears are fully developed at birth.

External Ear

The external ear is the only part of the ear that grows after birth. There are two parts to the external ear: the pinna and the external auditory canal. The pinna consists of an irregular plate of fibrocartilage tightly covered by skin and a thin layer of subcutaneous tissue. There are ridges and furrows on its lateral surface (Figure 3.1), which have all been named, and small rudimentary muscles that are attached posteriorly. The external auditory canal is a tortuous composite tube with an average length of 3.7 cm in the adult male. The skeleton of its outer half is cartilaginous, and the inner half is bone, primarily the tympanic bone. The canal is lined by skin that is thicker over cartilage and thin over bone. The skin of the cartilaginous canal contains hairs and special glands that secrete cerumen (wax). There is generous sensory innervation of the canal by branches of the fifth, seventh, and tenth cranial nerves.

TYMPANIC MEMBRANE (DRUMHEAD, EARDRUM). The tympanic membrane forms a common wall between the external canal and the middle ear. The membrane, which is fully developed at birth, is pearl-gray in color, semitranslucent, cone-shaped, concave laterally, and roughly oval (10 mm × 9 mm), with the consistency of loosely stretched cellophane. Its edges are thickened by an incomplete ring of fibrous tissue, which is called the annulus. The tympanic membrane has two parts: a small, triangular pars flaccida (Shrapnell's membrane) superiorly and the larger pars tensa (Figure 3.2). The pars tensa is composed of three distinct layers: an outer squamous epithelium, a middle fibrous layer with radial and circular fibers, and an inner mucosal layer (Figure 3.3). The long, thin handle of the malleus is imbedded in the upper half of the fibrous layer. At the superior end of the handle is the prominent, white lateral process of the malleus.

Middle Ear (Tympanum)

The middle ear is a flat, air-filled chamber that is enclosed by five bony walls (Figure 3.4). The sixth and lateral wall is the tympanic membrane. The middle ear is divisible into three areas: the epitym-

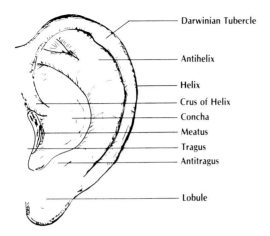

- Darwinian Tubercle
- Antihelix
- Helix
- Crus of Helix
- Concha
- Meatus
- Tragus
- Antitragus
- Lobule

Fig. 3.1.   The pinna (auricle). The plate of cartilage is molded into ridges and furrows, which are all named.

panum (attic) above the level of the tympanic membrane, the mesotympanum deep to the tympanic membrane, and the hypotympanum. The lumen, which is lined by a delicate, ciliated mucous membrane, is traversed laterally to medially by a chain of three small interarticulated bones—the malleus, the incus, and the stapes—and posteriorly to anteriorly by the slender chorda tympani nerve.

The medial wall of the middle ear is formed by the bony capsule of the inner ear. On this wall the basal turn of the cochlea creates a smooth bulge, which is called the promontory. There are two windows for communication between the middle and inner ears, both of which are sealed. At the posterosuperior edge of the promontory is the oval window, which is sealed by the footplate of the stapes, and at the posteroinferior edge is the round window. The round window is sealed by a fibrous membrane. Superior to the promontory is the horizontal part of the seventh cranial (facial) nerve, and superior to this, posteriorly, is the horizontal or lateral semicircular canal. The tensor tympani muscle arises in a bony semicanal superior to the eustachian tube, runs posteriorly to the midpoint of the horizontal facial nerve narrows to a tendon, takes a 90° turn, and

inserts into the neck of the malleus. These relationships are shown in Figure 3.5.

There are two important structures on the anterior wall of the middle ear: the tympanic orifice of the eustachian tube superiorly and the carotid canal inferiorly. In the posterior wall runs the vertical part of the facial nerve, to which is attached the tiny stapedius muscle, which is contained in a hollow pyramid of bone. The tendon of the stapedius muscle inserts into the neck and head of the stapes. Superiorly, the posterior wall has an opening, the aditus, that leads into the mastoid antrum, which communicates with the mastoid air cells. The roof of the middle ear is a thin plate of bone, the tegmen tympani, which separates the ear from the middle cranial fossa. The floor of the tympanum is formed by the bone of the jugular fossa, which contains the jugular bulb.

EUSTACHIAN TUBE. This composite tube connects the middle ear to the nasopharynx. It is 31 to 38 mm long in adults, runs downward and forward, and has two parts: a bony part (the protympanum) and a cartilaginous part, which are joined by a narrow isthmus. The cartilage is incomplete on its anterior surface, where the tube is completed by a membrane. The levator and tensor palatini muscles are attached along the length of the cartilage. The nasopharyngeal end of the cartilage forms an easily visible prominence (torus tubarius). The lumen of the tube is lined by a ciliated mucous membrane which is continuous with that of the middle ear and the nasopharynx. From its attachment to the cartilaginous tube, the tensor palatini muscle runs vertically downward, narrowing to a tendon that makes a 90° turn around the hamulus of the pterygoid plate and inserts into the aponeurosis of the soft palate. The tensor palatini muscle is innervated by the fifth cranial nerve, and the levator palatini is innervated by the tenth cranial nerve. Their contractions cause simultaneous stretching and elevation of the soft palate and opening of the eustachian tube.

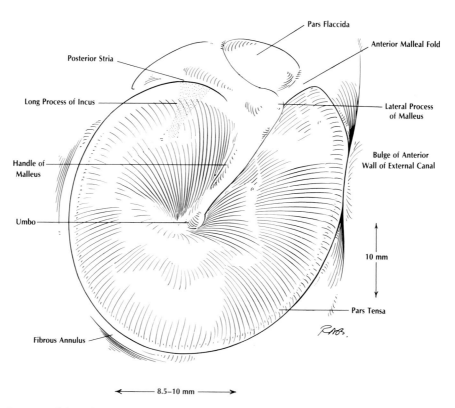

Lateral Wall of Epitympanum

Pars Flaccida

Anterior Malleal Fold

Posterior Stria

Long Process of Incus

Lateral Process
of Malleus

Handle of
Malleus

Bulge of Anterior
Wall of External Canal

Umbo

10 mm

Pars Tensa

Fibrous Annulus

8.5–10 mm

Fig. 3.2. Diagram of the right tympanic membrane. The handle of the malleus slants downward and posteriorly. The long process of the incus is just visible as a shadow behind the tympanic membrane. (From Karmody, C.S.: Anatomy and physiology of the ear. *In* Hearing and Hearing Impairment. Edited by L.J. Bradford and W.G. Hardy. New York, Grune & Stratton, Inc. 1979.)

OSSICLES. There are three tiny bones in the cavity of the middle ear: the malleus (hammer), the incus (anvil), and the stapes (stirrup) (Figure 3.5). The malleus articulates with the incus, and the incus articulates with the stapes. The bones are fully developed at birth and do not have the capacity for regeneration or repair; that is, any damage by trauma or infection is permanent.

The malleus has a handle, neck, and head. The incus has a triangular-shaped body. The apex of the triangle, or short process, sits in the aditus to the mastoid, and from the lower angle of the body a very delicate long process points downward and takes a 90° turn at its inferior end, which is called the lenticular process, to articulate with the head of the stapes. The head of the malleus and the body of the incus are in the epitympanum. Their articular surfaces are irregular, lined by cartilage, and meet in a firm diarthrodial joint that allows, at the most, only minimal slippage. The delicate stapes bone, shaped like a stirrup, has a head, neck, two crura (anterior and posterior), and a very thin footplate that fits into the oval window, with the joint sealed by a delicate annular ligament.

The seventh cranial (facial) nerve, which innervates the muscles of the face, passes through the temporal bone, first through the internal auditory canal and then in a

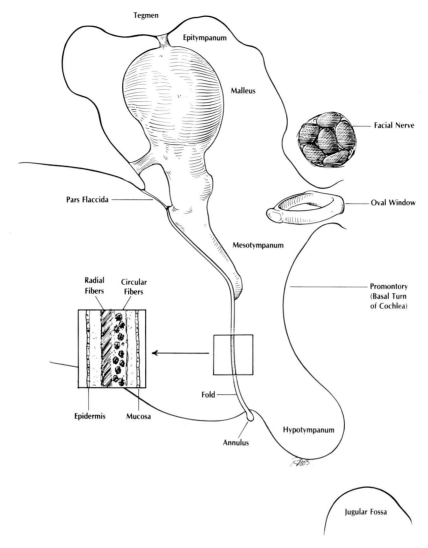

Fig. 3.3. Cross section of the middle ear in the vertical plane. The cavity of the middle ear (tympanum) extends above the limits of the external canal. The basal turn of the cochlea forms the promontory of the medial wall of the middle ear. (From Karmody, C.S.: Anatomy and physiology of the ear. *In* Hearing and Hearing Impairment. Edited by L.J. Bradford and W.G. Hardy. New York, Grune & Stratton, Inc., 1979.)

bony canal horizontally along the medial wall of the middle ear, turns downward to the posterior wall of the middle ear, leaves the temporal bone through the stylomastoid foramen, and enters the substance of the parotid salivary gland. In its vertical segment, the seventh cranial nerve supplies a motor nerve to the stapedius muscle and gives off the chorda tympani nerve, which runs forward and loops upward, crossing the middle ear between the malleus and incus. The chorda tympani is responsible for taste sensation on the ipsilateral half of the tongue and is secretomotor for the submandibular salivary gland.

Inner Ear

The inner ear is comprised of a system of channels and chambers (bony laby-

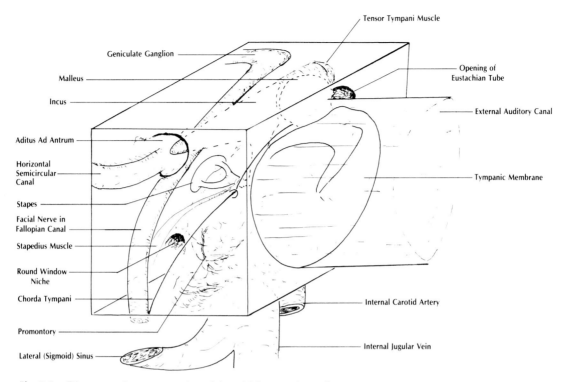

Tensor Tympani Muscle

Geniculate Ganglion

Malleus

Incus

Opening of
Eustachian Tube

External Auditory Canal

Aditus Ad Antrum

Horizontal
Semicircular
Canal

Tympanic Membrane

Stapes

Facial Nerve in
Fallopian Canal

Stapedius Muscle

Round Window
Niche

Chorda Tympani

Internal Carotid Artery

Promontory

Internal Jugular Vein

Lateral (Sigmoid) Sinus

Fig. 3.4. Diagrammatic representation of the middle ear. The walls are not as symmetric as illustrated.

rinth) hollowed into the densest bone in the body (otic capsule) (Figure 3.6). These channels are filled with fluid (perilymph), the composition of which is similar to that of cerebrospinal fluid. In the perilymph a corresponding closed system of delicate membranous tubes and sacs (membranous labyrinth) is suspended; these sacs are filled with fluid (endolymph) that contains a high level of potassium. The otic capsule has three layers: periosteal, endochondral, and endosteal. The endochondral layer contains islands of cartilage and has no regenerative capacity.

The inner ear is anatomically and functionally divided into two parts: the more primitive superior and posterior vestibular labyrinth (balance) and the anteroinferior cochlea (hearing). Both parts are joined to a common chamber, the vestibule, as shown in Figure 3.6.

COCHLEA. In the human the cochlea (snail) is a channel coiled into 2½ turns

around a central bony axis, the modiolus, which contains the spiral ganglion whose component cells are the cell bodies of the cochlear nerve. The turns are designated as basal, middle, and apical. The basal turn is the widest, has the greatest circumference, is closest to the stapes, is responsible for the perception of high frequencies, and bulges into the middle ear as the promontory.

The cochlear channel is subdivided into three compartments, called scalae (Figure 3.6). A central membranous cochlear duct, or scala media, contains endolymph. The two surrounding compartments, the scala vestibuli and the scala tympani, contain perilymph and communicate with each other at the apex of the cochlea. The scala vestibuli opens into the vestibule. At the basal end of the scala tympani there is a defect in the bony wall called the round window, which is sealed by the round window membrane.

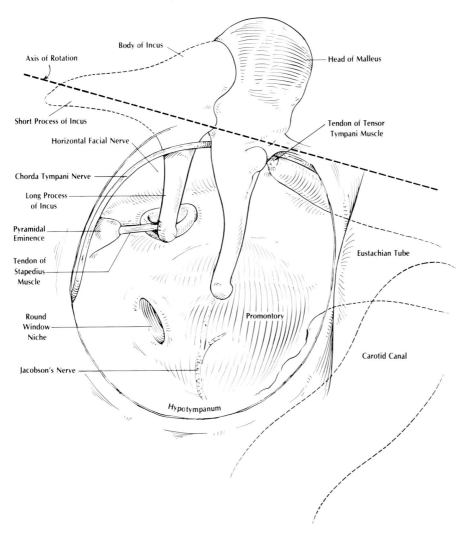

Fig. 3.5.   The medial wall of the middle ear. The tympanic membrane and lateral wall of the epitympanum are missing. The round window membrane is tucked away at the bottom of the round window niche. (From Karmody, C.S.: Anatomy and physiology of the ear. *In* Hearing and Hearing Impairment. Edited by L.J. Bradford and W.G. Hardy. New York, Grune & Stratton, Inc., 1979.)

The cochlear duct (scala media) is the essential hearing apparatus. It is roughly triangular when seen in cross section. The base of the triangle is the basilar membrane, which is comprised of fibers that extend from a tiny, hollow, bony partition to the spiral ligament, as shown in Figure 3.7. The fibers are longest at the apical end. The oblique side of the triangle is the delicate Reissner's membrane, which is two cells thick. The third side of the tri-angle contains a bed of capillaries, the stria vascularis.

The sensory cells of the hearing apparatus are massed together in the organ of Corti, which sits on the scala media surface of the basilar membrane. The organ of Corti is divided by a tunnel that is lined by two pillars of acellular material. On the inner side of the tunnel is a single row of hair cells, which is the inner hair cell; on the strial side of the tunnel are three rows

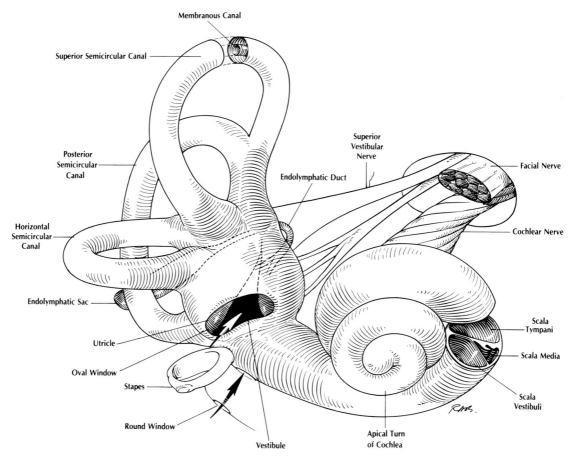

Fig. 3.6. Stylized diagram of the inner ear. There are two areas of deficit in the bony capsule of the inner ear that faces the middle ear: the oval window, into which fits the footplate of the stapes, and the round window, which is sealed by the round window membrane. The semicircular canals are disposed in the three dimensions of space. (From Karmody, C.S.: Anatomy and physiology of the ear. *In* Hearing and Hearing Impairment. Edited by L.J. Bradford and W.G. Hardy. New York, Grune & Stratton, Inc., 1979.)

of outer hair cells. In the human ear there are about 12,000 hair cells and 25,000 to 30,000 cell bodies in the spiral ganglion. An outer hair cell is an elongated cylindrical structure with rows of stiff cilia of different lengths (Figure 3.8). The base of the hair cells is flanked by the endings of the afferent and efferent nerves. The cilia are in contact with the undersurface of the tectorial membrane, a gelatinous structure that is firmly anchored to the limbus and draped over the organ of Corti, forming a barrier between the organ and the endolymph.

EFFERENT SYSTEM. A well-defined efferent system exists in the cochlea, in which cell bodies are in the superior olivary nucleus. Their axons form the olivocochlear bundle of Rasmussen, which follows the vestibular and cochlear nerves, passes through the spiral ganglion, and then crosses the tunnel of Corti to arborize around the bases of the outer hair cells.

BLOOD SUPPLY. The blood supply to the inner ear is provided by a single small vessel, the internal auditory artery, which originates from either the basilar or the anterior inferior cerebellar artery. This is

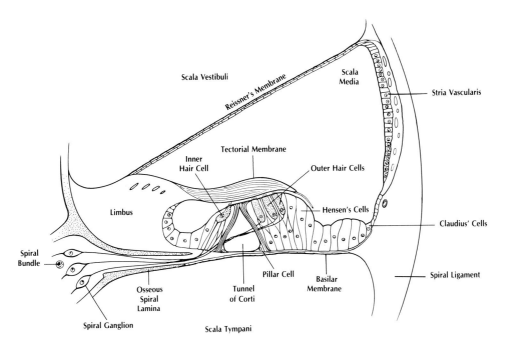

Fig. 3.7. The cochlear duct. The stria vascularis consists of fine capillaries and is probably responsible for homeostasis of the endolymph. There are three rows of outer hair cells and one row of inner hair cells in the organ of Corti. (From Karmody, C.S.: Anatomy and physiology of the ear. *In* Hearing and Hearing Impairment. Edited by L.J. Bradford and W.G. Hardy. New York, Grune & Stratton, Inc., 1979.)

an end artery and has no anastomosis with neighboring blood vessels.

The stria vascularis contains numerous capillaries through which there is an unusually fast flow of blood. The marginal cells at the endolymphatic surface of the stria are connected by tight junctions that form a barrier against endolymph.

CENTRAL CONNECTIONS. The fibers of the cochlear nerve run to the pons and terminate around the cells of the cochlear nucleus. Most of the ascending fibers leave the cochlear nucleus via the corpus trapezoideum. The trapezoid body connects contralateral olives; the fibers then ascend in the contralateral lemniscus to the inferior colliculus. The cells of the inferior colliculus give rise to tracts that terminate in the medial geniculate body. Fibers from the medial geniculate body then form the thalamic auditory relay, which runs to the auditory cortex. The position and extent of the auditory cortex cannot be stated

unequivocally but is traditionally considered to be represented in the anterior transverse temporal gyrus (Brodmann's area 41). There is extensive decussation of fibers, and both ears are represented on both sides of the cerebral cortex.

Running parallel with the ascending pathways is the descending, or efferent, system, the anatomy and functional organization of which is still being investigated.

VESTIBULAR LABYRINTH. The vestibular labyrinth is an essential part of the balancing system of the body. There are three semicircular canals disposed in the three dimensions of space, two vertical and one horizontal, and all are at right angles to each other, as shown in Figure 3.6. One end of each canal expands to accommodate a crest of sensory cells (the crista), which is topped by a gelatinous mass (the cupula), which is deflected by movements in the endolymph. In the vestibule of the

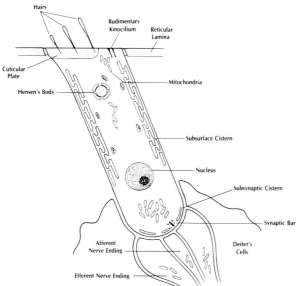

Fig. 3.8. Details of an outer hair cell. The cell is cylindrical, and its nucleus is eccentric. There is a thick cuticular plate at its endolymphatic surface, in which the cilia are embedded. Note the larger size of the terminal of the efferent nerve. (From Karmody, C.S.: Anatomy and physiology of the ear. *In* Hearing and Hearing Impairment. Edited by L.J. Bradford and W.G. Hardy. New York, Grune & Stratton, Inc., 1979.)

inner ear there are two structures that resemble sacs: the utricle, into which the semicircular canals open, and the saccule, which is connected to the cochlear duct. In the walls of the utricle and saccule are flattened areas (maculae), the internal surfaces of which are lined by sensitive hair cells that are surmounted by a gelatinous mass containing small crystals of calcium carbonate. This mass responds to gravitational forces, thereby stimulating the sensitive hair cells. Movement of the endolymph in the vestibular system can also be caused by a differential change in density, such as occurs with a change in temperature. This is achieved clinically by irrigating the ear canals with hot or cold water; this procedure is called the caloric test. Impulses from the vestibular system are transmitted along the superior and inferior vestibular nerves that run in the internal auditory canal to the brainstem.

Membranous ducts drain both the utricle and saccule. These ducts join to form the endolymphatic duct, which passes through the temporal bone in a posterior and lateral direction and opens into the endolymphatic sac. The endolymphatic sac is a flattened, closed chamber that lies between the posterior surface of the temporal bone and the dura. The sac is lined by an extensive cuboidal and columnar epithelium whose function is probably to reabsorb endolymph.

PHYSIOLOGY OF THE EAR

The human ear responds to sound stimuli from 16 to 20,000 Hz (cycles per second).

External and Middle Ears

The outer and middle ears have three primary functions: (1) to deliver sufficient sound energy to the inner ear for maximal sensitivity; (2) to protect the delicate inner ear against excessive energy input; and (3) to shape the overall frequency response of the ear. The pinna, a structure that is peculiar to mammals, is rudimentary in humans. In most mammals, however, the function of the pinna is to collect and deflect sound energy into the external canal. The external canal has the simple function of transmitting airborne sound to tympanic membrane, and has a peak resonance around 4 kHz.

TYMPANIC MEMBRANE. The tympanic membrane has three functions: (1) it protects the middle ear and round window; (2) it collects sound energy; and (3) because of its curvature, it functions as a small step-up transformer. As the membrane vibrates, a synchronous movement of the attached malleus occurs. The amplitude of motion is extremely small and has been compared to brownian movement. The malleus and the incus vibrate as a unit around an axis that runs through the anterior mallear ligament and the short process of the incus (Figure 3.5). The footplate of the stapes, which acts as a piston in the oval window, moves around a vertical axis.

TRANSFORMER MECHANISMS. Vibratory energy is transmitted poorly from one medium to another, and most of the energy is reflected at the interface of the various structures (e.g., between stapes footplate and perilymph). To counterbalance this loss of energy, it is necessary to increase the pressure levels of a sound at the interface by a transformer mechanism. The transformer action in the ear is accomplished at three levels: the pinna, external canal, and middle ear. The contributions of the pinna and external canal are slight. In the middle ear the transformer action occurs in three stages: (1) the curved-membrane mechanism of the tympanic membrane; (2) the lever action of the ossicles; and (3) the area ratio of the tympanic membrane to the stapes footplate. The three mechanisms together create an effective ratio of pressures between the footplate and the tympanic membrane of 87:1.

TYMPANIC MUSCLES AND PROTECTION OF THE INNER EAR. Despite the transformer action that increases sound pressure levels, mechanisms exist that protect the inner ear from excessive energy. This protection is achieved by contraction of the intratympanic muscles and by slippage at the incudomalleal joint, which occurs primarily at low frequencies. Sound is the stimulus for activity of the stapedius muscle by way of a reflex arc through the cochlea, cochlear nuclei, and seventh cranial nerve. This is a bilateral phenomenon, which can be excited by a stimulus of adequate intensity to the ipsilateral or contralateral ear (the stapedial reflex). The tensor tympani muscle in humans responds to sound stimuli with a comparatively long latency period.

EUSTACHIAN TUBE. In the normal state the middle ear and mastoid cell systems contain air at atmospheric pressure. The eustachian tube, because it opens into the nasopharynx, provides the main source of air, but some gaseous interchange occurs between the lumen and the mucosa of the middle ear. The eustachian tube at rest is closed but opens on swallowing by contraction of the tensor palatini and levator palatini muscles, which allows air to pass into the middle ear cleft. Obstruction of the eustachian tube causes gaseous absorption and an increase in negative pressure, which in turn induces transudation of serous fluid from the middle ear mucosa. The lumen of the eustachian tube is lined by a ciliated epithelium, which contributes to drainage from the middle ear.

DEFENSE MECHANISM OF THE MIDDLE EAR. A discussion of the physiology of the middle ear would be incomplete without reference to its defense mechanisms, which are mainly a function of its lining mucosa. The effusions of the middle ear include a potent collection of antibody-containing classes of immunoglobulins, specifically IgG, IgA, IgM, and IgD, and elevated levels of lysozymes. At the cellular level, infection of the middle ear results in a prompt and profuse outpouring of polymorphonuclear leukocytes. If the reaction is less severe, a substantial migration of macrophages and other phagocytic cells into the middle ear cleft occurs instead. The middle ear cleft, therefore, is capable of protecting itself, to some extent, from infection by small inocula of pathogens.

Inner Ear

FLUIDS OF THE INNER EAR. The composition of perilymph is similar to that of extracellular and cerebrospinal fluids in that it has a high sodium content. The composition of endolymph is similar to intracellular fluid with a content high in potassium and low in sodium.

Perilymph is probably a filtrate of or part of the cerebrospinal fluid, transported via the cochlear aqueduct, which connects the perilymphatic and subarachnoid spaces. The site of formation of endolymph is still unknown. The most popular theories suggest that endolymph is produced by either the stria vascularis, differential filtration of the perilymph by Reissner's membrane, or by secretion by the endolymphatic sac.

COCHLEA. The cochlea acts as a transducer, converting sound energy into neural activity for transmission to the brain, where it excites the sensation of hearing. Sound waves stimulate the organ of Corti by exciting movements of the cochlear fluids, which in turn causes motion of the basilar membrane and concomitant distortion of the hair cells. This distortion stimulates the hair cells to produce a chemical mediator, which initiates nerve impulses along the peripheral axon of the spiral ganglion cells and then along the cochlear nerve to the cochlear nuclei. Some degree of analysis of a sound into its components is performed peripherally. In its simplest concept this analysis is accomplished by frequency selection along the basilar membrane; this is the place/resonance theory first proposed by Helmholtz (1863). The basilar membrane is comprised of fibers of different lengths, shortest at the basal end and longest at the apical end. Each fiber has a natural resonance (i.e., a frequency at which it vibrates maximally); hence, the concept of frequency selection is based on the resonance of a given fiber. Bekesy (1928) proposed an alternate, but related, theory that was based on extensive experiments. His "traveling wave theory" states that as a sine wave progresses from the base to the apex of the cochlea, the whole basilar membrane vibrates at the frequency of the wave. The maximum amplitude of vibration, however, is at a specific point that is constant for a given frequency of stimulus. That is, amplitude maxima are frequency- and place-dependent, as originally suggested by Helmholtz. This implies that near threshold, hair cells in only a narrow range around the place of maximum displacement are stimulated enough to trigger nerve endings. In Bekesy's theory, therefore, sound waves travel along the scala vestibuli and cause movement in the scala media, which transmits motion to the scala tympani; this motion is, in turn, transmitted to the round window membrane, so that sound energy is dissipated back to the middle ear space. As a complex noise travels, its component waves stimulate the corresponding areas of the basilar membrane and organ of Corti (Figure 3.9). The final conscious interpretation of different frequencies and their reconstitution into a complex noise is accomplished by the higher centers of the brain.

ELECTRICAL ACTIVITY OF THE COCHLEA. The cochlea has resting electrical potentials: a positive potential of +80 mV in the endolymph (endolymphatic poten-

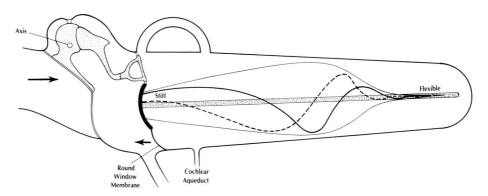

Fig. 3.9. Conceptual diagram of Bekesy's traveling wave. The amplitude of each wave is maximal at a given point on the basilar membrane depending on the frequency of the wave. (From Karmody, C.S.: Anatomy and physiology of the ear. *In* Hearing and Hearing Impairment. Edited by L.J. Bradford and W.G. Hardy. New York, Grune & Stratton, Inc., 1979.)

tial), a negative potential of −60 mV in the hair cells, and no (0) potential in the perilymph. Therefore the potential between the hair cells and the endolymph is 140 mV, which is a high differential across a cell membrane. Evidence indicates that the stria vascularis is ultimately responsible for the production and maintenance of the endolymphatic potential.

ELECTRICAL RESPONSE TO ACOUSTIC STIMULATION (EVOKED RESPONSE). At the present state of our knowledge, five electrical phenomena are recognized after acoustic stimulation: cochlear microphonic potentials, summating potentials, action potentials of the cochlear nerve, brainstem potential, and cortical potentials. The first four of these are recordable by electrodes placed in the vicinity of the ear, and the fifth electrical phenomenon is recorded from electrodes on the scalp.

Cochlear Microphonic Potential. This is an alternating current phenomenon. An electrical circuit that includes the inner ear responds to a sound stimulus with an almost totally faithful reproduction of the stimulus. The response is known as the cochlear microphonic (CM) potential and is maximal if one electrode is placed close to the cochlea (e.g., in the round window or on the promontory). The cochlear microphonic potential originates in the hair cells and has been used as an experimental and clinical tool.

Summating Potential. In addition to the alternating current cochlear microphonic potential, the organ of Corti generates a stimulus-related direct current potential, which is called the summating potential. This electrical phenomenon is still not very well understood.

Action Potential. Stimulation of the cochlea results in a burst of electrical energy along the acoustic nerve. Each fiber is stimulated by a narrow frequency range and its discharge of energy is related to the intensity of the stimulus. The action potential (AP) of the cochlear nerve is larger than the cochlear microphonic potential

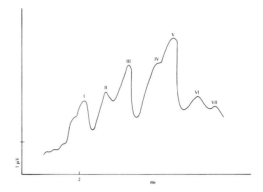

Fig. 3.10. Stylized diagram of an ideal brainstem-evoked response recorded from the vertex of the scalp with a reference electrode on the mastoid bone. Wave V is the largest and most constant.

and can be easily recognized. With advanced electronic and computerized averaging techniques, it is now possible to record the response activity of the cochlea and eighth nerve in a clinical setting, using electrodes in the external canal or on the promontory. This technique is known as electrocochleography, but it primarily records the action potential of the nerve.

Brainstem Potentials (Brainstem-Evoked Responses). The brainstem-evoked responses (BER) are the electrical responses of the eighth nerve and auditory nuclei of the brainstem to auditory stimuli. They are recorded by electrodes placed on the scalp and over the mastoid. These responses must be extracted from the background electrical activity of the brain by averaging computers. Calibrated clicks or pure-tone stimuli are usually used to elicit the responses, and the BER appears during the first 10 ms following stimulation. Normal responses consist of a pattern of five to seven recordable waves (Figure 3.10). At the present time, the latency of wave V is considered to be clinically significant. After adjustments for age and stimulus intensity, increased latency might indicate a pathologic process that is central to the cochlea.

Electrical response audiometry is the

only objective method of assessing hearing and is recordable even under general anesthesia. It is particularly useful for testing infants and children.

Cortical Potentials. With the advent of small averaging and summating computers, it is now possible to extract a cortical response to auditory stimuli from the background of electrical activity by the same technique that is used for brainstem action potentials.

The ear is anatomically simple and physiologically complex. The ability to receive, identify, analyze, reconstitute, and store in our memories the innumerable sounds that we hear even in a single day is truly amazing. In this chapter it was possible to give only the barest outline of anatomy and physiology. Much remains to be investigated and clarified in this area. In recent years a great deal of attention has been paid to electrical activity in the ear after auditory stimulation, and it is in this area that rapid advances are being made.

BIBLIOGRAPHY

Bast, T.H., and Anson, B.J.: The Temporal Bone and the Ear. Springfield, Illinois, Charles C Thomas, 1949.

Bekesy, G. von: Experiments in Hearing. New York, McGraw-Hill, 1960.

Brackman, D.E.: Electric response audiometry in clinical practice. Laryngoscope, 87:Suppl. 5, 1977.

Davis, H.: Priniples of electric response audiometry. Ann. Otol. Rhinol. Laryngol., 85:Suppl. 28, 1976.

Davis, H., and Silverman, R.S.: Hearing and Deafness. 3rd Ed. New York, Holt, Rinehart, and Winston, 1970.

Silverstein, H.: Biochemical studies of the inner ear fluids in the cat. Ann. Otolaryngol., 75:48–63, 1966.

Spoendlin, H.: The Organization of the Cochlear Receptor. Basel, Karger, 1966.

Tonndorf, J., and Khanna, S.M.: The role of the tympanic membrane in middle ear transmission. Ann. Otol. Rhinol. Laryngol., 79:743–753, 1970.

Wever, E.G., and Bray, C.W.: Auditory nerve impulses. Science, 71:215, 1930.

Chapter 4

TESTS OF THE AUDITORY APPARATUS

Hearing losses are classified into three types: conductive, sensorineural, and mixed.

Hearing tests are performed to measure the level of hearing, to determine the type of hearing loss, to guide further therapy, and to aid in differential diagnosis. Hearing tests are divided into two broad categories: clinical and instrumental. Clinical tests are by necessity only qualitative but are still valuable for quick assessment and for validating the results of instrumental tests.

CLINICAL TESTS

Voice

The examiner's voice is the first and most available test for hearing. Use the voice at different levels and at a standard distance (6 feet) away from the patient. The levels of voice are shout, conversational, and whisper.

Masking

Noise on one side of the head can be heard by the contralateral ear. There is only a small (5 dB) attenuation of intensity across the bone of the skull and a moderate (45 dB) attenuation by air conduction. Masking is the technique of blocking the function of one ear while the other ear is being tested. Masking is usually accomplished with a loud white noise produced by a Báránay noise box or an electrical device (Figure 4.1). Alternatively, the examiner may use the crackling sound of a piece of crumpled paper, or a small radio.

ABSOLUTE OR TOTAL DEAFNESS. Shouting through a speaking tube (ear trumpet) in the ear to be tested, while masking the contralateral ear, is still the best way of confirming a total, unilateral hearing loss.

Tuning Forks

Tests with tuning forks are used to distinguish between the various types of hearing losses. Although relatively unsophisticated, they are still reliable qualitative tests and are useful for validating instrumental examinations. A collection of tuning forks with frequency ranges of 128, 256, 512, 1024, 2048, and 4096 Hz (cycles per second) is desirable, but 256- and 512-Hz tuning forks are usually used for routine examinations. Hold the tuning fork by its stem and set it vibrating by striking it against a firm but cushioned surface (e.g., the heel of the hand or the kneecap). For tests of air conduction, the wide surface of the tine should be held about 2 cm away

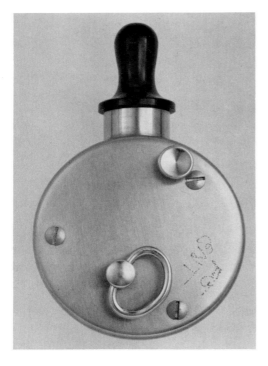

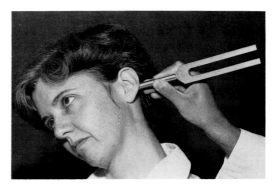

Fig. 4.3. Testing bone conduction with a tuning fork. The stem of the vibrating fork is pressed firmly against the mastoid bone.

Table 4.1. The Rinne Test

Positive (AC > BC)	Negative (BC > AC)
Normal hearing	Conductive loss
Sensorineural loss	False-negative (see text)

Fig. 4.1. A Báránay noise box. This instrument makes a loud noise and is used to mask one ear while the other ear is being tested.

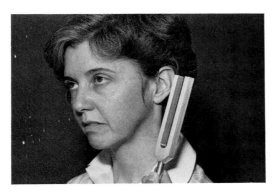

Fig. 4.2. Testing air conduction with a tuning fork. The broad surface of the tines are held 2 to 3 cm from the pinna.

from the pinna (Figure 4.2). For testing bone conduction, the stem end of the vibrating fork should be pressed firmly against the upper anterior part of the mastoid process (Figure 4.3). Because only a small attenuation of sound occurs across the skull, the opposite ear should be masked. Many tests with tuning forks have been described, but only four will be detailed here.

RINNE TEST. The Rinne test is useful for distinguishing between conductive and sensorineural hearing losses. Use a 256- or 512-Hz tuning fork. As originally described, the Rinne test compares the length of time the tuning fork is heard by air conduction with the length of time it is heard by bone conduction (Figures 4.2 and 4.3). Today, comparison is made between the intensity of perceived sound. The examiner wants to know whether air conduction or bone conduction is louder. Air conduction is heard better than bone conduction in patients with normal hearing or sensorineural hearing loss. This is known as a positive Rinne test. Patients with conductive hearing losses of greater than 20 to 25 dB hear bone conduction better than air conduction. This is a negative Rinne test. Therefore, a negative Rinne test is abnormal and indicates a conductive hearing loss. A false-negative result can be obtained if the tested ear is almost totally deaf and the contralateral ear is functioning much better. In this situation the better ear should be masked. The Rinne test is summarized in Table 4.1.

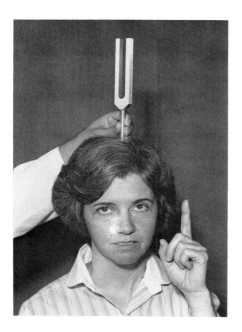

Fig. 4.4. The Weber test. The stem of the vibrating tuning fork is firmly applied to the midline of the vault of the skull or to the forehead. The patient indicates the side on which the sound is heard.

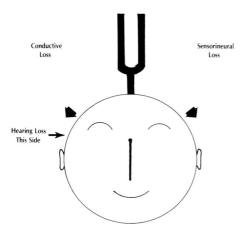

Fig. 4.5. The Weber test. There is a hearing loss on the right side. If the tuning fork is heard best on the right side, that indicates a conductive loss. If, however, the sound is referred to the left side, that suggests a sensorineural loss.

WEBER TEST. The Weber test is used to distinguish between conductive and sensorineural hearing losses. It is a comparatively crude test and is more useful for validating other tests. The stem of a vibrating 256- or 512-Hz tuning fork is pressed firmly against the vault of the head or on the forehead (Figure 4.4). Alternatively, the upper incisors or occiput can be used. Sound is heard best on the side with a conductive hearing loss (Figure 4.5). If, however, there has been a recent, absolute loss of hearing on one side, the sound will be lateralized to the remaining good side. Lateralization is lost if the absolute hearing loss is long-standing.

SCHWABACH TEST. This test is not used frequently today if instrumental tests are available. It compares the bone conduction of the patient with that of the examiner, assuming that the examiner's hearing is normal. The test gives a reasonable idea of cochlear function. A 512- or 256-Hz tuning fork should be used and the length of time that the vibrating fork is heard on the mastoid process of the patient compared to that of the examiner. The patient should be tested first, and when he stops hearing the fork, it should be transferred quickly to the mastoid process of the examiner. If the fork is still heard by the examiner, the patient's cochlear function is depressed (i.e., he probably has a sensorineural hearing loss). The following is an outline of the results of the Schwabach test:

Neutral = normal

Lengthened = conductive loss

Shortened = sensorineural loss

GELLE (BING) TEST. This test is used to determine a sensorineural or conductive hearing loss. If the stem of a vibrating turning fork is placed on the mastoid bone in a normal patient and the external canal is then occluded with a finger, the tuning fork will immediately seem louder. When the occlusion is removed, the loudness decreases. If a conductive hearing loss exists, occlusion of the ear canal will not cause a change in loudness.

INSTRUMENTAL TESTS (AUDIOMETRY)

Quantitative assessment of hearing became possible with the development of the audiometer, a piece of electronic equipment that produces pure tones at selected frequencies. Audiometry has now become a highly technical and rapidly advancing field, and in this chapter only the essentials will be outlined.

Physics

The first standardization of normal levels of hearing was based on a study of many thousands of young adults. This clinical base has subsequently been superseded by a more accurate, measurable standard.

The smallest sound that can be heard by the human ear at 1 kHz is at a pressure level of 0.0002 dynes/cm^2. All other levels of intensity are measured against this base, which is known as zero sound pressure level. Therefore, the zero level of an audiometer does not mean "no hearing"; it represents the smallest audible sound. The comparison of noise intensities is simplified by first determining their ratios and then calculating the $\log_{10}$ of these ratios. The unit measurements of hearing that are used in the clinical setting are the bel and decibel (dB). One bel represents a tenfold increase in sound energy. That is, where I_2 represents the sound to be tested and I_1 is the reference level, $I_2/I_1 = 10$. $\log_{10} 10 = 1$ bel $= 10$ dB. Alternatively, if only a doubling of sound energy occurs, $I_2/I_1 = 2$, then $\log_{10} 2 = 0.301$ bel $= 3.0$ dB.

> 10 dB/0 = 10 times the amount of energy
>
> 20 dB/0 dB = 100 times the amount of energy
>
> 60 dB/0 dB = 1 million times the amount of energy

Most audiometers are calibrated in decibels.

Tests are performed at frequencies of

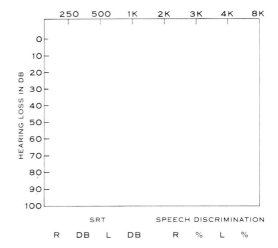

Fig. 4.6. Blank audiogram. Traditionally, frequencies are plotted on the horizontal axis and intensities are on the vertical axis. SRT = speech reception thresholds. Speech discrimination is scored by the percentage of phonetically balanced words that are correctly identified.

Table 4.2. Symbols Used in Audiometry

Side	Air Conduction	Bone Conduction
Right	O	<
Left	X	>

125, 250, 500, 1000, 2000, 4000, and 8000 Hz. Most speech sounds fall within the range of 500, 1000, and 2000 Hz; these are usually called the speech frequencies. An audiogram is plotted, and, by convention, frequencies are placed along the abscissa, with low frequencies to the left, and intensities are plotted along the ordinate, beginning at 0, with intensities increasing downward (Figure 4.6). Hearing loss is plotted downward from the 0 line. The right side is usually marked in red with circles, and the left is marked in blue with x's. Bone conduction is designated by open arrows, open to the right for the right side (<) and open to the left for the left side (>). Table 4.2 gives these symbols in tabular form.

The objective of pure tone audiometry is to determine the smallest sound that is audible at all test frequencies. This is the patient's hearing threshold.

Testing

A loud tone is first presented, and the patient indicates whether he hears it. The intensity is then reduced by 5-dB decrements until threshold is obtained. Air conduction and bone conduction levels are then plotted on an audiogram.

SPEECH DISCRIMINATION. The ability

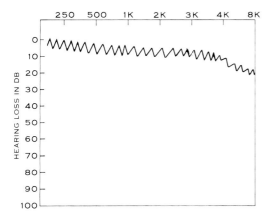

Fig. 4.7. Sweep audiometry. This is a self-test technique that is used for the rough testing of large numbers of people.

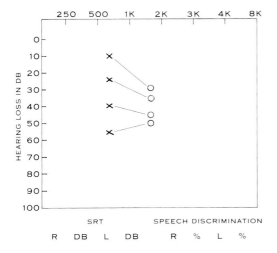

Fig. 4.8. Laddergram demonstrating recruitment. There is a hearing loss on the right side. Note that the perception of a 25-dB increase in intensity on the right side is matched by a 45-dB increase on the normal left side.

to understand speech is tested with phonetically balanced words and is expressed as a percentage. Normal speech discrimination is 80 to 100%.

SWEEP AUDIOMETRY. As described above, audiometry is performed manually by a technician one tone at a time. Sweep audiometry is a self-administered test in which the patient is presented with one frequency. When he indicates threshold, the audiometer automatically moves to the next frequency. This instrument was developed by Bekesy and is used with continuous or pulsed tones. Sweep audiometry is used in mass testing, as in industry and the military, because it takes less time and requires fewer personnel (Figure 4.7).

RECRUITMENT. Recruitment is an auditory phenomenon in which the perception of an increase in sound intensity is greater than the actual increase (Figure 4.8). This is typified by the patient who doesn't hear a voice at normal levels but then complains of shouting when a voice is slightly raised. Recruitment indicates a cochlear disorder.

Figures 4.9 to 4.12 are examples of typical audiograms, one of which is normal (Figure 4.9), one shows a conductive hear-

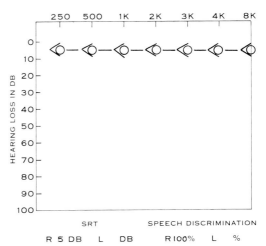

Fig. 4.9. Normal audiogram—right side. Audiometry is a subjective test, and human error accounts for a 10 to 15-dB range in thresholds.

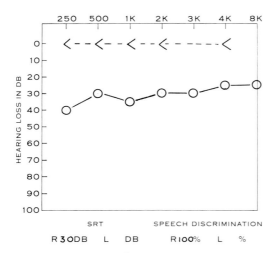

Fig. 4.10. Conductive hearing loss—right side. Bone conduction scores are normal. Thresholds by air conduction are elevated with greater losses in the lower frequencies.

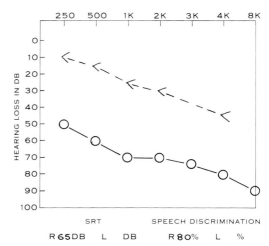

Fig. 4.12. Mixed hearing loss. In addition to the conductive loss (BC>AC) the bone conduction thresholds are elevated.

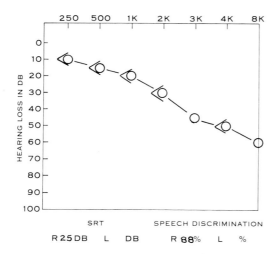

Fig. 4.11. Sensorineural hearing loss. This figure shows the most frequent pattern of sensorineural hearing loss. Thresholds of bone and air conduction are at the same levels, and the hearing loss is greater in the higher frequencies.

ing loss (Figure 4.10). Another illustrates a sensorineural hearing loss (Figure 4.11), and the last one shows a mixed hearing loss (Figure 4.12).

Special Tests

Special tests are used to distinguish between sensory and neural deafness.

SHORT INCREMENT SENSITIVITY INDEX (SISI). This test is positive in patients with cochlear loss. It consists of determining the short increments in intensity that the ear perceives. With a cochlear loss the ear perceives smaller increments.

TONE DECAY. Tone decay is based on the phenomenon that the ear loses its ability to hold a tone in the presence of a retrocochlear lesion. With normal hearing, a tone that is 25 dB above threshold will be heard for as long as it is presented. In neural deafness the same intensity of sound is heard for only a short time (i.e., the tone "decays").

BEKESY AUDIOMETRY. The response to sweep frequency audiometry changes, depending on the stimulus and pathologic process. Normally, tracings with pulsed and continuous tones are at the same levels. However, they diverge in different patterns with cochlear and retrocochlear disorders.

Tympanometry

Tympanometry is the technique of measuring intratympanic pressure. The pressures across the tympanic membrane should be balanced at atmospheric pressure. If, however, the pressure in the middle ear is abnormal, as occurs in certain diseased states, it should be possible to measure this abnormality.

Sound energy is reflected maximally from the normal tympanic membrane when pressures on both sides of the membrane are equal. If the pressure in the external canal is increased or decreased, the tympanic membrane becomes more fixed, and the amount of reflected energy decreases.

In tympanometry the external auditory canal is sealed by a hollow, soft-tipped probe, through which three tubes pass; one introduces a noise, the second receives reflected energy, and the third changes the pressure of the system (Figure 4.13). The objective of the test is to balance the pressures across the tympanic membrane, thereby obtaining an indication of the condition of the middle ear cleft. When noise is introduced and the reflected energy is measured, the maximum return of energy should be at zero (atmospheric pressure). If a negative pressure of -100 mm H_2O exists in the middle ear, maximum reflection will occur when pressure in the external canal is reduced to -100 mm H_2O. Therefore, the pressure in the external canal that is required to balance the system

indicates the condition of the middle ear. Changes in pressure and reflected energy are plotted on an X-Y recorder. Clinical studies suggest that tympanometric curves fall into a number of patterns (Figure 4.14), as follows:

Type A = normal
Type AS = stiff ossicular chain
Type AD = ossicular discontinuity
Type B = flat curve indicates fluid in the middle ear
Type C = negative pressure in the middle ear

STAPEDIAL REFLEX. Loud noise in one ear excites contraction of the stapedius muscle of the opposite ear, which can be recorded by tympanometry. This stapedial reflex requires functional integrity of a reflex arc that includes the acoustic nerve on one side and the seventh cranial nerve on the opposite side. The appropriate response will not occur if the normal pathways malfunction. The stapedial reflex is now one of the tests used to distinguish between sensory and neural hearing losses.

Evoked-Response Audiometry

Auditory stimuli incite a chain of electrical events along the auditory pathways. If the stimulus is consistent, the electrical events will be of a consistent pattern

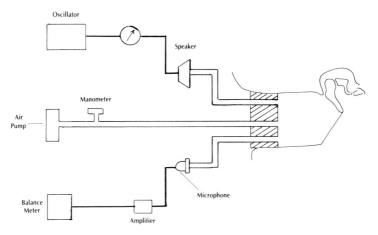

Fig. 4.13. Diagrammatic representation of a tympanometer (see the text for details). A good seal in the canal is essential.

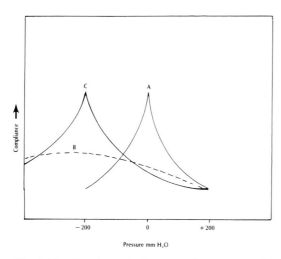

Fig. 4.14. The three classic types of tympanometric graphs. Type A will have a lower peak with increased stiffness (AS) and will be open at the top with discontinuity of the ossicular chain (AD).

against the background of brain activity. With modern techniques, it is possible to extract and record the electrical activity that is related to the auditory stimulation. Five waves are recordable from the region of the brainstem (Figure 3.10) and probably originate in the following areas:

Wave I—the cochlear nerve
Wave II—the cochlear nucleus
Wave III—the trapezoid body
Wave IV—the lateral lemniscus
Wave V—the inferior colliculus

Wave V is the largest and most constant. The latency of a given wave, usually wave V, is the length of time between onset of stimulus and the appearance of the wave. Latency increases with decrease in the intensity of the stimulus and is surprisingly uniform between normal right and left ears. Evoked-response audiometry is the only procedure that tests the hearing apparatus without requiring active patient participation and can be used even when the patient is under general anesthesia. It is useful in children, in malingering patients, and for the identification of more central problems because, with lesions along the

cochlear nerve and brainstem, electrical activity is prolonged and the latency of wave V is comparatively increased.

Tests for Malingering

Functional hearing loss is common. The following tests can be used to identify the malingerer.

REPEATED AUDIOMETRY. When audiometry is performed by a competent and patient person, the malingerer might find it difficult to reproduce identical levels.

STENGER TEST. If a noise is introduced in the right ear at 10 dB above threshold and a much louder noise is simultaneously played into the left ear, the noise in the left ear will cancel that in the right. Thus, the patient will not "hear" the right-sided noise. If, however, the left ear is truly deaf, the noise in the right will still be heard. This is the basis of the Stenger test to determine unilateral functional hearing loss.

LOMBARD'S TEST. If a patient is given a passage to read aloud and, during the reading, a noise is introduced into one ear, the intensity of his voice rises. Of course, if the ear is deaf, the patient's voice remains at the same pitch This phenomenon is used to investigate feigned unilateral hearing loss.

EVOKED-RESPONSE AUDIOMETRY. This is probably the most accurate and foolproof way of uncovering malingerers.

BIBLIOGRAPHY

Davis, H., and Silverman, R.S.: Hearing and Deafness. 4th Ed. New York, Holt, Rinehart, and Winston, 1978.
Feldman, A.S.: Acoustic impedance-admittance measurements. *In* Physiological Measures of the Audio-Vestibular System. Edited by L.J. Bradford. New York, Academic Press, Inc., 1975.
Gerber, S.E.: Introductory Hearing Science. Philadelphia, W.B. Saunders Co., 1974.
Jerger, J.: Clinical experience with impedance audiometry. Arch. Otolaryngol., 92:311–324, 1970.
Katz, J., Ed. Handbook of Clinical Audiology. Baltimore, The Williams and Wilkins Co., 1972.
Reger, S.: Differences in loudness response of the normal and hard of hearing ear at intensity levels slightly above threshold. Ann. Otol. Rhinol. Laryngol., 45:1029–1039, 1936.

Chapter 5

DISORDERS OF THE PINNA AND EXTERNAL AUDITORY CANAL

DISORDERS OF THE PINNA

The pinna and external auditory canal are, more often than not, afflicted simultaneously by the same problem. Separation of the two structures is, therefore, somewhat artificial and is done in this chapter only for clarity of description.

Congenital Anomalies

MICROTIA. Underdevelopment, which is the most frequent anomaly of the pinna, is known as microtia. The pinna might be completely absent or be represented by one or more tags of tissue. Microtia is a comparatively common congenital anomaly and is usually associated with anomalies of the external auditory canal, which can be aplastic, atretic, stenosed, or duplicated. Microtia is divided into four classes, with Type 4 representing complete aplasia (Figure 5.1).

PREAURICULAR SINUS. A preauricular sinus is a small pit that is characteristically positioned superior to the tragus where the helix meets the side of the head. Preauricular sinuses are particularly common in dark-skinned people and represent incomplete fusion of the hillocks of tissue that are the anlage of the pinna. The sinuses may be shallow or the tract might extend deeply toward the external canal. Recurrent infection is the only indication for surgical excision of a preauricular sinus.

Traumatic Disorders

The pinna is easily damaged by mechanical and environmental forces. Blunt trauma, such as occurs in boxing, causes a soft-tissue or subperichondrial hematoma (Figure 5.2). If the hematoma is allowed to be absorbed slowly, the cartilage calcifies and the soft tissues thicken to form a "cauliflower ear." Therefore a hematoma should be evacuated as soon as possible by making a curvilinear incision and a small rubber drain should be kept in place until drainage ceases. A firm pressure dressing is applied.

Subperichondrial effusions may also occur spontaneously and are treated in the same way or by repeated aspiration.

FROSTBITE. Because of its exposed position and tenuous blood supply, the pinna is particularly prone to frostbite. Initially, there is no pain, the pinna becomes white, and then quickly becomes pink. The skin vesiculates and later sloughs (Figure 5.3). It is unwise to further traumatize the skin

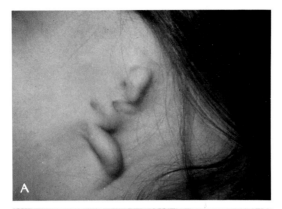

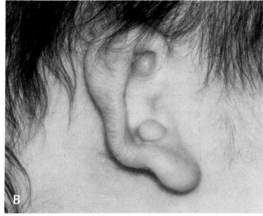

Fig. 5.1. Microtia. Microtia is a congenital maldevelopment of the pinna. There are many variations of anomalies, two of which are shown here.

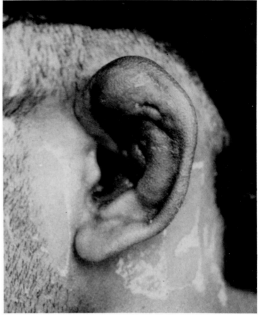

Fig. 5.2. Subperichondrial hematoma of the pinna secondary to trauma. The upper lateral surface of the pinna is swollen and tender.

by vigorous rubbing. Warm the pinna rapidly with warm water and use analgesics, if necessary. Topical antibiotics and warm, wet compresses are helpful.

KELOIDS. A keloid is a grossly hypertrophic scar, which is more common in dark-skinned people. Keloid formation is a hazard of piercing the lobule of the ear (Figure 5.4). They present as a slowly expanding and usually painless mass. Small keloids are treated by intralesional injections of corticosteroids (triamcinolone). Larger keloids must first be excised; subsequently, the scar is periodically infiltrated with corticosteroids.

GOUTY TOPHI. Patients with gout may develop small excrescences on the pinna, which are collections of crystals of uric acid. These nodules are removed surgically only if they are cosmetically unacceptable to the patient.

Malignant Neoplasms

SQUAMOUS CELL CARCINOMA. Squamous cell carcinoma is the most frequent malignancy of the pinna. It presents as a painless ulceration with rolled edges, usually on the rim of the helix. Small lesions are treated by primary excision. Larger lesions might respond to radiation therapy.

BASAL CELL CARCINOMA. Basal cell carcinomas are more insidious than the squamous variety, have the typical pearly, umbilicated form (but may be ulcerated), and are treated by surgery or radiation therapy.

Inflammatory Disorders

ALLERGIC DERMATITIS. Allergic dermatitis of the pinna is caused by hair-

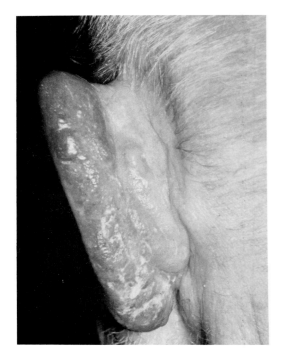

Fig. 5.3. Frostbite of the pinna in a 73-year-old indigent man.

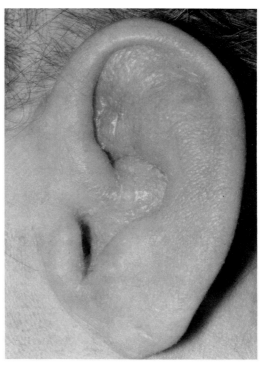

Fig. 5.5. Chronic allergic dermatitis of the pinna. The skin is thick and weeping, but it is not tender.

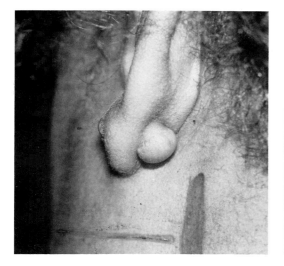

Fig. 5.4. Keloid of the lobule of the ear in a young black woman that developed after piercing.

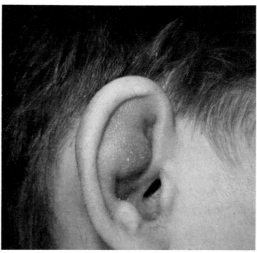

Fig. 5.6. Perichondritis of the pinna. This red, tender swelling of the pinna developed postoperatively.

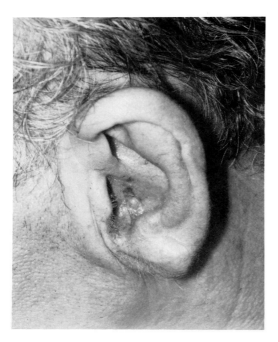

Fig. 5.7. Herpetic lesion of the pinna. Characteristic, painful vesiculations convert into superficial ulcerations, as shown here. The patient depicted in this figure also had facial paralysis.

sprays, earrings, and other agents. The skin is swollen, reddened, and might weep profusely but is not tender (Figure 5.5). The condition responds rapidly to the administration of topical corticosteroids in the form of a cream, ointment, or lotion.

INFECTIONS OF THE PINNA. BACTERIAL INFECTIONS. Infections of the pinna are usually secondary to trauma. The most severe form is a perichondritis from Pseudomonas aeruginosa. The pinna is red, hot, swollen, and very tender (Figure 5.6). Pus collects deep to the perichondrium. The condition is treated with intravenous antibiotics and wide surgical drainage, if necessary.

VIRAL INFECTIONS. *Herpes Zoster Oticus (Ramsay Hunt Syndrome)*. This disorder is a polyneuropathy of the seventh, eighth, and in rare cases, the ninth cranial nerves, which is caused by the herpes zoster virus. This viral infection can have wide variation in its clinical manifestation. Facial

paralysis occurs, which is preceded by or concomitant with painful vesicular lesions of the pinna and external auditory canal (Figure 5.7). The cochlear and vestibular nerves might also be involved, with associated hearing loss and vertigo. Even the vagus nerve can be affected, with associated hoarseness and dysphagia.

The treatment of herpes zoster oticus is supportive and symptomatic. Dusting the skin with boric acid powder is helpful, and analgesics are used, as necessary.

DISORDERS OF THE EXTERNAL AUDITORY CANAL

Congenital Anomalies

Congenital anomalies of the external auditory canal, the pinna, and middle ear usually occur together but without a set pattern of relationship. For instance, the pinna might be grossly deformed, while the external canal is nearly normal, and vice versa. The anomalies of the external auditory canal are classified as follows.

1. Aplasia—the canal has not developed. The condyle of the mandible is displaced posteriorly and articulates with the anterior face of the mastoid process.
2. Atresia—the tympanic bone is present but has failed to canalize. The position of the external auditory canal is represented by a block of bone or bone and soft tissue.
3. Stenosis—the external auditory canal has developed but its lumen is small and frequently tortuous. Stenosis of the external auditory canal is common in patients with Down's syndrome.
4. Duplication—in duplication anomalies the anlage of the external auditory canal has split into two fractions: one develops into a normal canal and the other forms a tract that ends blindly close to the periauriclar skin, sometimes taking a variable course through the parotid gland. Pa-

tients with duplication anomalies present with recurrent infections.

Cerumen (Earwax)

Cerumen is a protective substance. There are two basic types: the soft, brown sticky variety found in blacks and caucasians (80%) and a dry, rice-like, scaly type found primarily in people belonging to mongoloid races (20%). Cerumen is secreted by the ceruminous glands, which are modified sebaceous glands in the skin of the cartilaginous external canal. Cerumen consists of a mixture of triglycerides and contains lysozymes. It has mild antibacterial activity and is a vehicle for the removal of epithelial debris, which migrates slowly away from the tympanic membrane.

If epithelial migration fails, if cerumen production is excessive, or if the lumen of the canal is too small, cerumen might completely occlude the canal. The patient then complains of a painless blockage of the ear and has a partial conductive hearing loss. The wax should be removed. There are two techniques for removing cerumen: directly, with a small curette (Figure 1.3), or by irrigation. In the direct method, good exposure with a speculum of adequate size and lighting by a head mirror or headlight are necessary. Very gently use a small curette. Irrigation is performed with a

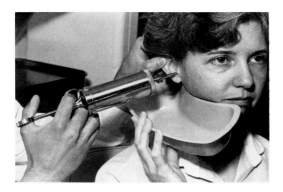

Fig. 5.8. Irrigating the external ear canal. The water is directed to the posterior wall of the canal. It is reflected back by the tympanic membrane and displaces cerumen or foreign bodies.

rounded or soft-tipped, large syringe or dental irrigator with water at body temperature. The jet of water is directed in a posterosuperior direction to separate the cerumen from the canal skin (Figure 5.8). If the plug of cerumen is too hard for easy removal, it should first be softened by the daily use of drops of warmed olive oil, hydrogen peroxide, or triethanolamine polypeptide oleate-condensate (Cerumenex). Irrigation and softeners should not be used if a perforation of the tympanic membrane is suspected.

External Otitis

External otitis (otitis externa, swimmer's ear, Singapore ear) is an inflammation of the skin of the external auditory canal, which might be allergic or infective.

ALLERGIC EXTERNAL OTITIS. Allergic external otitis is usually associated with an allergic reaction of the pinna. The specific allergens are generally difficult to identify but can be cosmetic products such as hairsprays and hair tints. An allergic reaction to fungal spores might be the cause of some cases of chronic external otitis. Neomycin, a common ingredient in many topical ear preparations, can cause a "contact dermatitis." The treatment is to avoid the allergen and apply a topical corticosteroid, such as 0.1% betamethasone, as a cream or ointment.

INFECTIVE EXTERNAL OTITIS. Infective external otitis can be either localized (furuncle) or diffuse.

LOCALIZED CONDITIONS (FURUNCLES). Abscesses are caused by infection of the hair follicles of the external auditory canal by Staphylococcus aureus. These abscesses are usually small and extremely painful. The skin is swollen, pink, turgid, shiny, and exquisitely tender. The rest of the external canal and the tympanic membrane are normal. A tender enlargement of the ipsilateral high jugular lymph node might develop. Systemic antibiotics are rarely indicated. Warm compresses are soothing, and insertng a wick that has been soaked with glycerin into the ear canal is helpful. Topical drops containing an antibiotic and a corticosteroid might hasten resolution, and analgesics should be used liberally.

DIFFUSE CONDITIONS. *Viral External Otitis.* Acute viral external otitis is uncommon and usually presents with very painful vesicles. The vesicles vary in size and appearance, are usually small (about 3 mm in diameter), yellow and transparent, and are filled with clear fluid (Figure 5.9). They are more common in the bony canal and on the tympanic membrane (myringitis bullosa). Therapy is symptomatic, and warmed irrigations are soothing. Rupturing the vesicles might relieve the pain.

Myringitis Bullosa. Myringitis bullosa is an acutely painful vesiculation of the squamous epithelium of the tympanic membrane. This disorder was originally thought to be caused by a viral infection of the tympanic membrane. There is evidence, however, that many cases are secondary to underlying otitis media.

Bacterial External Otitis (Swimmer's Ear, Singapore Ear). Bacterial infection is the most frequent cause of diffuse external

otitis. The organism usually involved is Pseudomonas aeruginosa, but Streptococci and Staphylococci are occasionally contributing organisms. Bacterial external otitis is common in hot, humid climates, in the summer months, and after swimming.

The patient first complains of itching, which is followed in a few hours or a day or two by wetness in the canal and, sometimes, by pain. The moisture varies from a minimal, almost undetectable, amount to frank otorrhea. The discharge is cream-

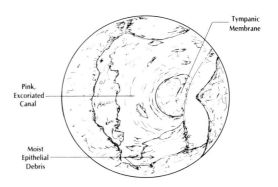

Fig. 5.10. Diffuse bacterial external otitis. The skin of the canal is pink, edematous, and inflamed. There is a large amount of epithelial debris.

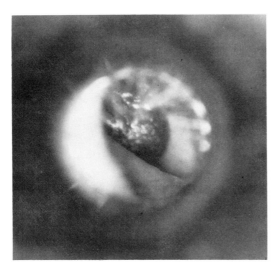

Fig. 5.9. Vesicle in the skin of the external ear canal. The bleb is filled with serosanguineous fluid. This painful condition is probably caused by viral infection.

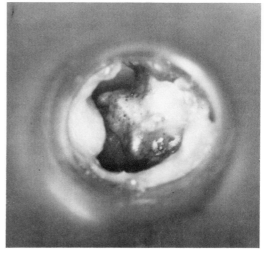

Fig. 5.11. Fungal external otitis caused by Aspergillus. The large mass of debris is gray in color with numerous black spots (sporangiophores) on its surface.

colored or yellow. The canal contains a variable amount of moist epithelial debris that might block the lumen, causing secondary hearing loss (Figure 5.10).

Before beginning treatment, take a sample for bacteriologic study. Next, thoroughly clean the canal using fine suction or cotton-tipped probes under direct vision. Magnification is useful. Topical preparations, particularly drops, are helpful. These preparations should contain a topical antibiotic, such as neomycin, polymyxin, and colistin, and a corticosteroid, such as hydrocortisone. If the infection is severe, insert a wick that has been soaked with eardrops. Analgesics can be used, if necessary.

Fungal External Otitis. Fungal external otitis occurs less frequently than bacterial external otitis. The presenting symptom is usually itching, followed by pain, otorrhea, and hearing loss. The hearing loss is caused by an accumulation of epithelial debris and purulent material. The lumen of the canal is filled with thick sheets of white or gray membranous material (resembling wet blotting paper). The skin of the canal is red and excoriated. Aspergillus infection is characterized by the presence of numerous black sporangia on the epithelial debris (Figure 5.11).

Fungi require moisture and an alkaline medium to live. Treatment is more effective after the canal has been thoroughly cleaned and dried. Then, use topical preparations that are slightly acid; drops of 10% acetic acid with or without hydrocortisone are effective. Other antifungal agents are also useful, such as gentian violet as drops, iodochlorhydroxyquin (Vioform) cream, and drops of m-cresylacetate 25% (Cresylate). Swimming is not allowed.

Fulminating (Malignant) External Otitis. Fulminating external otitis is an infection that occurs in middle-aged or elderly diabetics. It is a fast-spreading, tenacious, and highly resistant infection by species of Pseudomonas. Initially, only the cartilaginous canal is affected. The infection subsequently spreads into the surrounding soft tissues, involving the facial nerve and mastoid bone and finally extending intracranially.

Painful swelling of the cartilaginous canal occurs with little otorrhea, and the diabetes becomes difficult to control. The discharge must be cultured and the appropriate antibiotic administered intravenously in high doses. Gentamicin, tobramycin, and carbenicillin are generally used in different combinations, and treatment must be continued for 2 weeks after the infection is eradicated because of the tendency for it to recur. Necrotic tissue should be excised only if absolutely necessary. Even with the most vigorous treatment, a number of patients with this condition will die.

Neoplasms

BENIGN. Exostoses are small, asymptomatic, smooth, white excrescences in the bony external auditory canal. The usual site is the roof of the canal close to the tympanic membrane, but larger, more diffuse excrescences are found on the pos-

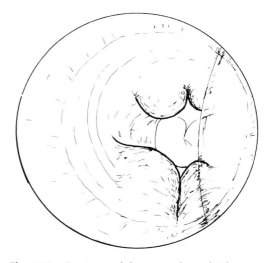

Fig. 5.12. Exostoses of the external canal. There are two smooth, hard, white, round masses on the roof of the canal close to the tympanic membrane. Two more diffuse bony thickenings are also found on the floor of the canal.

terior and anterior walls (Figure 5.12). Swimming in cold water allegedly predisposes one to exostoses of the ear canal. Exostoses cause problems if they grow large enough to cause blockage of the canal. They are removed only if they cause frequent symptoms such as external otitis or hearing loss.

MALIGNANT. Malignant tumors of the external auditory canal are rare. The most frequent type is a squamous cell carcinoma. The patient complains of symptoms that are identical to those of an external otitis but which are recalcitrant to the usual forms of management. A granular mass might be visible or there might be an area of thickened skin with serous drainage. A neoplasm should be suspected in any patient who has an external otitis that is unresponsive to the usual forms of medication. A biopsy usually establishes the diagnosis. Small lesions are treated by wide surgical excision, including removal of all of the skin and part of the bone of the external canal. Larger lesions require more extensive treatment, either radical surgery and/or radiation therapy.

BIBLIOGRAPHY

Arndt, K.A.: Manual of Dermatologic Therapeutics. 2nd Ed. Boston, Little, Brown, and Co., 1978, pp. 25–31.

Chandler, J.R.: Malignant external otitis: Further consideration. Ann. Otol. Rhinol. Laryngol., 86:417–428, 1977.

Crabtree, J.A., Britton, B.H., and Pierce, M.K.: Carcinoma of the external auditory canal. Laryngoscope, 86:405–415, 1976.

DiBartolomeo, J.R.: Exostoses in the external auditory canal. Ann. Otol. Rhinol. Laryngol., 88(Suppl. 61): 1979.

Karmody, C.S.: Classification of the anomalies of the first branchial groove. Otolaryngol. Head Neck Surg., 87:334–338, 1979.

Senturia, B.H., Marcus, M.D., and Lucente, F.E.: Diseases of the External Ear. 2nd Ed. New York, Grune and Stratton, 1980.

Senturia, B.H.: External otitis, acute diffuse. Ann. Otol. Rhinol. Laryngol., 82(Suppl. 8):1–23, 1973.

Tanzer, R.C., and Edgerton, M.T. (eds.): Symposium on Reconstruction of the Auricle. St. Louis, C.V. Mosby Co., 1974, pp. 150–160.

Wanamaker, H.A.: Suppurative perichondritis of the auricle. Trans. Am. Acad. Ophthalmol. Otolaryngol., 76:1289–1291, 1972.

Chapter 6

DISORDERS OF THE MIDDLE EAR

Most disorders of the middle ear result in a conductive hearing loss, and traumatic and inflammatory problems of the middle ear are frequently associated with temporary or permanent perforation of the tympanic membrane.

CONGENITAL ANOMALIES

The middle ear is frequently involved in congenital anomalies of the first and second branchial arch apparatus. Anomalies may individually or collectively involve the ossicles, the facial nerve, and even the cavity of the middle ear.

Ossicles may be fused together, a part or all of an ossicle might be missing, or there might be gross deformation of an ossicle. The malleus and incus are frequently fused together. The long process of the incus and the stapes are more likely to be deformed. The stapes might consist of a single crus, or the footplate might be fused to the edges of the oval window. All of these anomalies result in a conductive hearing loss.

The fallopian canal might be widely dehiscent, particularly in its horizontal segment, and expose the facial nerve. Alternatively, the facial nerve might take an abnormal course, sometimes across the promontory. The facial nerve might also split in two and wrap around the stapes.

None of these anomalies necessarily causes dysfunction of the facial nerve. Dysplasia of the nerve is often associated with anomalies of the middle ear and mandible. Frequently, obvious or subtle congenital dysfunctions of the facial musculature exist that suggest various degrees of dysplasia of the facial nerve. The lower third of the face is most often affected.

TRAUMATIC PROBLEMS

Mechanical trauma of the middle ear can occur directly via the ear canal or be secondary to fracture of the temporal bone. Fractures of the temporal bone are discussed in Chapter 7. Injury to the middle ear by way of the ear canal is caused accidentally by cotton-tipped swabs, pencils, and other instruments that are used to clean or scratch the ear canal. The tympanic membrane, ossicles, and facial nerve are all at risk, and almost all injuries result in a conductive hearing loss. The commonest middle ear injury is perforation of the tympanic membrane. The ossicles might be fractured or dislocated, and, of these three bones, the incus is the most frequently involved. The crura of the stapes, and, in rare cases, the footplate of the stapes might be fractured. Dislocation of the footplate into the vestibule results in a sensorineural hearing loss. Fractured ossicles do not mend, but the associated conductive hearing loss can be corrected by surgically repositioning or replacing the affected bone to restore continuity of the sound-conducting mechanism.

Trauma to the facial nerve is discussed in Chapter 9.

IDIOPATHIC PROBLEMS

Otosclerosis

Otosclerosis is a genetically determined, dominant, proliferative, invasive bony condition of the otic capsule that afflicts 4% of Caucasians. Clinical symptoms, however, occur in only 0.5% of the population and are more frequent in females.

At a point on the medial aspect of the anterior edge of the oval window, around the fissula ante fenestram, the bone of the otic capsule changes. The bone becomes more vascular (otospongiosis), grows faster, loses its architecture, and slowly invades the rest of the otic capsule and the footplate of the stapes. As a result, the stapes becomes fixed, causing a conductive hearing loss. Later, the bone matures, becoming less vascular and more sclerotic (otosclerosis) (Figure 6.1). Otosclerosis usually progresses slowly. A conductive hearing loss frequently presents during the teenage years and progresses over many years. There is a characteristic pattern to the hearing loss. In the early stages a greater loss occurs in the lower frequencies, and

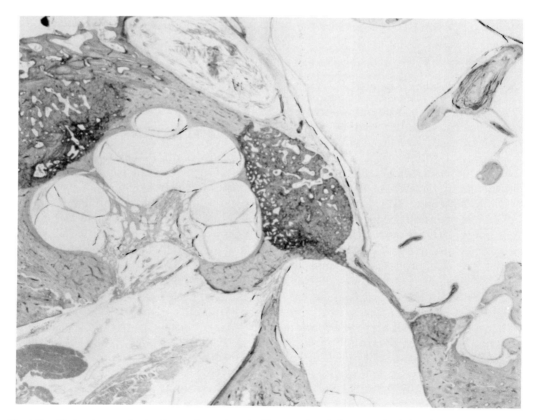

Fig. 6.1. Photomicrograph of a focus of otosclerosis. The otosclerotic bone on the left is disorganized and more vascular than the normal otic capsule that can be seen at the lower right corner of the field. The footplate of the stapes is invaded and fixed by the otosclerosis.

bone conduction thresholds are near normal except for a dip at 2000 Hz (Carhart's notch) (Figure 6.2). Much later, cochlear function is affected so that a purely conductive loss becomes mixed. Speech discrimination scores are usually within normal limits.

There is no known treatment for otosclerosis. The hearing loss, however, can be handled in one of two ways: either with a hearing aid or by surgery (a stapedectomy) (see Chapter 23). In a stapedectomy the fixed stapes bone is removed and replaced by a prosthesis. Some evidence exists to suggest that large doses of sodium fluoride over a long period of time might hasten maturation and slow the progression of otosclerosis.

INFLAMMATORY DISORDERS (OTITIS MEDIA)

Otitis media is probably one of the most ubiquitous diseases that afflicts mankind. It has a particularly high incidence in the Mongoloid and Caucasian races, Eskimos, and North American Indians.

By definition, otitis media is any inflammation of the middle ear. Inflammation of the middle ear always results in effusion of fluid into the tympanum. Otitis media is more common in children, with a peak incidence between the ages of 2 and 6 years. One or more factors contribute to inflammatory disease of the middle ear mucosa: (1) infection (bacterial or viral, rarely fungal); (2) allergy; (3) nonspecific mucosal disease (e.g., Wegener's granulomatosis); and (4) obstruction of the eustachian tube. Obstruction of the eustachian tube plays an integral part in otitis media but its precise role is as yet undetermined. For instance, it is not known whether obstruction of the tube occurs before, simultaneous with, or after the infection. What is known, however, is that a purely mechanical dysfunction of the tube will result in a collection of transparent, amber-colored, nonpurulent fluid. Acute otitis media is usually related to upper respiratory tract infections.

Clinically, otitis media can be divided into two broad categories: serous otitis media and suppurative (infective) otitis media. Both categories have acute and chronic forms.

Serous Otitis Media

By definition, serous otitis media (also called catarrhal otitis, seromucinous otitis, and "glue ears") is a nonsuppurative otitis media that is characterized by the accumulation of a nonpurulent effusion in the middle ear. The most significant effect of serous otitis media is a conductive hearing loss. The magnitude of the loss varies, depending on the type of fluid and whether the middle ear is partially or completely filled with effusion. Serous otitis media is a generic term that includes a number of different entities. At least three subcategories of effusion have been recognized:

1. Serous, which has an amber-colored, serous fluid that is bacteriologically sterile.
2. Thick, mucoid, tenacious "glue ear."

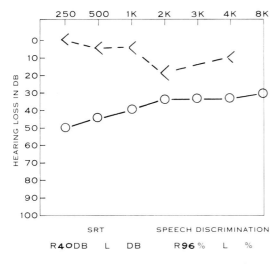

Fig. 6.2. Audiogram of a 45-year-old woman with otosclerosis. A moderate conductive hearing loss has resulted. The dip in the bone conduction threshold at 2000 Hz is a typical Carhart notch.

Few bacteria can be cultured from this material.

3. Mucopurulent, which has a thick, cream-colored effusion that is usually under pressure.

SEROUS EFFUSIONS. This condition is caused by an effusion of serous transudate into the middle ear. Serous fluid is common in viral infections of the upper respiratory tract, allergies, and mechanical malfunction of the eustachian tube. The patient complains of blockage of the ear and diminished hearing. The tympanic membrane has a yellow color and, if the middle ear is only partially filled, air-fluid levels and bubbles can be seen (Figure 6.3). The air-fluid level will change with variations in the position of the head. A conductive hearing loss of 15 to 40 dB occurs. The mucosa of the middle ear is usually flat and minimally thickened. Acute serous otitis media can present with otalgia, hyperemia of the tympanic membrane, and rapid development of effusion. Otalgia usually subsides spontaneously. Treatment is with oral and topical nasal decongestants. Effusions that persist for more than 3 months are treated by placement of a ventilating tube (see Chapter 22).

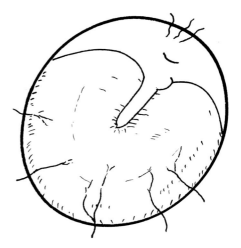

Fig. 6.4. Drawing of the tympanic membrane in chronic mucopurulent serous otitis media ("glue ear"). The tympanic membrane is usually slate-colored and might be slightly full or retracted.

MUCOID EFFUSIONS (GLUE EARS). The causative factors of glue ears are unknown, but recent studies indicate that it is a low-grade, inflammatory response to infection. The primary symptom is conductive hearing loss at a 25 to 40 dB level. Neither pain nor evidence of active infection is usually associated with glue ears. The tympanic membrane is slate-colored, thickened, and retracted, with prominence of the handle of the malleus, loss of the light reflex, and grossly diminished mobility (Figure 6.4). After myringotomy, the effusion does not flow out spontaneously but remains in the tympanum and must be removed by suction. The tenacity of the material makes aspiration difficult.

Treatment is with oral and topical nasal decongestants because antibiotics will not clear up established glue ears. If the effusion persists, myringotomy is performed, the effusion is aspirated, and a ventilating tube is inserted through the incision (see Chapter 22).

MUCOPURULENT EFFUSION. This cream-colored effusion is less common, contains many polymorphonuclear leukocytes, and probably represents a partially treated or smoldering, acute sup-

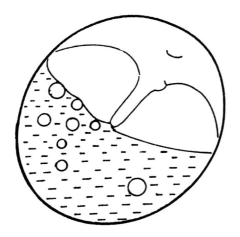

Fig. 6.3. Serous otitis media. There is a pale yellow, watery fluid, and bubbles of air can be seen in the middle ear. An air-fluid level is shown but is not always visible.

purative otitis media. Effusions may persist for weeks after an episode of acute otalgia and fever.

The tympanic membrane is full (i.e., bulges slightly) and hyperemic with prominent, radially disposed vessels, and a 30 to 40 dB conductive hearing loss develops. After myringotomy, the fluid wells out of the tympanum. The mucosa of the middle ear is markedly edematous. Treatment is by oral and topical nasal decongestants and appropriate antibiotics such as amoxicillin, 20 mg/kg/day in divided doses for 10 days. If conservative management fails, myringotomy is performed and a ventilating tube is inserted.

Serous otitis media is generally thought to predispose to ossicular necrosis, particularly of the long process of the incus; however, the culprit behind ossiculolysis is most likely suppuration rather than the presence of a nonsuppurative effusion.

Decongestants are used in the treatment of serous otitis media to reduce mucosal edema in the hope that this will open the lumen of the eustachian tube. Their efficacy is doubtful.

Acute Suppurative Otitis Media

Acute suppurative otitis media occurs when there is a bacterial infection of the mucosa of the middle ear. The bacteria that are usually involved are Streptococcus pneumoniae, Hemophilus influenzae, group A Streptococcus pyogenes, and Staphylococcus aureus (in rare cases); more recently, anaerobic bacteria have also been identified. Obstruction of the eustachian tube is probably a predisposing factor. Exactly how the bacteria get into the mucosa of the middle ear is unknown. The mode of entry could be by direct ascent up the eustachian tube, a direction which is opposite to ciliary action, or by hematogenous or lymphatic spread.

Acute, severe pain, hearing loss, fever and leukocytosis are associated with acute suppurative otitis media. The pain is excruciating and responds poorly to the usual analgesics. A child with this disease usually has a very high fever that might rise to 40°C, rapidly becomes toxic, pulls at his ears, and usually screams because of the severity of the pain. A purulent effusion accumulates extremely rapidly, within even minutes, in the middle ear. The tympanic membrane is at first pink, hyperemic, edematous, bulging, loses its luster and its light reflex, and might even be vesiculated. The usual landmarks are obscured (Figure 6.5). The skin of the external auditory canal is hyperemic and might be vesiculated, but is usually not infected. A concomitant tenderness over the mastoid process might occur. The tympanic membrane bulges because of the accumulation of fluid under pressure in the middle ear. One area of the membrane, usually either the center or in the antero-inferior quadrant, eventually becomes whitish, and, under continued pressure the tympanic membrane ruptures spontaneously through this area. A sudden gush of blood-tinged, purulent fluid follows, with immediate relief of pain. The mucosa of the middle ear is grossly inflamed, hyperemic, edematous, and is infiltrated with polymorphonuclear leukocytes (Figure 6.6). The effusion in the cavity of the middle ear is thick, yellow, might even be blood-tinged, and contains many polymorphonuclear leukocytes.

Acute suppurative otitis media should be treated immediately with high doses of antibiotics. Most of the organisms involved are sensitive to penicillin, ampicillin, amoxicillin, and erythromycin, but ampicillin and amoxicillin (20 mg/kg/day orally in divided doses) have become the agents of choice in young children because they are effective against H. influenzae. In addition, oral and topical nasal decongestants should be used and analgesics given liberally. A warm pack applied to the ear is soothing. Warm anesthetic solutions (Auralgan) instilled into the ear canal are also helpful. If the tympanic membrane continues to bulge significantly and the

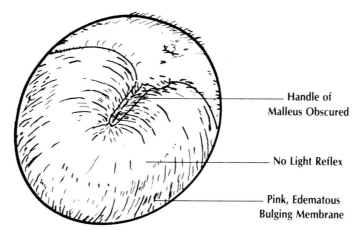

Handle of
Malleus Obscured

No Light Reflex

Pink, Edematous
Bulging Membrane

Fig. 6.5. Drawing of the tympanic membrane in acute suppurative otitis media. The membrane bulges and is red because of intense hyperemia. The landmarks, specifically the lateral process of the malleus, are obscured.

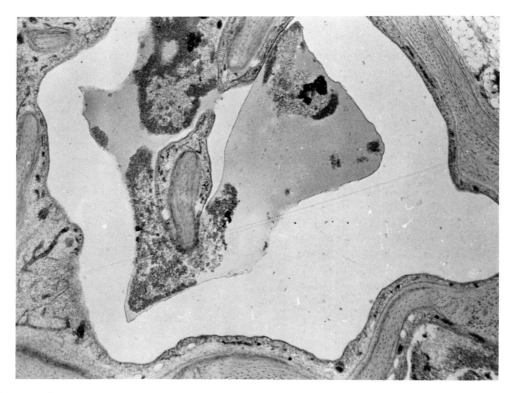

Fig. 6.6. Photomicrograph of the middle ear in acute suppurative otitis media. The mucosa is thickened and edematous, with dilated blood vessels and infiltrated with polymorphonuclear leukocytes. There is pus in the lumen.

pain increases instead of subsiding over 24 to 48 hours, a wide myringotomy should be performed.

ACUTE NECROTIZING OTITIS MEDIA. This condition is a fulminating infection that characteristically occurs in association with scarlet fever and measles but also in debilitated patients.

The inflammatory process is severe and causes dissolution of the tympanic membrane and ossicles, particularly the long process of the incus. Necrotizing otitis media must be treated early and vigorously with large doses of antibiotics, and myringotomy should be done earlier rather than later.

VIRAL OTITIS MEDIA. The role of viruses in otitis media is not clear. They probably predispose the mucosa of the middle ear to secondary infection by bacteria. Clinically, it is impossible to differentiate between viral and bacterial otitis media.

IDIOPATHIC HEMOTYMPANUM. This condition has been partially misnamed. Idiopathic hemotympanum is merely a type of serous otitis media in which hemosiderin is present in the effusion, probably as a result of the disintegration of a comparatively small number of red blood cells. The characteristic finding is a blue-black appearance of the tympanic membrane. The membrane is retracted and its mobility is limited. The causes, symptoms, and treatment of idiopathic hemotympanum are the same as for serous otitis media. A true hemotympanum (i.e., frank hemorrhage into the middle ear) is found with fractures of the temporal bone and sometimes in blood dyscrasias such as leukemia and thrombocytopenic purpura. No specific treatment is required; the blood in the middle ear usually clears with time.

CHOLESTEROL GRANULOMA. A cholesterol granuloma is a reddish-brown, painless mass of granulation tissue that, histologically, contains cholesterol-like crystals and foreign-body giant cells. The size of the mass varies considerably and might be tiny or might fill the middle ear and mastoid cells. A cholesterol granuloma is formed after spontaneous hemorrhage into the mucosa. The symptoms depend on the size of the lesion. Substantial conductive hearing loss can develop. Cholesterol granuloma is part of the spectrum of otitis media but usually requires surgical removal.

BAROTRAUMATIC OTITIS. A sudden relative increase in atmospheric pressure causes the eustachian tube to be closed or even locked. The resulting negative pressure in the tympanum causes acute otalgia, a serous or even blood-tinged effusion, and a conductive hearing loss. Barotrauma occurs in rapidly descending airplanes and in scuba diving. Intercurrent upper respiratory tract infection predisposes one to barotraumatic otitis. Treatment is with systemic and topical nasal vasoconstrictors. Myringotomy might be necessary for severe otalgia. Prophylaxis is by chewing gum, repeatedly swallowing or using oral or topical nasal decongestants half an hour before the anticipated descent of the aircraft.

SYSTEMIC DISEASE AND OTITIS MEDIA. Any systemic disease, such as Wegener's granulomatosis, that particularly affects the upper respiratory tract might present as acute otitis media. These episodes, however, do not respond to the usual therapeutic measures. Diagnosis might require biopsy of the mucosa of the nose or nasopharynx.

MYRINGOTOMY. Myringotomy is the technique of opening the tympanic membrane, usually by incision. The tympanic membrane is anesthetized locally by infiltration of the external canal, by iontophoresis, or by the use of topical agents such as phenol; general anesthesia may be necessary. Infants and very young children usually require no anesthesia. Incisions are either radial in the anteroinferior quadrant or horizontal across the inferior half of the tympanic membrane (Figure 6.7). Horizontal incisions are used for wide drain-

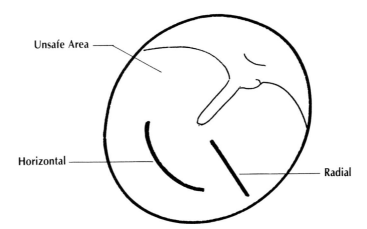

Fig. 6.7. Incisions for performing myringotomy. The horizontal incision gives a wide opening and, therefore, better drainage. Incisions must not be placed in the posterosuperior quadrant.

age. Incisions should not be made in the posterosuperior quadrant because of danger to the incus, stapes, and chorda tympani. If indicated, the fluid in the middle ear is first sampled for culture and sensitivity studies. The contents of the middle ear are then aspirated using a fine suction. A biflanged ventilating tube is frequently inserted through the incision, leaving one flange outside (see Figure 22.1). This technique ventilates the tympanum and reduces the tendency for fluid to accumulate.

Chronic Suppurative Otitis Media

Chronic suppurative otitis media is a generic term that assumes a long-standing perforation of the tympanic membrane, chronic otorrhea, and, usually, a conductive hearing loss.

There are two main types of chronic suppurative otitis media, which seldom occur simultaneously in the same patient. They are benign catarrhal otitis and chronic otitis with cholesteatoma. A comparison of the main clinical findings of these two disorders is given in Table 6.1.

CHRONIC CATARRHAL OTITIS MEDIA. Chronic catarrhal otitis media (also called catarrhal otitis, chronic secretory otitis media, and chronic tubotym-

panitis) is characterized by a mucoid otorrhea that increases in the presence of upper respiratory tract infections. The quality and quantity of the drainage varies from patient to patient and from time to time. It is usually thick, clear to yellow in color, and has a slight odor.

Chronic catarrhal otitis media usually begins in childhood after an episode of acute otitis media. Obstruction of the eustachian tube is the basic cause of catarrhal otitis. The cause of the obstruction might be scarring, allergy, or adenoid hypertrophy.

In chronic catarrhal otitis media the tympanic membrane is thickened and scarred and a central perforation exists (Figure 6.8), through which the discharge exudes. The mucosa of the middle ear is granular, edematous, and might be polypoid. A conductive hearing loss develops, the magnitude of which depends on the size and position of the perforation and whether the ossicles are damaged.

TREATMENT. Thoroughly examine the nose and nasopharynx. Culture the aural secretions, have sensitivity studies performed, and administer the appropriate antibiotics. Topical otic drops that contain antibiotics (neomycin, Polymyxin) and a corticosteroid are helpful. An antihistamine-decongestant preparation might be

Table 6.1. Clinical Differentiation in Chronic Suppurative Otitis Media

	Benign	Cholesteatoma (potentially dangerous)
Discharge:	Mucoid	Purulent, malodorous
Site of disease:	Eustachian tube	Superior half of middle ear, epitympanum, and mastoid process
Tympanic membrane:	Perforation of the pars tensa, usually central	Perforation of the pars flaccida or posterosuperior marginal perforation of pars tensa
Mucosa:	Edema with gland formation	Ectopic squamous epithelium
Cholesteatoma:	No	Yes
Bone erosion:	Ossicles only	Ossicles and mastoid
Polyp:	Uncommon	Frequent
Roentgenograms:	Clouding of mastoid cells and sclerosis	Underdeveloped sclerotic mastoid, frequently with erosion of the periantral area and scutum
Treatment:	Medical, sometimes surgical	Primarily surgical

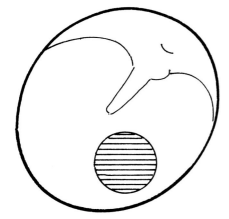 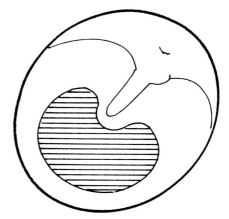

Fig. 6.8. Types of central perforations usually associated with chronic catarrhal otitis media.

useful, particularly if an allergy of the upper respiratory tract is suspected. If the middle ear mucosa becomes excessively polypoid, remove the redundant tissue with fine-cupped forceps.

Exenteration of the mastoid cells and a tympanoplasty are occasionally successful, especially if episodes of severe, superadded bacterial infection occur and if there is even a partial patency of the eustachian tube.

Chronic Suppurative Otitis Media With Cholesteatoma

A cholesteatoma is a sac of ectopic squamous epithelium. Cholesteatomas usually

develop in the superior half of the middle ear and frequently extend posteriorly into the mastoid process.

If, during an episode of acute otitis media, the tympanic membrane becomes perforated at its edge (marginal) or through the pars flaccida, squamous epithelium tends to grow into the middle ear space forming a "sac" in which keratin accumulates. This sac is known as a cholesteatoma because of the original erroneous concept that it was a tumor with a high cholesterol content.

The patient complains of a small amount of a yellow or green, foul-smelling discharge and a hearing loss. The ear canal is

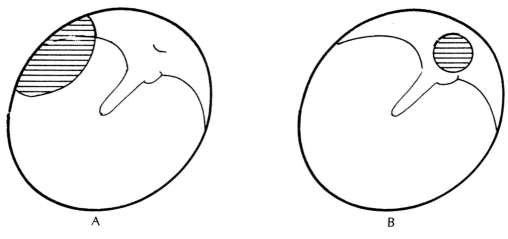

A   B

Fig. 6.9. *A.* Marginal perforation in the posterior superior segment of the pars tensa. *B.* Perforation in the pars flaccida.

usually moist but might also be dry or lined by thick, greenish-brown crusts, which must be removed before the pathologic process can be properly assessed. Squamous epithelium sheds keratin, which accumulates in the cholesteatoma sac as sheets of soft, shiny, chalk-white material. If this keratin is completely removed, the underlying "cholesteatoma matrix" (squamous epithelium) is seen as a smooth, gray, shiny layer. In some patients there is a perforation of the pars flaccida, from which drains a purulent otorrhea and keratin flakes protrude. Alternatively, a marginal perforation might develop, usually in the posterosuperior quadrant of the pars tensa (Figure 6.9). Here, the squamous epithelium is plastered onto the chorda tympani, the long process of the incus and the stapes, and other parts of the medial wall of the middle ear. Cholesteatomas tend to erode bone, either by pressure or by enzymatic action. The inferior edge of the scutum, which is the lateral wall of the epitympanum, and the long process of the incus are particularly vulnerable (Figure 6.10). Similarly, a cholesteatoma will cause expansion of the mastoid antrum. Because the expansion is slow, an osteoblastic reaction occurs in the surrounding bone. Ra-

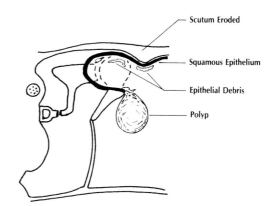

Scutum Eroded

Squamous Epithelium

Epithelial Debris

Polyp

Fig. 6.10. Diagrammatic representation of a cholesteatoma. The skin of the superior bony external canal has grown through a perforation in the pars flaccida into the epitympanum, forming a sac that is filled with keratinous debris. A polyp partially obscures the tympanic membrane.

diologically, the cavity looks smooth with a sclerotic border (Figure 6.11).

AURAL POLYPS. Cholesteatomas also stimulate the formation of red, vascular polyps in the middle ear. Aural polyps tend to protrude through the perforation in the tympanic membrane, extend into the external canal, and usually indicate the presence of a cholesteatoma.

TREATMENT. Cholesteatomas are potentially dangerous because of their propensity to erode bone in the presence of active

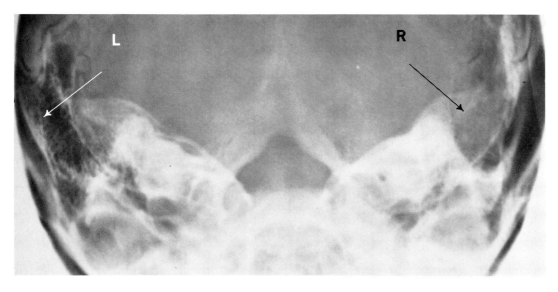

Fig. 6.11. Roentgenogram of the right mastoid of a patient with chronic suppurative otitis media with cholesteatoma. There is a large defect in the mastoid with sharply defined edges. *(Left arrow)* Normal mastoid. *(Right arrow)* Defect in mastoid.

infection. Cultures usually produce heavy growth of Pseudomonas aeruginosa and Proteus organisms. However, evidence exists to suggest that the organisms are primarily saprophytes that depend on the presence of keratin debris.

The treatment of chronic suppurative otitis media with cholesteatoma depends on the size and accessibility of the cholesteatoma. If the "mouth" of the cholesteatoma is wide and the cholesteatoma itself is small, removal of all keratin debris, usually by suction, will substantially reduce or eliminate the infection. Alternatively, if the bulk of the cholesteatoma is inaccessible, its removal by a surgical procedure is necessary. Surgery usually entails a mastoidectomy. Before surgery, however, the ear should be thoroughly cleaned and topical medication (solutions) containing antibiotics and a corticosteroid should be used. A solution containing neomycin, Polymixin, and hydrocortisone, three drops twice daily, is effective. This cleansing and topical therapy is carried out for a few weeks with the

objective of eliminating as much of the infection as possible. Systemic antibiotics are usually unnecessary but should be prescribed if the patient has a great deal of purulence and pain.

Mastoidectomy (see Chapter 22 for more detail). Mastoidectomy is a surgical procedure of exenteration of the mastoid process for the removal of diseased tissue and drainage of the cellular system. There are basically two types of mastoidectomies: simple and radical. Two incisions are used for mastoidectomies. The first is a postauricular incision that is 2 to 3 mm posterior to the postauricular sulcus, and the second is an "endaural" incision that begins just anterior to the crus of the helix and runs inferiorly into the posterior external auditory canal.

In the simple mastoidectomy the intercellular bony septa of the mastoid are removed, creating a single cavity. The aditus ad antrum is widened, and the posterior wall of the bony external canal is kept intact (Figure 6.12). In a radical mastoidec-

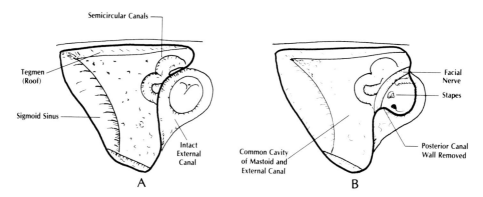

Fig. 6.12. (A) Simple and (B) radical mastoidectomies. The heavy black lines outline the cavities that are created.

tomy the mastoid cells are exenterated and the posterior canal wall is removed so that the cavity of the mastoid process and the lumen of the external auditory canal are joined into a common chamber. The bone overlying the vertical segment of the facial nerve is preserved in the deep canal as the "facial ridge." The tympanic membrane, malleus, incus, and mucosa of the middle ear are removed. In a modified radical mastoidectomy the tympanic membrane and ossicles are preserved.

If it is possible during the mastoidectomy, the hearing apparatus should be reconstructed with a tympanoplasty (see Chapter 22).

Complications of Otitis Media

The same complications may occur with acute or chronic otitis media but are more common with chronic disease. The complications can be divided into two broad categories: those that are confined to the temporal bone and those that go beyond the temporal bone (Figure 6.13).

COMPLICATIONS CONFINED TO THE TEMPORAL BONE. The following is a list of the complications that are confined to the temporal bone:

1. Permanent perforation of the tympanic membrane.

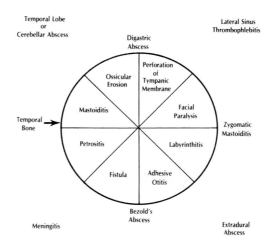

Fig. 6.13. Plan of the complications of otitis media. Complications may be confined to the temporal bone or spread beyond the temporal bone.

2. Erosion of the ossicles of the middle ear.
3. Labyrinthine fistula.
4. Dysfunction of the seventh cranial nerve (see Chapter 9).
5. Labyrinthitis (see Chapter 8).
6. Necrosis of the mucosa with extensive adhesions—adhesive otitis.
7. Mastoiditis.
8. Abscess in the apex of the petrous part of the temporal bone.

COMPLICATIONS BEYOND THE TEMPORAL BONE. INTRACRANIAL EXTENSION. The following is a list of the complications that extend intracranially:

1. Thrombophlebitis of the lateral venous sinus with secondary otitic hydrocephalus and abscess in the occipital musculature.
2. Extradural abscess or pachymeningitis.
3. Meningitis from infection of the subarachnoid space.
4. Abscess of the temporal lobe or cerebellum.

EXTRACRANIAL EXTENSION. The following is a list of the complications that extend extracranially, which are usually secondary to mastoiditis:

1. Spread of infection into the upper sternocleidomastoid muscle—Bezold's abscess.
2. Zygomatic matoiditis.
3. Spread of infection into the digastric muscle—Citelli's abscess.

PERMANENT PERFORATIONS OF THE TYMPANIC MEMBRANE. Perforations of the tympanic membrane may occur in either the pars flaccida or pars tensa. Most acute perforations heal spontaneously; however, they persist when the mucocutaneous edges heal prematurely because this aborts the natural drive to complete closure.

Perforations of the pars tensa may be either central or marginal. Perforations of the pars flaccida are usually associated with cholesteatoma and erosion of the scutum.

CENTRAL PERFORATIONS. Central perforations do not involve the fibrous annulus of the tympanic membrane. They are the commonest type of perforation, occurring most frequently in the anteroinferior quadrant (Figure 6.8). Central perforations tend to be either small and round or larger (one-third to one-half of the tympanic membrane) and kidney-shaped. Central perforations are rarely associated with cholesteatoma.

MARGINAL PERFORATIONS. Marginal perforations involve any margin of the tympanic membrane, at which point the annulus is lost. They are much more common in the posterosuperior quadrant (Figure 6.9). Marginal perforations are usually associated with the ingrowth of squamous epithelium into the middle ear, which might form a cholesteatoma. They are more frequently associated with erosion of the ossicular chain than are central perforations.

EROSION OF THE OSSICLES. Erosion of the ossicles is more common with chronic otitis media but might occur with acute infections. The incus is most frequently eroded, particularly the lower end of the long process and the lenticular process. Next in order of frequency are the head and crura of the stapes. The footplate is relatively resistant. The malleus is also comparatively resistant but its component parts might be involved: the handle with benign chronic otitis and the head with cholesteatoma (Figure 6.14).

FISTULA OF THE OTIC CAPSULE (LABYRINTHINE FISTULA). Labyrinthine fistulae are usually secondary to cholesteatoma. Most "fistulae" of the otic capsule are really not fistulae in the true sense of the word. That is, no free communication occurs between the spaces of the labyrinth and the mastoid cells. Fistulae are areas of bony erosion beneath the matrix of the cholesteatoma, which cause symptoms because of the loss of the bony

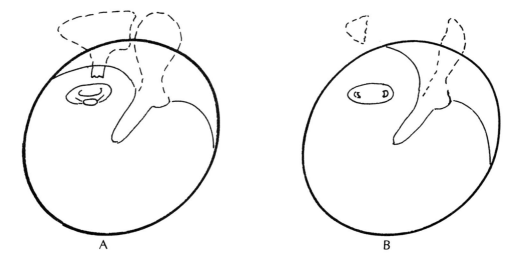

Fig. 6.14. Diagram of different types of erosion of the ossicles. *A.* The long process of the incus is missing. The rest of the ossicles are intact.
B. Severe erosion of the incus, the crura of the stapes, and the head of the malleus has occurred.

protection of the labyrinthine spaces. The eroded area remains sealed by the cholesteatoma. The most frequent site is on the horizontal semicircular canal, but fistulae can also occur on the superior and posterior semicircular canals, on the promontory, and through the footplate of the stapes.

The patient, who has a history of chronic otitis media, suddenly complains of dizziness. Spontaneous onset of vertigo, nausea, and vomiting might develop, or the patient might only experience a sensation of imbalance, or symptoms might be induced only by stimulation (e.g., forceful pressure on the tragus). Sensorineural hearing loss might accompany the disorder, but hearing could also be unaffected. The diagnosis is made by history and by performance of a fistula test.

FISTULA TEST. In the fistula test the pressure in the external auditory canal is deliberately altered. Fistula tests are performed with the same instruments that are used for pneumatic otoscopy: a closed system consisting of an aural speculum that is sealed at one end and fitted with a small rubber bulb for altering pressure (see Fig-

ure 1.1). Siegle's specula are made specifically for this purpose. A tight seal must exist between the speculum and the external canal. Positive pressure is gently created by manipulating the rubber bulb, and the patient's eyes are monitored by the examiner or, preferably, by an assistant.

In the presence of a fistula altering the pressure causes an immediate sensation of dizziness and might induce nystagmus, which is a positive fistula test. The fistula test might also be positive in the absence of chronic otitis media; for example, in congenital syphilis and in a post-traumatic perilymph leak caused by a fractured or dislocated stapes footplate.

Tuning fork tests and an audiogram should also be performed. Erosion of the horizontal semicircular canal can be demonstrated by polytomography and computed tomography.

A labyrinthine fistula not only causes debilitating vestibular symptoms but is a potential pathway for infection of the labyrinth. A fistula must, therefore, be considered for urgent treatment, although in some patients fistulae may exist for a long time without causing labyrinthitis. After an appropriate course of antibiotics to reduce bacterial contamination, a mastoidectomy is performed, the cholesteatoma carefully removed, and the fistula covered with a free graft of temporalis fascia.

MASTOIDITIS. Acute mastoiditis is an infection of the mastoid cell system that occurs secondary to acute or chronic otitis media. Of course, the mastoid cellular system can be involved to some extent in every episode of acute otitis media. The patient first complains of all the symptoms of an acute otitis media. Pain, however, persists even after spontaneous rupture of the tympanic membrane. Fever persists and even increases, and signs of systemic toxicity are present. The postauricular area is first tender, then swells and becomes erythematous. The postauricular sulcus is blunted and the pinna is displaced forward. The points of maximum tenderness are over the tip of the mastoid or over the cribriform area, which is posterior to the posterosuperior quadrant of the external meatus. The swelling increases and eventually becomes fluctuant because the infection spreads beyond the mastoid cortex, forming a subperiosteal abscess. Eventually, the abscess might rupture through the skin. While these clinical events are evolving, parallel changes are occurring in the radiologic picture (Figure 6.15.). At first, the mastoid process looks uniformly cloudy because the cells are filled with fluid. Later, the intercellular septa dissolve to form a coalescent mastoiditis.

The sequence described above can be altered and even aborted by vigorous treatment with antibiotics. Uncontrolled mastoiditis, particularly if a subperiosteal abscess develops, requires mastoidectomy for drainage.

ADHESIVE OTITIS MEDIA. Adhesive otitis media is a condition in which the tympanic membrane or its replacement

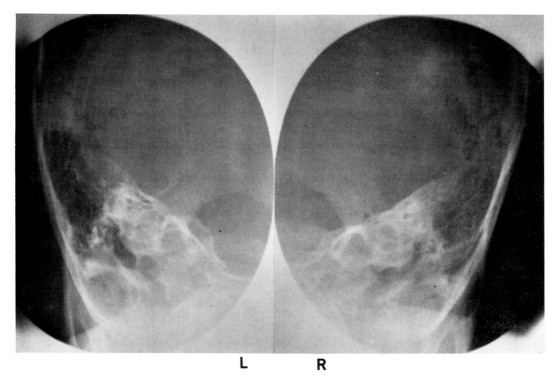

L   R

Fig. 6.15. Roentgenograms of a patient with acute mastoiditis on the right side. The air-cell system is present but is hazy because of the accumulation of fluid. Later, the intercellular septa dissolve to give a coalescent mastoiditis.

adheres to the surface of the promontory. This occurs when the mucosa of the middle ear is severely damaged by infection. The tympanic membrane then becomes plastered against and firmly adherent to the structures on the medial wall, rendering it immobile. The handle of the malleus stands out in bold relief and is pulled medially. A conductive hearing loss results.

THROMBOPHLEBITIS OF THE LATERAL SINUS. Infection of the mastoid might spread to the lateral venous sinus. The sinus thromboses, and the thrombosis might develop into suppurative thrombophlebitis, or the thrombosis might spread and cause increased intracranial pressure (otitic hydrocephalus).

Septic thrombophlebitis is characterized by a spiking fever that rises and falls rapidly (''picket fence''). The patient quickly becomes toxic. A lumbar puncture reveals clear cerebrospinal fluid, sometimes under slightly increased pressure. Pressure over the ipsilateral jugular vein in the neck does not increase the cerebrospinal fluid pressure (Queckenstedt's test). Treatment is with large doses of intravenous antibiotics, such as ampicillin and dicloxacillin, and immediate exploration and drainage of the infected sinus via a mastoidectomy.

MENINGITIS. Meningitis is a fairly common complication of acute otitis media, especially in children. The usual causative organisms are Hemophilus influenzae and pneumococcus. Meningitis occurs very rapidly after the onset of otitis media. Usually, the child complains of otalgia and has all the symptoms of acute otitis media. The inital symptoms are followed within 24 hours by increasing fever, headache, toxicity, and lethargy. The neck is stiff and a positive Kernig's sign is present. A lumbar puncture confirms the diagnosis. Treatment must be vigorous with the appropriate antibiotics. For infection by Hemophilus influenzae, intravenous ampicillin or chloramphenicol is useful. If the meningitis is caused by pneumo-coccus, intravenous penicillin (1 g every 4 hours) is usually adequate.

CEREBRAL ABSCESS. Cerebral abscess is more frequently a complication of chronic suppurative otitis media. The patient complains of acute exacerbation of a chronic otitis media; that is, otorrhea is increased. This is followed by increasing headache and fever. The neck is not stiff and Kernig's sign is absent. Papilledema might develop. A lumbar puncture yields clear fluid under moderate pressure, with a lymphocytosis and normal levels of lactose and glucose. Diagnosis is confirmed by angiography or computed tomography and can be made earlier if the physician is alert to its possibility. In the early stages of cerebritis vigorous antibiotic therapy might abort the process, but if an abscess develops, it must be drained.

DISORDERS OF THE EUSTACHIAN TUBE

The lumen of the eustachian tube is narrow and lined by a ciliated columnar epithelium. The normal eustachian tube is closed at rest but opens on swallowing. The primary function of the eustachian tube is ventilation of the middle ear, with a subsidiary function of drainage. The infant's eustachian tube is short, wide, and horizontal, with cartilage that is softer and compressible; all of these factors predispose the middle ear to contamination. The eustachian tube, however, matures and becomes longer, more rigid, and oblique as the child grows.

The patency of the eustachian tube can be assessed by the Valsalva maneuver, in which the patient blows the tightly closed nose and mouth, which causes the tympanic membrane to bulge outward. The patient feels the movement, and the examiner may see it. Alternatively, the same increased pressure can be achieved by forcing air through the nostril while the nasopharynx is closed by swallowing. Tympanometry is an elegant method of assessing the patency of the eustachian tube.

Obstruction of the Eustachian Tube

The narrow lumen of the eustachian tube is easily obstructed by inflammatory conditions such as allergy or infection. Patency may also be compromised by neoplasms in the nasopharynx and by dysfunction of the levator or tensor palatine muscles.

These muscles have abnormal anatomy and function in all patients with cleft palates. Consequently, 70 to 90% of patients with cleft palates have effusions in their middle ears during the first year of life.

Patulous Eustachian Tube

This disorder is caused by an excessively patent eustachian tube. The lumen remains patent at rest and the pressure of the nasopharynx is transmitted to the middle ear. The patients complain of a sensation of fullness or pressure in the ear and autophony (this is a condition in which the patient's voice sounds hollow, as though he is "talking in a drum or echo chamber"). Hearing, however, is unaltered. The symptoms subside when the patient assumes a recumbent position because of the increase in peritubal congestion. The eustachian tube might become patulous when the patient experiences a rapid loss of weight, such a occurs after treatment for congestive heart failure.

On examination, the tympanic membrane might show spontaneous to and fro movement when the patient breathes through his nose. This is the only diagnostic sign of a patulous eustachian tube. Treatment is by insufflating the eustachian tube with irritating powders, such as salicylic acid, or inserting a ventilating tube.

NEOPLASMS OF THE MIDDLE EAR

Neoplasms of the middle ear are comparatively uncommon, and most tumors are benign.

Benign Tumors

TUMORS OF THE GLOMUS BODIES. By far the commonest neoplasm of the

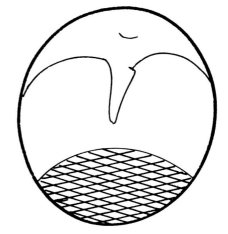

Fig. 6.16. Diagrammatic representation of a glomus jugulare tumor. A pink, pulsatile mass is present in the hypotympanum, behind the tympanic membrane.

middle ear is a tumor of the glomus bodies. These tumors are really chemodectomas. Glomus bodies are microscopic masses that are found in the adventitia of the jugular bulb (glomus jugulare), on the promontory of the middle ear (glomus tympanicum), along the arch of the aorta, and in the beds of the fingernails. Glomus bodies consist of clumps of specialized cells: the "chief cells" and sinusoidal blood vessels, both of which are also the components of glomus tumors. Glomus tumors therefore bleed easily and profusely. In the middle ear neoplasms arise from the glomus jugulare or glomus typanicum.

SYMPTOMS. The characteristic symptom of a glomus tumor of the middle ear is pulsatile tinnitus, which is synchronous with the pulse. A conductive hearing loss develops as a result of ossicular involvement or obstruction of the eustachian tube. As the glomus tumor grows further, a widening of the jugular foramen occurs, the ninth, tenth, eleventh, and twelfth cranial nerves become involved, and the facial nerve slowly becomes compressed. Glomus jugulare tumors, however, may grow to a substantial size before becoming symptomatic.

PHYSICAL FINDINGS. There is a pink vascular mass in the middle ear, usually be-

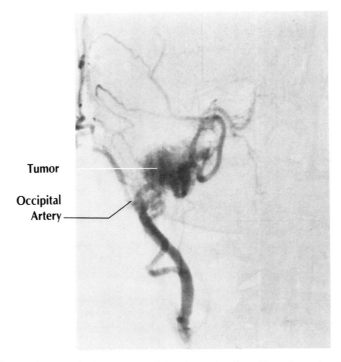

Tumor

Occipital
Artery

Fig. 6.17. Subtraction angiogram of a large tumor of the glomus jugulare. The primary feeding vessels arise from the occipital artery.

hind an intact tympanic membrane (Figure 6.16). The mass may blanch when positive pressure is applied with a pneumatic otoscope. Most tumors of the glomus jugulare develop in the hypotympanum and may grow laterally to involve the floor of the bony external canal. Only a small part of the tumor is visible on otoscopy.

INVESTIGATION. An audiogram should be done. Routine roentgenograms, including views of the jugular foramen, and multidirectional tomography are helpful. Angiography or computed tomography with an intravenous contrast medium are more useful for delineating the position and extent of the neoplasm (Figure 6.17).

PATHOLOGY. A biopsy should be considered only if absolutely necessary and then only under ideal comditions. The histologic picture is characteristic, with clumps of cells (Zellen Bollen) interspersed between blood-filled sinusoidal vessels.

TREATMENT. Surgery is the treatment of choice for tumors of the glomus bodies. Glomus tympanicum tumors can usually be totally removed by a transcanal approach. Glomus jugulare tumors require much more extensive surgery, and preoperative embolization of feeder vessels is helpful. Radiation therapy might control unresectable tumors.

Meningiomas occasionally erode into and present in the middle ear.

Malignant Tumors

Malignant tumors of the middle ear and mastoid process are rare. Most are squamous cell carcinomas and are usually of substantial size by the time they become symptomatic. Bleeding from the ear, pain, hearing loss, and dysfunction of the facial and lower cranial nerves are possible symptoms of a malignant tumor.

The middle ear and/or the mastoid process is filled with a granular, friable tumor that bleeds easily, but which is sometimes indistiguishable from an inflammatory polyp. Diagnosis is made by biopsy, and radiologic studies are done to determine the extent of the neoplasm. Treatment is by wide resection of the temporal bone or radiation therapy and/or chemotherapy. The prognosis is grave.

CAUSES OF OTALGIA

The following is an outline of the causes of otalgia:

1. Origin in the ear (positive otologic examination)
   a. External ear
      —perichondritis of the pinna
      —furuncle
      —external otitis (bacterial; fungal)
      —herpes zoster oticus (initial examination might be negative)
      —impacted cerumen (rarely causes pain)
      —frostbite of the pinna
      —malignant neoplasms
   b. Middle ear
      —otitis media
      —mastoiditis
      —neoplasms
      —petrositis
      —extradural abscess
2. Origin from outside the ear (negative otologic examination)
   a. Periauricular
      —temporomandibular joint
      —Bell's palsy (early stage)
      —temporal arteritis (vascular)
      —carotidynia (vascular)
      —pre- and postauricular lymphadenitis
      —parotitis (mumps; suppurative parotitis)
      —neoplasms (parotid; infratemporal fossa)
      —infected branchial cleft anomalies
   b. Distant sources (referred otalgia)
      —see Chapter 14
   c. Inflammatory or neoplastic lesions.
      —nasal cavity
      —paranasal sinuses
      —oral cavity
      —nasopharynx
      —oropharynx
      —hypopharynx
      —larynx
      —cervical esophagus

BIBLIOGRAPHY

Bernstein, J.M., and Reisman, R.: The role of acute hypersensitivity in secretory otitis media. Trans. Am. Acad. Ophthalmol. Otolaryngol., 78:120–127, 1974.

Bluestone, C.D., and Beery, Q.C.: Concepts in the pathogenesis of middle ear effusions. Ann. Otol. Rhinol. Laryngol., 85(Suppl. 25):135–139, 1976.

Brookler, K.M., and Birken, E.A.: Surface tension-lowering substance of the eustachian tube. Laryngoscope, 81:1671–1673, 1971.

Freidman, I., and Graham, M.D.: The ultrastructure of cholesterol granuloma of the middle ear. An electron microscope study. J. Laryngol. Otol., 93:433–442, 1979.

Healy, B.G., and Teele, D.W.: The microbiology of chronic middle ear effusions in children. Laryngoscope, 87:1472–1478, 1977.

Lewis, D.M., Schram, J.L., Lim, D.J., et al.: Immunoglobulin E in chronic middle ear effusions. Ann. Otol. Rhinol. Laryngol., 87:197–202, 1978.

Lim, D.J., and Birck, H.: Ultrastructural pathology of the middle ear mucosa in serous otitis media. Ann. Otol. Rhinol. Laryngol., 80:838–853, 1971.

Liu, Y.S., Lim, D.J., Lang, W., and Birck, H.C.: Chronic middle ear effusions. Arch. Otolaryngol., 101:278–286, 1975.

Maxim, P.E., Sprinkle, P.M., and Veltri, R.W.: Chronic serous otitis media: An immune-complex disease. Trans. Am. Acad. Ophthalmol. Otolaryngol., 84:234–238, 1977.

McCabe, B., Sade, J., and Abramson, M.: Cholesteatoma, First International Conference. Birmingham, AL, Aesculopus, 1977.

Mravec, J., Lewis, D.M., and Lim, D.: Experimental otitis media with effusion: An immune-complex-mediated response. Trans. Am. Acad. Ophthalmol. Otolaryngol., 86:258–268, 1978.

Politzer, A.: Atlas der Beleuchtungs Bilder des Trommelfells. Vienna, William Braumuller, 1896.

Recent advances in middle ear effusions. Ann. Otol. Rhinol. Laryngol., 85(Suppl. 25): 1976.

Schuknecht, H.F.: Pathology of the Ear. Chapter 5. Cambridge, Massachusetts, Harvard University Press, 1974.

Toynbee, J.: On the muscles that open the eustachian tube. Proc. Roy. Soc. Med., 6:286, 1853.

Chapter 7

DISORDERS OF THE COCHLEA

Disorders of the cochlea frequently involve the vestibular labyrinth and vice versa. Therefore, separation of the disorders of the cochlea and the vestibular system is artificial and is done here only for the sake of clarity and ease of description. Some overlap is inevitable.

Disorders of the cochlea cause sensorineural hearing loss and tinnitus. Most sensorineural hearing losses are more pronounced in the higher frequencies (Table 7.1).

CONGENITAL DEAFNESS

Congenital sensorineural hearing loss is fairly common. It can be either hereditary or acquired. Hereditary hearing loss can be dominant or recessive, and both dominant and recessive types might be isolated defects or they might be associated with other anomalies into well-defined syndromes of symptoms (e.g., Waardenburg's syndrome). Both dominant and recessive types are frequently associated with pigmentary or renal abnormalities. Acquired congenital hearing loss is usually secondary to an intrauterine catastrophe occurring in the first trimester. The commonest causative factor is a transplacental viral infection from maternal rubella or the cytomegalovirus. Other viruses probably cause similar problems. Hyperbilirubinemia, neonatal anoxia prematurity, and

drugs such as thalidomide also cause hearing losses (Table 7.2).

Symptoms

The observations of the parents are always correct until they are disproven. If the parents suspect a hearing loss, more often than not the child is found to have a hearing loss. The child with a hearing loss shows no response to environmental noises but constantly monitors the surroundings with his eyes. He sleeps deeply, does not babble readily, and develops speech slowly or not at all. Older children are prone to temper tantrums because of frustration.

Examination

A thorough physical examination is essential, noting all congenital anomalies. Carefully assess the ears and vigorously treat any effusions in the middle ears. Simple tests of hearing are helpful but are not diagnostic. Loud noises are made preferably behind the child and away from his field of vision. The normal response of infants and young children to loud noise is a startle reflex. In the infant a sudden jerking motion of the upper limbs occurs; this is called the Moro reflex. In older children the response might be a cessation of activity, a blink reflex, a cry, or a turning of the head towards the noise.

78

Table 7.1. Comparison of the Features of Conductive and Sensorineural Hearing Losses

	Conductive hearing loss	Sensorineural hearing loss
Pathology:	External auditory canal; middle ear	Cochlea; cochlear nerve; brainstem
Physical examination:	External canal and tympanic membrane might be abnormal	Normal external auditory canal and tympanic membrane
Tuning forks:	Rinne—negative	Rinne—positive
	Weber—heard on "deaf" side	Weber—lateralized to better side only in severe unilateral loss
Audiogram:	Bone conduction—usually normal	Bone conduction—elevated threshold
	Air conduction—elevated threshold (i.e., BC and AC are separated)	Air conduction—elevated threshold (BC and AC are at same levels)
	Loss—greater in low frequencies	Loss—usually greater in high frequencies
Speech discrimination:	Excellent	May be depressed
Recruitment:	None	Possible
Radiology:	Might reveal pathologic process	Frequently negative

Table 7.2. Etiology of Sensorineural Deafness

Disorder	Cause
Congenital and perinatal	
Genetic	Waardenburg's syndrome (deafness, heterochromia iridis, white forelock)
	Usher's syndrome (deafness and retinitis pigmentosa)
	Chromosomal abnormalities (e.g., Turner's syndrome)
Acquired	Intrauterine viral or treponemal infection (rubella, cytomegalovirus, syphilis)
	Teratogenic factors (e.g., thalidomide)
	Intrauterine toxins (e.g., quinine, hyperbilirubinemia)
	Prematurity
	Neonatal anoxia
Traumatic	
Mechanical	Fractures of the temporal bone
	Severe cerebral concussion
	Iatrogenic
	Loud noise (acoustic trauma)
Chemical (ototoxicity)	Aspirin (reversible)
	Quinine
	Aminoglycosides
	Ethacrynic acid
Inflammatory	
Infectious	Bacterial (suppurative labyrinthitis)
	Secondary to otitis media, meningitis, Viral labyrinthitis (e.g., mumps, Syphilis)
Autoimmune	Wegener's granulomatosis
Neoplastic	Acoustic neuroma
	Meningioma
	Leukemia
Idiopathic	Presbycusis (may be familial)
	Otosclerosis
	Progressive familial sensorineural deafness

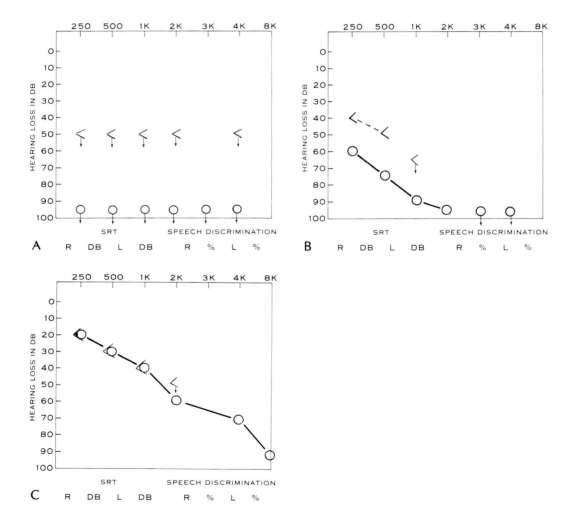

Fig. 7.1. Audiometric patterns frequently seen in congenital hearing loss. In general, the high-frequency responses are compromised and residual hearing is confined to the lower frequencies (B and C). A represents absolute deafness.

Attempt audiometry with the child on his parent's lap and with free-field noises (i.e., without head phones). The child's reaction should be monitored by a trained observer. Behavioral audiometry may have to be repeated a number of times before acceptable results are obtained (Figure 7.1). Electrical (evoked) response audiometry is most helpful in these cases (see Chapter 4).

Treatment

As soon as a child is diagnosed as having a significant hearing loss, hearing aids should be fitted; arrangements must also be made for the child's education. Hearing-impaired children need special help to develop speech and language. The parents and other family members are the most important factors in the progress of these children and should be encouraged to participate actively. All children should be examined periodically to ensure that their ears are functioning maximally. It is especially important to look for the presence of middle ear effusions. Most of these children are of normal intelligence and grow into useful citizens.

TRAUMATIC DISORDERS

Trauma to the inner ear might be either mechanical or chemical. Mechanical trauma to the cochlea can be secondary to loud noise (acoustic trauma) or secondary to fracture of the temporal bone or severe head injuries.

Acoustic Trauma

Noise-induced hearing loss has been recognized for many generations (boilermaker's deafness) and is probably becoming more common because of the general increase in the level of environmental noise, particularly in factories. Most noise-induced hearing losses begin with a characteristic maximum loss at 4000 Hz (Figure 7.2). Two types of noise may cause a hearing loss: a sudden and explosive noise or exposure to high-intensity noise over a

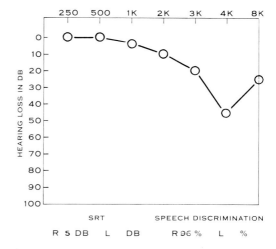

Fig. 7.2. Typical audiogram of early noise trauma. The hearing loss is maximal at 4000 Hz, and a smaller loss occurs at 8000 Hz. With continued exposure, the hearing loss increases and spreads to the middle frequencies.

long period of time. Hearing loss secondary to explosions is fairly common among infantry personnel.

High-level noise is common in factories, mines, airfields, rock and roll music, busy traffic intersections, and so on. Exposure to high-intensity noise during an 8-hour working day results in a temporary shift in the auditory threshold, which recovers within a few hours. If, however, this exposure is repeated every day over a number of months or years, permanent damage occurs to the cochlea. Initially, a characteristic loss is isolated at 4000 Hz, but with continued exposure the loss spreads to the adjacent frequencies. The United States Office of Safety and Health Administration recommends that the upper limit of ambient noise be 90 dB. Even at this level, continuous exposure for an 8-hour day over a period of 20 years will cause an appreciable hearing loss. The management of acoustic trauma is primarily preventive. Machines should be sound-dampened and workers must be provided with, and encouraged to use, protectors such as earplugs, headphones, mufflers, and so on.

Chemical Trauma (Ototoxicity)

Ototoxicity refers to trauma to the inner ear by various substances, which are usually ingested or given parenterally. For a long time, aspirin and quinine were the only ototoxic drugs that were in common usage, but drug ototoxicity has become more frequent with the development of new agents. With the exception of aspirin, most ototoxic agents cause permanent sensorineural losses, which are more severe in the higher frequencies. The following is a list of the more commonly used ototoxic drugs:

1. Aspirin—aspirin causes a high-pitched tinnitus and a flat sensorineural hearing loss when the serum salicylate level rises to around 30 mg/100 mL. Hearing returns to normal when aspirin is withdrawn. This is one of the few situations in which a sensorineural hearing loss is reversible.

2. Aminoglycosides—most, if not all, of the aminoglycoside antibiotics are both ototoxic and nephrotoxic. The most commonly used aminoglycosides are gentamicin, tobramycin, kanamycin, neomycin, and streptomycin. Gentamicin causes sensorineural hearing losses and loss of vestibular function. Streptomycin may damage the vestibular system if it is used in large doses or if the patient has an idiosyncratic reaction to the drug. Dihydrostreptomycin, used extensively in the past, is much more toxic to the cochlea, as is kanamycin. All of these agents damage the hair cells of the organ of Corti, the cristae of the semicircular canals, and the macula utriculi (Figure 7.3).

3. Diuretics—a close relationship exists between renal and cochlea physiology; similarly, most nephrotoxic agents are also ototoxic. Two diuretics in particular depress auditory function: furosemide causes a tem-

porary sensorineural hearing loss, and ethacrynic acid causes a permanent hearing loss. Ototoxicity, however, only occurs when high doses are given intravenously and is heightened by concomitant renal dysfunction.

4. Quinine—quinine was first used to treat malaria. It is now more commonly used in various cold medicines and tonics. In moderate to large oral doses quinine causes tinnitus and a permanent sensorineural hearing loss. Quinine can also cross the placental barrier and affect the developing fetus.

Fractures of the Temporal Bone

It is appropriate at this point to discuss fractures of the temporal bone in more detail. Temporal bone fractures are always secondary to severe head trauma and are either longitudinal along the axis of the petrous bone or transverse across the axis (Figure 7.4). Longitudinal fractures follow the thin tegmen mastoidea and tegmen tympani and extend into the squamous temporal bone. They usually do not involve the inner ear. Transverse fractures follow the windows and canals of the inner ear, particularly the oval and round windows and the internal auditory canal. Therefore, transverse fractures usually result in sensorineural hearing losses and vestibular dysfunction, while longitudinal fractures might not. In addition, transverse fractures may damage the facial nerve (see Chapter 9).

Following a head injury, bleeding might occur from the external auditory canal. Alternatively, the skin of the external auditory canal becomes ecchymotic and blood is present in the middle ear behind an intact tympanic membrane (hemotympanum). If the fracture is extensive and the dura and tympanic membrane are torn, a cerebrospinal fluid otorrhea develops. Facial paralysis might be obvious when the patient awakens, and he may complain of

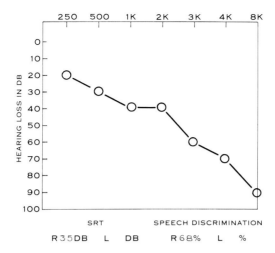

Fig. 7.3 Typical audiometric and pathologic findings in antibiotic ototoxicity caused by gentamicin. A precipitous fall occurs in the thresholds for the higher frequencies.

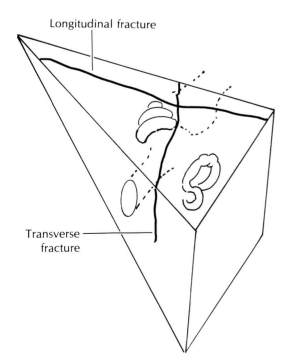

Fig. 7.4. Composite diagram of the types of fractures of the temporal bone. Longitudinal fractures are more common.

an ipsilateral hearing loss and dizziness. True vertigo and nystagmus may be present if the inner ear or internal auditory canal is damaged. Displacement or fractures of the ossicles are fairly common with longitudinal fractures. All patients with suspected injury to the temporal bone should have audiometry and vestibular tests performed as soon as possible, and function of the facial nerve must be documented.

Treatment is initially anticipatory. Bleeding and cerebrospinal fluid otorrhea usually stop spontaneously within 7 to 10 days. If facial paralysis is identified immediately after injury, the facial nerve should be explored and repaired as soon as possible. Leakage of perilymph or cerebrospinal fluid should be stopped surgically if it does not cease spontaneously. Ossicular discontinuity is usually caused by displacement of the incus, fracture of the long process of the incus, or fracture of the stapedial crura. These can be treated at a later date by exploratory tympanometry and repositioning of whatever has been displaced.

INFLAMMATORY DISORDERS OF THE INNER EAR (LABYRINTHITIS)

The term labyrinthitis is much abused. A true inflammation of the labyrinth is uncommon and is certainly not the major cause of dizziness. Meniere's disease is not caused by labyrinthitis. There are three types of labyrinthitis: serous, suppurative (bacterial) and viral.

Serous Labyrinthitis

This condition is uncommon and is somewhat similar to sympathetic arthritis. Serous labyrinthitis is caused by an inflammatory process adjacent to the labyrinth such as otitis media. The level of protein in the perilymph increases as does the volume of endolymph (endolymphatic hydrops). The patient complains of dizziness, and a moderate sensorineural hearing loss develops; of course, otitis media or surgical trauma are predisposing factors. Vigorous treatment of the primary problem usually results in reversal of the vertigo and hearing loss.

Suppurative Labryrinthitis

Bacterial invasion of the inner ear occurs through a defect of the otic capsule, such as a fistula of the semicircular canal, or via the subarachnoid space in meningitis (Figure 7.5). Suppurative labyrinthitis is catastrophic to the inner ear. The patient becomes extremely ill, unusually toxic, vertiginous, and has a profound ipsilateral sensorineural hearing loss. Treatment is with intravenous antibiotics and surgery, as indicated. The vertigo subsides, but the hearing loss is permanent. For this reason, pneumococcal and meningococcal meningitis can cause profound, sometimes bilateral, deafness. Suppurative labyrinthitis is sometimes followed by a partial or total ossification of the lumen of the inner ear, which is called labyrinthitis ossificans (Figure 7.6).

Viral Labyrinthitis

Infection of the inner ear by viruses is comparatively common and probably ac-

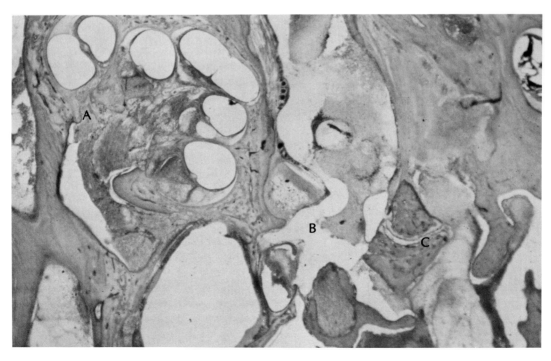

Fig. 7.5. Suppurative labyrinthitis. A purulent exudate permeates all turns of the cochlea. *A.* Cochlea. *B.* Middle ear. *C.* Malleus and incus.

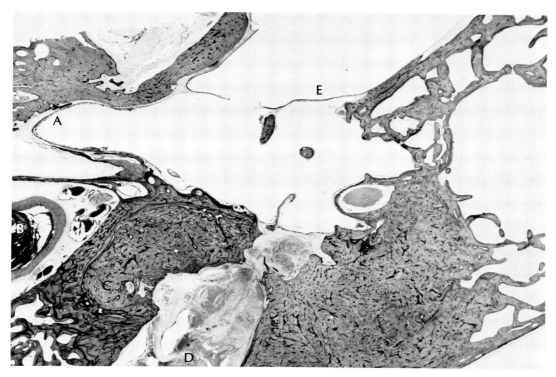

Fig. 7.6. Labyrinthitis ossificans. The cochlea has been filled in with bone and only a few strands of nerve fibers are present. *A.* Middle ear. *B.* Internal carotid artery. *C.* Ossified cochlea. *D.* Internal auditory canal. *E.* Tympanic membrane.

counts for most cases of sudden deafness. Viral labyrinthitis can occur at any age, even in utero, which causes congenital deafness. A viral infection can cause vestibular and/or auditory symptoms. That is, the patient might develop only a hearing loss, a hearing loss and vertigo, or vertigo only (vestibular neuronitis). Postnatal viral labyrinthitis has been associated with mumps, measles, herpes, adenoviruses, and chickenpox, but not necessarily with a well-defined preceding or accompanying illness.

Viral infection of the cochlea causes death of the hair cells of the organ of Corti. The tectorial membrane becomes encapsulated by a thin layer of cells and loses contact with the organ of Corti. Viral labyrinthitis is treated empirically in its early stages with vasodilators and high doses of corticosteroids.

SUDDEN DEAFNESS. Sudden partial or total sensorineural hearing loss is, fortunately, usually unilateral. The sudden deafness might be caused either by a viral infection or a vascular occlusion, but the evidence favors a viral origin. Sixty percent of patients will recover spontaneously (partially or completely) within 2 weeks of the onset of the deafness. Sudden deafness should be treated vigorously in the early stages with vasodilators and corticosteroids, although the value of therapy is still controversial.

DEGENERATIVE DISORDERS

Presbycusis

This form of deafness is caused by aging and is the most prevalent cause of sensorineural hearing loss. Around the age of 40 years all humans begin to lose their

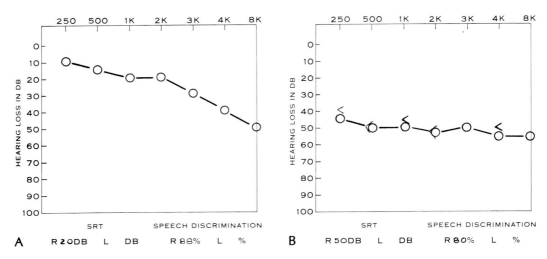

Fig. 7.7. Typical audiometric patterns in presbycusis. (A) Hearing loss is more marked in the higher frequencies because of selective degeneration of the organ of Corti. (B) Flat type hearing loss caused by degeneration of the stria vascularis.

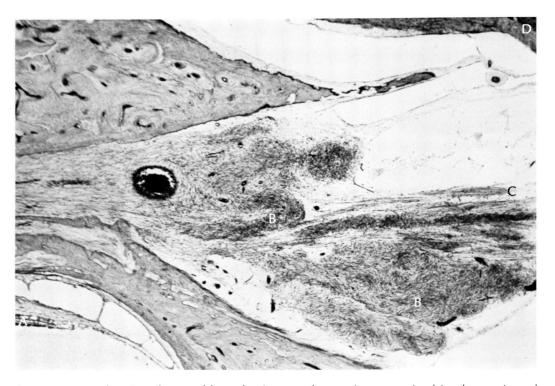

Fig. 7.8. Horizontal section of temporal bone showing an early acoustic neuroma involving the superior and internal auditory vestibular nerves. A characteristic whorling pattern is present. The utricular macula is in the lower left-hand corner, and the facial nerve is in the upper right of the field. *A.* Utricular macula. *B.* Tumor. *C.* Superior vestibular nerve. *D.* Facial nerve.

hearing, initially in the higher frequencies. In the early stages the hearing loss is mild, but it progresses with time and might even involve the middle frequencies. Typical audiograms of presbycusis are shown in Figure 7.7. A concomitant, but much slower, fall occurs in speech discrimination, and tinnitus is a frequently associated symptom.

Presbycusis can be classified as sensory, neural, or metabolic, caused by degeneration of the organ of Corti, cochlear nerve, and stria vascularis, respectively. Degeneration of the stria vascularis is reflected by a flat audiometric curve with comparatively good speech discrimination.

A definite familial pattern exists in presbycusis, which is particularly obvious when the hearing loss begins at a comparatively younger age. Patients with advanced presbycusis can be helped by the use of the appropriate type of hearing aid.

IDIOPATHIC DISORDERS

Functional Deafness (Malingering)

Functional deafness is common. The patient may complain of a total or partial hearing loss, which might be unilateral or bilateral. Patients malinger for many reasons, usually to obtain some form of compensation or avoid distasteful situations. Malingering is common among armed forces personnel. Occasionally, deafness might be a truly psychosomatic problem.

Tinnitus

Tinnitus is a spontaneous, internally generated noise, which is usually heard in one ear, but can also be heard in both ears. Almost any condition that causes malfunctioning of the auditory end-organ might cause tinnitus, but the commonest cause is age-related degeneration (presbycusis). Other causes are biochemical changes (e.g., from aspirin), Meniere's disease (see Chapter 8), trauma (acoustic or chemical), and labyrinthitis. Tinnitus can be either objective or subjective. Subjective tinnitus is by far more common. Subjective tinnitus might be described by the patient as a buzzing, whistling, or, sometimes, a hollow seashell-type sound.

Objective tinnitus is a noise that can be heard by both the patient and physician. This form of tinnitus usually derives from one of two sources: the vascular system or from muscle contraction. Vascular tinnitus is usually pulsatile and synchronous with the pulse. Glomus tumors, aneurysms along the carotid system, and other vascular malformations cause a pulsatile tinnitus that can be heard with a stethoscope and which abates when pressure is applied to the feeding vessels. The tinnitus of muscular contraction is usually a most annoying clicking noise caused by clonic activity of the tensor tympani or tensor veli palatini muscles (palatal myoclonus). Treatment is difficult, but tranquilizers and muscle relaxants might be helpful.

Patients with tinnitus complain bitterly about the persistent noise. They may or may not complain of a hearing loss, even when there is concomitant mild hearing loss. Subjective tinnitus is more noticeable in the quiet moments after retiring at night.

Tinnitus demands a thorough examination of the ears, head and neck, throat, and nasopharynx, including auscultation of the ears and audiometry. Roentgenograms of the temporal bones, including views of the internal auditory canals, serologic studies, and basic laboratory data should be obtained, as necessary. Unilateral tinnitus, particularly in younger patients, might herald an acoustic neuroma and requires investigation.

There is no known cure for tinnitus. An external masking noise might help.

NEOPLASMS OF THE INTERNAL AUDITORY CANAL

Primary neoplasms originate on the nerves in the internal auditory canal but

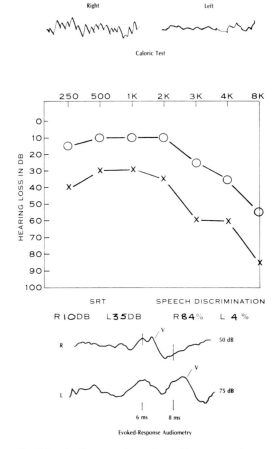

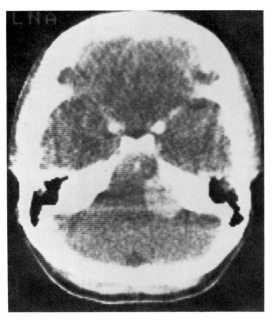

Fig. 7.10. Acoustic neuroma (schwannoma). Computed tomography with an intravenous contrast medium outlines a large tumor in the left cerebellopontine angle. This technique is not reliable in detecting tumors that are smaller than 2 cm in diameter.

Fig. 7.9. Audiogram of a patient with an acoustic neuroma. The speech discrimination scores are low when compared with pure tone thresholds. Brainstem audiometry shows an increase in the latency of wave V. The caloric response is depressed on the involved side.

have not been reported in the cochlea or the vestibular labyrinth.

Acoustic Neuroma

An acoustic neuroma (also called an acoustic schwannoma or a vestibular schwannoma) is a benign, usually slow-growing neoplasm that originates on one of the divisions of the eighth cranial nerve, most frequently from the superior vestibular nerve. The tumor consists of Schwann's cells arranged in whorls with characteristic patterns of nuclei, which are

known as Antoni A and Antoni B types. In the type A pattern the nuclei are sometimes parallel in palisades; in type B the pattern is more haphazard (Figure 7.8). Most of these tumors begin in the intracanalicular parts of the nerves and, therefore, compress and cause dysfunction of the other contents of the internal auditory canal. A slowly progressive dysfunction of the vestibular nerves is easily compensated for and might be asymptomatic. Dysfunction of the cochlear nerve presents as a unilateral, slowly progressive hearing loss, which is characterized by an abnormal loss of the ability to understand speech. Thus, a discrepancy exists between the threshold for pure tones and the scores for speech discrimination. The threshold for pure tones might even be nearly normal, while the ability to understand speech is grossly depressed in that ear. The response to caloric stimulation is reduced or absent. As the tumor enlarges, the facial nerve and the fifth cranial nerve might be involved and cause facial paralysis and facial parethesia, respectively. Occasionally, facial pain or otalgia is present. Large tumors distort the brainstem and cause increased intracranial pressure. Acoustic neuromas usually grow slowly but may expand suddenly from an interstitial hemorrhage, causing instant compression of the brainstem or even death from coning.

INVESTIGATIONS. A thorough neurologic examination, including a detailed examination of all cranial nerves, should be performed. The ipsilateral corneal reflex might be depressed. The following audiologic tests are necessary (see Chapter 4):

1. Pure tone audiometry—the threshold and pattern of hearing loss are highly variable. The audiogram might be flat with a minimal loss (Figure 7.9), might be sloping with a primarily high frequency, or hearing may be absent.
2. Speech discrimination—speech discrimination is usually abnormally depressed.
3. Tone decay—tone decay increases because of the inability of the ear to "hold a tone." That is, the ear becomes easily fatigued.
4. Stapedial reflex—the reflex is prolonged or absent on the affected side.
5. Evoked-response audiometry—brainstem evoked-response audiometry usually demonstrates an increase in the latency of wave V when compared with the unaffected side.
6. Caloric tests—caloric tests are mandatory and usually show a depressed or completely absent response to caloric stimulation on the affected side.

All of the audiologic and caloric tests must be performed because no single test is diagnostic. Each test contributes to the overall diagnostic situation.

7. Radiographic studies—widening of the internal auditory canal is demonstrated by routine radiologic studies and by polytomography. Contrast radiography is sometimes necessary for confirmation. Acoustic neuromas are best identified by computed tomography using intravenous iodinated contrast material (Figure 7.10). Small tumors are demonstrated by computed tomography and oxygen (air) introduced into the subarachnoid space for contrast. When the patient's head is placed in the proper position, air rises into the internal auditory canal. This is prevented if a tumor is present in the canal.

TREATMENT. Surgery is the only therapeutic modality. Smaller tumors are more easily removed by approaches either through the mastoid process, the middle cranial fossa, or the occiput. Larger tumors require a posterior craniotomy.

BIBLIOGRAPHY
Friedman, I.: Cochlear pathology in viral disease. Adv. Otorhinolaryngol., 20:155–177, 1973.
Gacek, R.R.: Diagnosis and management of primary tumors of the petrous apex. Ann. Otol. Rhinol. Laryngol., 84:(Suppl. 18): 1975.
Goodhill, V. (ed): Ear Diseases, Deafness, and Dizziness. Chapter 14. Hagerstown, Maryland, Harper and Row, 1979.
Jerger, J., and Jerger, S.: Audiologic comparison of cochlear and eighth nerve disorders. Ann. Otol. Rhinol. Laryngol., 83:275–285, 1974.
Konigsmark, B.W., and Gorlin, R.J.: Genetic and Metabolic Deafness. Philadelphia, W.B. Saunders, Co., 1976.
Prado, S., and Paparella, M.M.: Sensorineural hearing loss secondary to bacterial infection. Otol. Clin. North Am., 11(No. 1):35–42, 1978.
Schuknecht, H.F.: Pathology of the Ear. Chapter 10. Cambridge, Massachusetts, Harvard University Press, 1974.
Weber, H.J., and Pirkey, W.B.: Selection of hearing aids. Otol. Clin. North Am., 2(No.1):173–186, 1978.

Chapter *8*

THE VESTIBULAR SYSTEM

The equilibrating system of the human is an extraordinary, finely tuned composite of four basic parts: the vestibular apparatus, the eyes, the proprioceptive mechanisms, and the brain, which functions as a coordinating and control center.

Each part of the system is represented bilaterally, with each side making an exactly equal but opposite contribution. Each component sends a constant stream of tonic impulses to the brain, so that the individual's orientation in space is being carefully monitored at all times.

The developing human brain learns by experience, beginning immediately after birth, and eventually becomes programmed to accept certain head positions and body postures. When the position of the head or body changes suddenly, or when one side of the equilibrating system suddenly dysfunctions, the resting impulses to the brain immediately become unequal. The brain interprets this inequality of impulses as different sensory phenomena, initially as a sense of imbalance or loss of spatial orientation. If the abnormal signals are continuous and if sufficient magnitude exists, a sensation of rotation, called vertigo, develops. Corrective measures are instituted instantly to bring the body back to its usual alignment. These measures might include movements of the eyes back to a set position (nystagmus) in an attempt to stabilize the visual field. Concomitantly, the muscles of the neck, limbs, and trunk alter their tonicity with the objective of achieving a posture that is acceptable to the brain based on previous experience.

Sudden severe dysfunction of the labyrinth, therefore, causes subjective sensations of vertigo, a sense of imbalance, and falling. In addition, there are symptoms of dysfunction of the autonomic nervous system, specifically nausea, vomiting, sweating, and, possibly, diarrhea. Objectively, nystagmus, past-pointing, and ataxia occur.

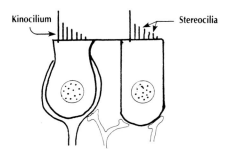

Fig. 8.1. The two types of hair cells found in the macula of the utricle: the flasked-shaped type I and cylindrical type II. Kinocilia and stereocilia are identified at the surface of the cells. The cilia are covered by the gelatinous otolithic membrane that contains crystals of calcium carbonate.

PHYSIOLOGY OF THE VESTIBULAR SYSTEM

The vestibular system of the inner ear is an essential part of the balancing mechanism of the body. The semicircular canals respond to angular acceleration (rotation), and the utricle and saccule respond to linear acceleration (gravity). The canals, therefore, help to orient and coordinate the position of the head, and the otolithic organs contribute to posture by controlling muscle tone.

The cristae of the semicircular canals and the maculae of the utricle and saccule contain hair cells. These hair cells have a kinocilium and stereocilia. All the kinocilia on a crista are oriented in the same direction (Figure 8.1). In the utricle they are oriented toward a central line (Figure 8.2). In the saccule they are directed away from the central line (striola) (Figure 8.2). Deflection of stereocilia toward the kinocilium causes an increase in neural firing along the vestibular nerve. Therefore, as would be expected, the cristae of the semicircular canals respond positively to stimulation in one direction and negatively in the opposite direction.

If the head (i.e., the semicircular canals) is suddenly rotated in one direction, inertia causes the movement of the endolymphatic fluid to lag behind. The result is that the cristae are stimulated as though from the opposite direction. If rotation continues at a constant rate, endolymph will catch up with the wall of the canal, and deflection of the cristae will diminish and the sense of rotation ceases. The process is reversed if rotation is suddenly stopped.

The function of the semicircular canals was first studied by Ewald, who described the following phenomena when endolymph is in motion:

1. Stimulating the horizontal semicircular canal induces a horizontal nystagmus. Stimulation of the vertical semicircular canal causes a vertical nystagmus.
2. The direction of the slow component of nystagmus is always in the direction of the flow of endolymph. Thus, if the right horizontal semicircular canal is placed in a vertical position with the ampullated end superiorly, cooling and increasing the density of the endolymph will produce a convection current in a downward direction away from the crista (ampullofugal); in this situation the current will be to the right, the fast component of the nystagmus will be in the opposite direction (to the left). Therefore, a cold stimulus to the right horizontal semicircular canal induces a nystagmus to the left, and a warm stimulus induces a nystagmus to the right.

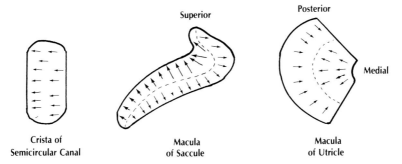

Fig. 8.2. Diagram illustrating the direction of ciliary activity in the saccule, utricle, and crista of the semicircular canals.

3. In the horizontal canal the maximum effect occurs with flow toward the ampulla.
4. In the vertical canals the maximum effect occurs with flow away from the ampulla.

The functions of the utricle and saccule are much more complex and are still not well understood. It is possible that the saccule has no vestibular function. The utricle responds to gravitational stimuli and, therefore, is important in the maintenance of body posture. The utricle is probably a major source of tonic impulses to the musculature.

TESTING THE VESTIBULAR SYSTEM

First, a thorough neurologic examination is performed with special attention to gait, coordination, the presence or absence of spontaneous nystagmus, the Romberg test, and past-pointing.

Spontaneous Nystagmus

Nystagmus is a rhythmic movement of the eyes, with each cycle characteristically consisting of fast and slow components. Nystagmus can be in a horizontal or vertical direction, or it might be rotatory. By convention, the direction of nystagmus is designated by the direction of the fast component. Thus, if the fast component is to the right, the nystagmus is said to be right-beating. Nystagmus occurs whenever the fine tuning of the body's balancing system is upset, and can be either spontaneous or induced.

All labyrinthine dysfunctions cause spontaneous nystagmus. The horizontal semicircular canal is most often involved, and, therefore, horizontal nystagmus is more frequent. The examiner holds his finger 3 feet in front of the patient's eyes and moves the finger to one side to a maximum angle of 30° from the midline. Moving the finger any further laterally might induce false movements. Note and document any nystagmus. Repeat the process with the finger on the other side, superiorly and inferiorly. Spontaneous nystagmus is classified as first, second, or third-degree. First-degree nystagmus occurs only when the eyes look in the direction of the fast component. Second-degree nystagmus occurs when the eyes are looking straight ahead. Third-degree nystagmus is noted when the eyes are turned in the direction of the slow component.

Past-Pointing

Labyrinthine dysfunction causes a sensation of motion even of fixed objects. On pointing to an object, particularly with the eyes closed, the patient tries to compensate for this movement and will point "past" the object. The direction of past-pointing is usually opposite to that of the nystagmus.

Positional Tests

Positional tests are designed to test for labyrinthine dysfunction that occurs when the patient's head is in different positions. Theoretically, these tests are supposed to stimulate the semicircular canals. In practice, however, a number of other structures are stimulated: the proprioceptors of the cervical muscles and joints, intracranial centers, and even the vertebral arteries might be partially occluded.

To perform positional tests, have the patient sit upright on a bed. Instruct the patient to keep his eyes open at all times so that any nystagmus can be noted. Ask the patient to lie down suddenly, keeping his head straight. If no nystagmus occurs, have the patient turn his head quickly to the right and keep it there for 1 minute. If nystagmus occurs, note the direction and duration. Repeat the procedure with the patient's head to the left.

Caloric Tests

Caloric tests are performed by stimulating convection movements in the endolymph of a semicircular canal; this is achieved by changing the temperature in

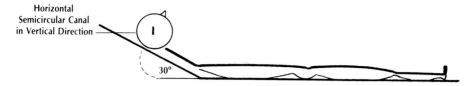

Fig. 8.3. Patient position during caloric tests. The head and neck are elevated 30° from the horizontal, and the head is extended on the neck. The objective is to bring the horizontal semicircular canal into vertical alignment.

the external auditory canal. The horizontal semicircular canal is usually stimulated, which causes horizontal nystagmus. Cold or hot stimuli can be used, and the usual media are water or air. Ice water (0.5 mL at 0°C) stimulates a violent response, which is qualitative. Hallpike and Fitzgerald (1942) found that water at 7°C above and below body temperature is both comfortable and effective. Standardizing the stimulus by using a constant volume of water and timing the response from the onset of stimulation quantifies the response. Usually, the ear canal is first irrigated with 400 mL of water at 30°C and again with water at 44°C. Have the patient lie with his head elevated slightly and his chin pointing 30° upward so that the horizontal canal is perpendicular (Figure 8.3). Irrigate the external canal with a slow flow of water through a rubber-tipped nozzle. Monitor the nystagmus directly with the help of Frenzel glasses or by electronystagmography. Frenzel glasses are 20-diopter lenses, which are set in a frame that has a low-intensity light source. The patient cannot see through the glasses, but the examiner can see the patient's eyes. Electronystagmography is an electronic technique that records the potentials between the cornea and retina, which changes with all movements of the globe (Figure 8.4). A tracing is obtained (electronystagmogram). This can be examined, measured, and stored. By convention, the parameter that is measured is the angular speed of the slow component of nystagmus.

Torsion Swing

The torsion swing is not a commonly used method of testing the vestibular system and is available in only a few medical centers.

Baranay Chair

A Baranay chair is a special chair designed to rotate at specific speeds. The chair is rotated 10 times in 20 seconds, then stopped suddenly, and the after-rotation nystagmus is recorded. After a resting period, the procedure is reversed. This type of chair is expensive and is available primarily in research centers.

DISORDERS OF THE VESTIBULAR SYSTEM

Sudden, severe dysfunction of the labyrinth causes subjective sensations of vertigo, a sense of gross imbalance, and falling. Nausea and vomiting, sweating, and, possibly, diarrhea are symptoms of autonomic malfunction. Objectively, nystagmus, past-pointing, and ataxia are present.

Traumatic Disorders

Injury to the vestibular system can occur either mechanically or chemically.

MECHANICAL TRAUMA. Mechanical trauma might occur from a fracture of the temporal bone. Direct insult to the inner ear is caused by transcanal foreign objects (e.g., pencils, sticks, etc.). Damage is also possible during surgical procedures such as stapedectomy and mastoidectomy. During mastoidectomy, injuring the horizontal semicircular canal is always a possibility.

CHEMICAL TRAUMA. Chemical damage (ototoxicity) to the labyrinth is usually

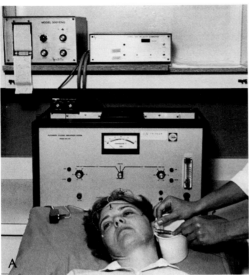

Fig. 8.4. *A.* Electronystagmography. The patient is lying in the position that was shown in Fig. 8.3. Electrodes are attached to the forehead and around the eyes, and water at 30°C and 44°C is circulated in the external auditory canals. *B.* Normal electronystagmogram after stimulation of the right ear. Note the direction of nystagmus in opposite directions with cold and hot stimuli.

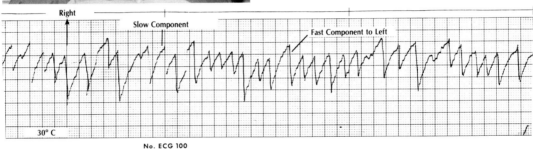

Right

Slow Component

Fast Component to Left

30° C

No. ECG 100

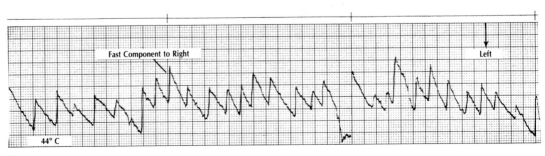

Fast Component to Right

Left

44° C

B

If the disease is bilateral and severely debilitating, the use of a vestibulotoxic agent is highly successful in ablating the attacks of vertigo. For this purpose, streptomycin can be used at a dosage of 3 g/day for about 5 days, then gradually reducing the dosage, using caloric tests to monitor vestibular function. Therapy is stopped when vestibular activity ceases. The only disadvantage to this form of therapy is that the patient is left with nonfunctioning labyrinths that cause considerable difficulty with orientation in wide-open spaces or in the dark.

Vertigo

POSITIONAL VERTIGO. Positional vertigo is induced by placing the head in certain positions such as turning to the right or left while lying supine. The patient complains of a sense of rotation that might last for only a few seconds or might persist for longer and be accompanied by nausea and vomiting. The condition may remit spontaneously for long periods of time, only to recur later. The only reasonable explanation for positional vertigo that has been expounded so far is that utricular otoliths, which are dislodged by trauma, gravitate into the posterior semicircular canals and adhere to the cupula of the crista (cupulolithiasis).

Positional tests should be performed, as described earlier in this chapter, and a complete neurologic examination must be completed. Generally, the nystagmus that is elicited is fatigable (i.e., will subside after repeated testing). Positional vertigo might be caused by a more central lesion.

In these patients symptoms are progressive, and the nystagmus is indefatigable.

Positional vertigo is treated by counseling the patient to avoid the provocative positions and by reassurance. Severe cases may benefit from sectioning the singular nerve that supplies the posterior semicircular canal.

VERTIGO OF CENTRAL ORIGIN. Almost every major intracranial condition can cause vertigo. There are, however, no specific features that distinguish central from peripheral vertigo. The diagnosis of vertigo of central origin eventually depends on the identification of associated neurologic deficits. Vertigo might be the presenting symptom in thrombosis of the posterior or anterior cerebellar artery, vertebrobasilar arterial insufficiency caused by atherosclerosis, arthritis of the cervical spine, multiple sclerosis, neoplasms of the cerebellopontine angle, and many other problems.

BIBLIOGRAPHY

Alford, B.R.: Report of subcommittee on equilibrium and its management. Trans. Am. Acad. Ophthalmol. Otolaryngol., 76:1462–1464, 1972.

Aschan, G.: Clinical vestibular examinations and their results. Acta Otolaryngol. (Stockh.) Suppl., 224:56, 1967.

Coats, A.C.: Electronystagmography. *In* Physiological Measures of the Audio-Vestibular System. Edited by L.J. Bradford. New York, Academic Press, Inc. 1975.

Dix, M., and Hallpike, C.: The pathology, symptomatology, and diagnosis of certain common disorders of the vestibular systems. Ann. Otol. Rhinol. Laryngol., 61:987, 1952.

Goodhill, V. (ed.): Ear Diseases, Deafness, and Dizziness. Chapter 10. Hagerstown, Maryland, Harper and Row, Inc., 1979.

Vosteen, K.J., et al. (eds.): Meniere's Disease. New York, Thieme-Stratton, Inc., 1981.

Chapter 9

DISORDERS OF THE SEVENTH CRANIAL (FACIAL) NERVE

Paralysis or other dysfunctions of the facial musculature cause severe problems of cosmesis and functions, which can be readily understood by studying its anatomy.

ANATOMY

The facial nerve begins at the ipsilateral facial nucleus in the pons. Contributions from both cerebral cortices synapse on each facial nucleus, but most of the innervation from the contralateral cortex goes to the frontalis muscle. As it leaves the pons, the nerve is joined by the small autonomic nervus intermedius (nerve of Wrisberg). The facial nerve then traverses the internal auditory canal to lie superior to the cochlea, where the nerve is separated from the dura of the middle cranial fossa by a thin flake of bone. At this point, the geniculate ganglion arises, from which the greater superficial petrosal nerve exits through the anterior surface of the temporal bone to eventually enter the vidian canal. The facial nerve then turns 90° (first genu), enters the middle ear, and runs horizontally in the bony fallopian canal between the horizontal semicircular canal and the oval window. It then turns downward (second genu) into its vertical part, sends a small branch to the stapedius mus-

cle, gives off the chorda tympani, and leaves the temporal bone through the stylomastoid foramen (Figure 9.1). The facial nerve then turns again to run anteriorly, entering the parotid gland where it splits into upper (zygomaticofrontal) and lower (cervicofacial) divisions. The network within the parotid gland is called the pes anserinus ("goose's foot"). The upper-division nerve supplies the frontalis and orbicularis oculi muscles. The lower division supplies the orbicularis oris, depressor anguli oris, and platysma muscles (Figure 9.2). The chorda tympani carries taste sensation from the anterior two-thirds of the tongue and secretomotor fibers to the submandibular salivary gland. The greater superficial petrosal nerves are secretomotor nerves to the lacrimal gland and nasal mucosa. The functions of the facial nerve are as follows:

1. Motor to the facial and postauricular muscles.
2. Sensory to a small part of the posterior bony external auditory canal.
3. Secretomotor to the lacrimal, nasal, and submandibular glands (greater superficial petrosal nerves and chorda tympani).
4. Protect the inner ear (stapedius muscle).

100

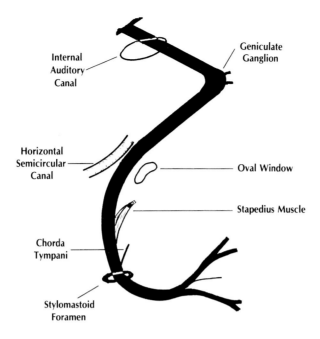

Seventh Cranial Nerve

Fig. 9.1. Stylized diagram of the facial nerve and its branches.

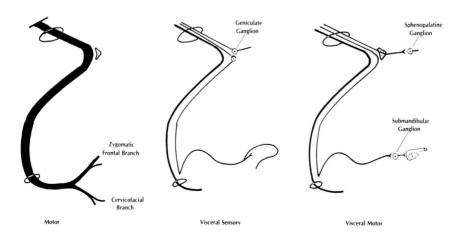

Fig. 9.2. Diagrammatic representation of the major components of the facial nerve. A small somatosensory nerve is also present, which innervates the skin of the posterior bony external canal close to the tympanic membrane.

5. Carry the visceral sensation of taste from the anterior tongue (chorda tympani).

SYMPTOMS AND PHYSICAL FINDINGS

Central Versus Peripheral Dysfunction

CENTRAL LESION. A lesion of the motor cortex will result in contralateral hemiparesis or hemiplegia, which includes the corresponding side of the face. Because the frontalis muscle has bilateral innervation, a central lesion causes paralysis of the voluntary function of only the lower two-thirds of the face. The frontalis, secretomotor, and visceral sensory divisions retain normal functions. In addition, with a central lesion the "paralyzed" side moves with involuntary emotional stimuli such as laughing. On the other hand, a peripheral lesion of the facial nerve causes paralysis of the entire ipsilateral face (Figure 9.3).

PERIPHERAL LESIONS (Figure 9.4). A lesion of the facial nerve in the internal auditory canal results in the following ipsilateral phenomena:

1. Paralysis of the facial musculature, which causes sagging of the face, nonclosure of the eyelids and mouth,

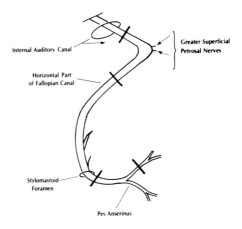

Fig. 9.4. Diagram showing the common sites of injury to the facial nerve. The site of injury can be determined by careful examination.

Bell's phenomenon (a turning upward and outward of the ipsilateral globe on attempted closure of the eye), and drooling during meals, particularly on taking fluids.
2. Collapse of the nasal ala.
3. Dryness of the eye, which, together with the inability to close the eyelids, could result in exposure keratitis.
4. Cessation of secretion of the submandibular salivary gland.
5. Depression of taste on the ipsilateral tongue.
6. Reduction of nasal secretion.
7. Hyperacusis for high-frequency auditory stimuli.

A lesion along the horizontal or vertical part of the nerve, distal to the geniculate ganglion, causes total paralysis of the face, but tearing remains normal. Submandibular salivary gland function and taste on the ipsilateral tongue are depressed.

A lesion at the stylomastoid foramen, distal to the takeoff of the chorda tympani, causes total facial paralysis. Tearing, submandibular salivary gland function, and taste remain normal.

A lesion in the substance of the parotid gland might cause segmental paralysis of the face. Lesions along the course of the

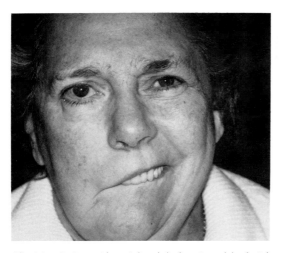

Fig. 9.3. Patient with peripheral dysfunction of the facial nerve.

facial nerve seldom cause spasm of the facial musculature.

Examining the Patient with a Dysfunction of the Facial Nerve

A thorough examination will determine the site of the disorder. To assess the function of the different parts of the facial nerve, different tests are performed.

GREATER SUPERFICIAL PETROSAL NERVE (LACRIMATION). Schirmer's test measures lacrimation. Place two strips of filter paper of equal width, thickness, and length on the conjunctival surface of the lower eyelids. Compare the length of wetness along the strips after 1 to 5 minutes.

CHORDA TYMPANI (SUBMANDIBULAR GLAND AND TASTE). To assess the function of the chorda tympani, examine the flow of saliva from Wharton's duct. Clinical observation is usually adequate, but plastic catheters can be inserted into the ducts to measure the volume of saliva. To test for taste, dry the patient's tongue and touch first the abnormal side, then the normal side with a cotton-tipped applicator that has been moistened with a solution of salt or sugar. Avoid an excess of solution. An alternative method is the use of an electrical stimulus (a gustometer).

MOTOR FUNCTIONS. To determine the function of the stapedius muscle, perform the stapedius reflex test (see the section on tympanometry in Chapter 4). The degree of dysfunction of the motor nerve can be roughly assessed by comparing the strengths of a galvanic current, applied just inferior to the lobule of the pinna, which is required to stimulate the normal and abnormal sides. Electromyography of the facial muscles also indicates the activity of the nerve and is probably more accurate than percutaneous galvanic stimulation

DISORDERS OF THE FACIAL NERVE

All patients with a dysfunction of the facial nerve must be submitted to a thorough examination of the neurologic system.

Congenital Disorders

Partial or total paralysis of the face occurs fairly frequently from the anomalous development of the facial nerve.

Traumatic Disorders

Trauma to the facial nerve occurs directly or secondary to a fracture of the temporal bone. Direct trauma is caused by penetrating transcanal injuries or during mastoid surgery. The horizontal segment and second genu are particularly vulnerable in these injuries. Fractures of the temporal bone are either longitudinal or transverse to the axis of the petrous bone. Longitudinal fractures traverse the length of the bone, usually on the superior surface. Involvement of the facial nerve is relatively uncommon but nevertheless does occur. Transverse fractures frequently cause injury to the facial nerve in the internal auditory canal or in its horizontal part. If paralysis occurs immediately after injury, a neurotmesis is probably present. Routine and computed tomographic roentgenograms help to identify the site of injury. The nerve should be explored as soon as possible and the severed ends approximated or a graft interposed. Paralysis occurring 24 to 48 hours after a head injury is caused by edema and should be treated expectantly.

Inflammatory Disorders

OTITIS MEDIA. Paralysis of the facial nerve can occur in either acute or (more frequently) chronic suppurative otitis media. In acute disease a severe infection usually develops, with involvement of the perifacial mastoid cells. Treatment is with vigorous antibiotic therapy and early drainage by myringotomy or mastoidectomy. Facial paralysis is more common with cholesteatoma that erodes into the fallopian canal, especially the horizontal part. Treatment is immediate mastoidectomy and decompression of the nerve by removal of the cholesteatoma.

HERPES ZOSTER OTICUS (RAMSAY HUNT SYNDROME). Herpes zoster oticus is a herpetic infection of the nerves that traverse the temporal bone (i.e., the seventh and eighth cranial nerves). Initially, an acute pain develops that involves the pinna and/or the postauricular area and the deep external canal. Within a day or two a vesicular eruption of the skin of the external canal, pinna, and postauricular area occurs. Frequently, facial paralysis accompanies the infection. If the eighth nerve is involved, an additional, sudden loss of hearing and vertigo may develop. Treatment is primarily supportive. Keep the skin lesions dry with boric acid powder. Corticosteroids are not indicated. Surgical decompression of the facial nerve is of questionable value.

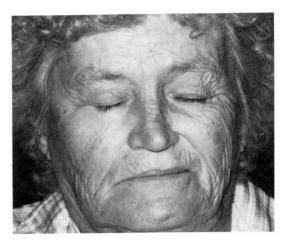

Fig. 9.5. Synkinesia of the left side of the face. The axons of the regenerating facial nerve have grown into all the muscles of the face. The result is a loss of selective contraction and simultaneous mass contraction of the facial musculature.

Idiopathic Disorders

BELL'S PALSY. Bell's palsy is an idiopathic, usually unilateral dysfunction of the facial nerve. There is, however, mounting evidence that Bell's palsy is but a part of a viral polyneuropathy that might involve many cranial nerves simultaneously.

SYMPTOMS. A sudden (usually overnight) onset of facial paralysis occurs. Ipsilateral otalgia might precede paralysis by 1 to 2 days. The patient first notices a twisting of the face on smiling, an inability to close the ipsilateral eye, and a change in the speech pattern because of laxity of the cheek. The site and degree of paralysis vary from very mild paresis to total dysfunction of all components of the nerve.

All patients with Bell's palsy should be thoroughly investigated to determine if there are other causes of dysfunction of the facial nerve. Detailed roentgenograms of the temporal bones are necessary to rule out the presence of disease (e.g., cholesteatoma, tumor).

TREATMENT. In the absence of a definitive cause, the treatment of Bell's palsy is empiric. Function, however, might return spontaneously at one of three levels: (a) completely, without residuum; (b) com-

pletely, but with synkinesia (Figure 9.5); or (c) partially, with permanent paresis. Function also might not return at all. Eighty-five percent of patients with Bell's palsy recover complete function without residuum. Unfortunately, there are no reliable guidelines as to which patient with complete paralysis has a poor prognosis. Generally, the longer the paralysis persists the worse the prognosis.

Vasodilators, such as nicotinic acid, antibiotics, and corticosteroids have been tried empirically to treat Bell's palsy. Corticosteroids (e.g., prednisone, 10 mg four times daily), might be valuable if administered within the first 3 days of onset of Bell's palsy. Blocking the cervical sympathetic chain with a local anesthetic has been tried on the etiologic basis of vascular spasm. Decompression of the facial nerve by opening widely the entire length of the fallopian canal is advocated as treatment for severe cases of Bell's palsy. Nerve conduction is monitored sequentially twice daily after the onset of facial paralysis. Rapid deterioration of nerve conduction is taken as indication for decompression.

BILATERAL FACIAL PARALYSIS. Simultaneous bilateral facial paralysis is a rare phenomenon. It can be congenital, as in Möbius' syndrome. Simultaneous acquired bilateral facial paralysis is sometimes seen in fractures of the skull. Metachronous bilateral facial paralysis can be idiopathic (Bell's palsy) or secondary to a systemic disease, such as sarcoidosis or the Melkersson-Rosenthal syndrome.

SYNKINESIA (MASS MOVEMENT). Synkinesia is the phenomenon of loss of selectivity of facial muscular activity. That is, if the patient attempts to close only one eye, his eyelids and other parts of his face contract simultaneously. Synkinesia is caused by a loss of direction of the regrowing axon, so that some of the axons that should innervate the orbicularis oculi may innervate the orbicularis oris. Therefore, geographically distant muscles are activated simultaneously (Figure 9.5).

REANIMATION OF THE FACE. Continuing facial paralysis presents problems of cosmesis and function. A variety of techniques, however, have been designed to address this problem. Nerve to nerve anastomosis usually entails joining the cut end of the hypoglossal nerve to the peripheral end of the facial nerve. Muscle transfer techniques are useful and consist of suturing various muscles, such as the temporalis, to the facial musculature. More recently, cable grafts have been used, which are free-nerve grafts that join the normal side to the paralyzed side.

FACIAL SPASM. Involuntary spasm of the facial muscles is an uncommon phenomenon of unknown etiology. The condition usually afflicts middle-aged adults and can be a severe cosmetic problem, sufficient to cause withdrawal from society. Currently, the usual treatment is selective partial section of the peripheral branches of the facial nerve.

BIBLIOGRAPHY

Adour, K.K., Wingerd, J., Bell, D.N. Manning, J.J., Hurley, J.P.: Prednisone treatment for idiopathic facial paralysis. N. Engl. J. Med., 287:1268–1272, 1972.

Adour, K.K.: Facial paralysis. Trans. Am. Acad. Ophthalmol. Otolaryngol., 75:1284–1301, 1971.

Alford, B.B., et al.: Diagnostic tests of facial nerve function. Otol. Clin. North Am., 7:331–342, 1974.

Bell, C.: The Nervous System of the Human Body. Washington, D.C., Duff Green, 1833, pp., 46–51.

Diamond, C., and Frew, I.: The Facial Nerve. Oxford, Oxford University Press, 1979.

Donaldson, J.A., and Anson, B.J.: Surgical anatomy of the facial nerve. Otol. Clin. North Am., 7:289–308, 1974.

Harker, L.A., and McCabe, B.F.: Temporal bone fractures and facial nerve injury. Otol. Clin. North Am., 7:425–431, 1974.

Kettel, K.: Peripheral Facial Palsy. Copenhagen, Munksgaard, 1959.

Chapter 10

THE NOSE AND PARANASAL SINUSES

ANATOMY

The external nose consists of two fused nasal bones superiorly and four alar cartilages inferiorly. For further anatomic details and nomenclature see Figure 10.1.

There are two nasal passages, which are separated by a central vertical septum containing cartilage anteroinferiorly and bone posterosuperiorly. Both passages have anterior and posterior openings (choanae). Both passages are lined by ciliated respiratory mucoperichondrium that contains mucus-secreting cells and glands. The anterior nares leads to a skin-lined vestibule containing hairs (vibrissae). The posterior openings (choanae) open into the nasopharynx. The cribriform plate forms the roof of the nose, while the hard palate forms the floor. The lateral wall of the nose is a partition between the maxillary and ethmoid sinuses and the nasal passages. There are three turbinates on each lateral wall: superior, middle, and inferior. The inferior turbinate is the largest and most vascular (Figure 10.2)

The turbinates are scroll-like, thin plates of bone that are covered by a thick mucosa. The bone and mucosa contain longitudinal blood vessels, resembling channels, through which blood passes rapidly. The olfactory area is lined by a yellowish mucosa that covers the roof and parts of the adjacent walls to the level of the superior turbinates. There are four paranasal sinuses on each side. The frontal and sphenoid sinuses straddle the midline, but the ethmoid and maxillary sinuses are more laterally placed. The respiratory mucoperichondrium (schneiderian membrane) is somewhat thinner in the sinuses. Each sinus has at least one ostium into the nose. The ostia of the maxillary and sphenoid sinuses are not in the most dependant positions; that is, they are not in the best place for drainage. Secretions in the nose and sinuses, however, are transported by ciliary action (Figure 10.3).

The maxillary and ethmoid sinuses are present at birth. The frontal and sphenoid sinuses develop later. At the age of 5 years the maxillary sinus is 5 ml in volume and increases to about 20 ml in adults (Figure 10.4); however, considerable variation in the size of the sinuses exists among adults.

The nasal septum is composed of a skeleton of a large quadrilateral plate of cartilage anteriorly and the thin perpendicular plate of the ethmoid bone and the vomer posteriorly (Figure 10.5). The maxillary crest contributes inferiorly. Both sides of the septum are covered by a thin mucoperichondrium.

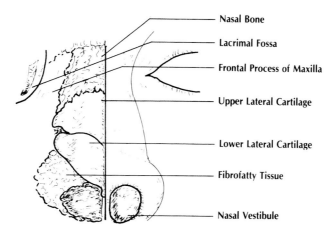

Fig. 10.1. Diagrammatic representation of the external skeleton of the nose. The skin has been removed from the right half of the nose to expose the nasal bones and alar cartilages.

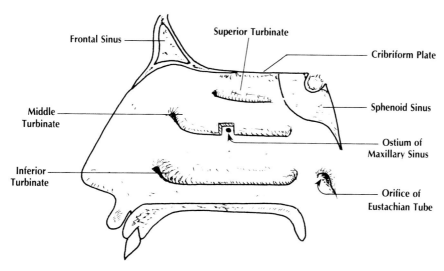

Fig. 10.2. The lateral wall of the nose. A section of the middle turbinate has been removed to show the ostium of the maxillary sinus.

PHYSIOLOGY OF THE NOSE

The nose has three main functions: to conduct air, to condition inspired air, and for olfaction. Olfaction will be discussed later. Air conduction is self-explanatory, and the volume of air that passes is controlled by the size (i.e., the degree of turgidity) of the turbinates. A natural rhythm occurs in nasal breathing: one nasal passage opens while the other closes by engorgement of the turbinates. The schnei- derian membrane is extraordinarily efficient. Every breath of air is warmed, humidified, and cleansed of particulate matter; inspired air at the laryngeal level is at body temperature, almost 90% humid, and virtually free of solid particles. The nose secretes up to 1 L of fluid per day, which is layered as a thin film on the surface of the mucosa. This film has a pH of 7, is continuous from the anterior nose to the nasopharynx, and is in constant motion, propelled toward the nasopharynx by

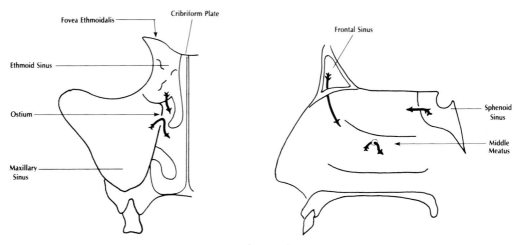

Fig. 10.3.   Sagittal and coronal sections to illustrate the pathways of drainage from the sinuses; only the sphenoid sinus does not empty into the middle meatus.

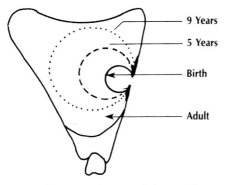

Fig. 10.4.   Changes in the size of the maxillary sinus with age. At birth the sinus is a small, slit-like cavity.

ciliary action. Larger particles are strained by vibrissae in the nasal vestibule, and small particles stick to the mucosal film. Nasal secretion contains lysozymes and immunoglobulins that protect the nose against bacterial contamination.

The nose is an adaptable organ that continues to function with remarkable efficiency in most environments. Certain characteristics of the nose, however, are genetically determined. For example, the thin, narrow, Caucasian nose is more suited to colder climates, while the broader, wider, Negroid nose is better adapted to hot, humid, tropical climates.

Evidence exists to suggest that the nose also plays a part in, and is partially controlled by, sexual stimuli. The core of the inferior turbinate is similar to the cavernous tissue of the genitalia.

DISORDERS OF THE NOSE

Congenital Anomalies

Congenital anomalies of the nose are common because the nose is always affected by clefting of the lip and palate. Clefting of the lip is caused by failure of the median and lateral nasal processes to fuse. The cleft usually extends into the floor of the nasal vestibule. The alae nasi are hypoplastic and collapsed. The hard palate forms the floor of the nose, and clefting of the palate causes a defect into the nasal passages and, in rare cases, into the maxillary sinuses. The nasal septum is usually shortened vertically. These anomalies initially cause difficulty in feeding, which usually improves as the child grows older. Cleft lips are repaired within a few months after birth, while cleft palates are usually repaired around the age of 1 to 2 years. The ideal time for repair, however, seems to be around the age of 3 years. Repair techniques are detailed in more specialized publications.

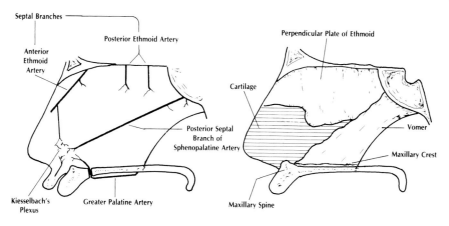

Fig. 10.5. Stylized diagrams of the blood supply and skeleton of the nasal septum. The perpendicular plate of the ethmoid is thin and easily fractured.

CHOANAL ATRESIA. Atresia of the posterior choanae of the nasal passages results from the failure of the buccopharyngeal membranes to dissolve. Atresia might be unilateral or bilateral. Bilateral choanal atresia causes respiratory distress in the newborn immediately after birth because the neonate is an obligatory nasal breather who also has a comparatively large tongue that fills the oral cavity. Choanal atresia is, therefore, a dire emergency and a potentially fatal problem in the newborn. Feeding is particularly difficult. Diagnosis is easily confirmed by the lack of misting on a shiny object held in front of the anterior nares and by the inability to pass a small catheter transnasally into the naso- and oropharynx. Contrast radiography with a radiopaque solution in the nasal cavity defines the level of obstruction.

TREATMENT. An airway must be provided immediately. This can be accomplished with an oral airway or with a McGovern's nipple, which is specifically designed for this purpose. Sooner or later, the atresia must be opened. Surgical manipulation is easier and safer if it can be postponed for a few weeks or months, during which time the child requires careful, dedicated nursing. Alternatively, if immediate intervention is necessary, the obstructing plates are perforated, usually by transnasal instrumentation, either blindly by feel or with microsurgical techniques. The openings are splinted with silicone tubes that extend from the anterior nares to the oropharynx and are sutured in place for 6 weeks. Thereafter, periodic dilatations are necessary. In the older child an alternative transpalatal approach can be used to open the choanae.

MIDLINE NASAL DERMOID. At birth there is a tiny pit in the midline of the cartilaginous nasal dorsum, from which small hairs may protrude. The orifice leads into a skin-lined tract that extends for variable distances through the alar cartilages into the septum and toward the cribriform plate. If the tract becomes infected, intermittent or constant drainage might develop from the external punctum. Midline dermoids may cause meningitis and should be completely excised.

ENCEPHALOCELES. Congenital defects in the cribriform plate or floor of the anterior cranial fossa predisposes to prolapse of the meninges into the nasal cavity, resulting in the formation of a meningocele or meningoencephalocele. Therefore, any intranasal mass in a neonate or young child should be respected and must not be incised without prior investigation.

CONGENITAL HEMANGIOMAS. Congenital hemangiomas may present in the nose as obstructing masses, or they may cause epistaxis.

DISORDERS OF THE EXTERNAL NOSE

Inflammatory Conditions

BACTERIAL INFECTIONS. The venous system of the external nose connects to the angular veins, which drain directly into the cavernous sinuses. Therefore, infections of the nasal skin have the potential for causing thrombophlebitis of the cavernous sinuses. Staphylococcal infections are particularly dangerous.

Furuncles of the skin of the external nose and nasal vestibule should be treated with antistaphylococcal agents, such as dicloxacillin, 250 mg four times daily, and warm compresses to hasten resolution. The lesions should not be massaged or squeezed, and, therefore, topical salves are not recommended.

LEPROSY. Although the incidence of leprosy is declining worldwide, the disease is still endemic and afflicts large numbers of people in Africa, Southeast Asia, and parts of South America. Leprosy may present with generalized thickening of the skin of the face (leonine facies). The nose becomes thicker and bulbous. A painless, slowly progressive ulcer might develop on the dorsum of the nose and erode the skeletal framework. Eventually, the whole external nose disappears. Diagnosis is confirmed on growing Hansen's bacilli (Mycobacterium leprae), by inoculating tissue fluid into the interdigital webs of the armadillo. Leprosy is treated with dapsone, given orally. The disease is minimally contagious.

Neoplasms

BENIGN NEOPLASMS. Benign neoplasms of the external nose are rare. Even sebaceous cysts are uncommon on the nose.

RHINOPHYMA (PFUNDNASE). Although this is not a neoplasm, it should be discussed here. Rhinophyma is a red, nodular, glossy, bulbous, gross thickening of the skin of the cartilaginous nose, which is caused by excessive hypertrophy of the sebaceous glands. Rhinophyma usually occurs in middle-aged males, is associated with chronic alcoholism, and is preceded by long-standing acne rosacea ("whiskey nose"). The problem is primarily cosmetic, although there are occasional episodes of superadded infection. Rhinophyma is treated by paring off the redundant tissue with a razor or by dermabrasion. More normal skin regenerates and covers the raw area.

MALIGNANT NEOPLASMS. Two types of malignancies involve the external nose: basal cell carcinoma and squamous cell carcinoma.

BASAL CELL CARCINOMA. Basal cell carcinomas present as circular, shallow ulcers with firm, pearl-gray, bumpy margins, which are surrounded by an indurated zone. The central area might be only depressed and not ulcerated (Figure 10.6). Microscopically, basal cell carcinomas extend for substantial distances beyond their borders.

Most basal cell carcinomas are asymptomatic, grow slowly, and almost never

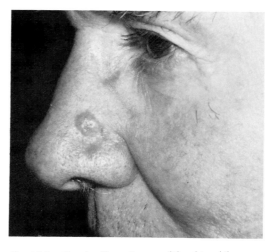

Fig. 10.6. Basal cell carcinoma of the skin of the nose. The lesion is round and characteristically umbilicated.

metastasize. They will, however, erode into bone and cause symptoms because of involvement of adjacent structures. Basal cell carcinomas are best treated by excision, with careful monitoring of the margins of resection by rapid frozen sections. Small lesions are easily excised along with an appropriate margin of normal tissue. The defect is closed primarily or with a variety of tissue flaps. Larger lesions require more extensive surgery and reconstructive maneuvers. Alternatively, radiation therapy might be successful.

SQUAMOUS CELL CARCINOMA. Squamous cell carcinoma of the skin of the external nose and face is more prevalent in fair-skinned people who are exposed to sunlight. Lesions begin as flat, crusted areas with ill-defined margins. The center ulcerates and becomes unsightly. Light-related cancer of the skin can be multifocal; hence, all exposed areas should be thoroughly examined. Squamous cell carcinoma metastasizes to the regional lymph nodes. Small lesions should be excised with an adequate margin of normal tissue. Larger lesions may be treated with radiation therapy.

INFLAMMATORY DISORDERS OF THE NASAL MUCOSA

The schneiderian membrane is a continuous, ciliated mucosa that lines the nose and paranasal sinuses. Therefore, any disease that affects the nose almost always involves the sinuses, and vice versa.

Allergy plays an important active or background role in rhinosinusitis. Allergy and viral infections of the upper respiratory tract are frequent precursors of bacterial rhinosinusitis. With chronic irritation, the mucosa, particularly that of the ethmoid sinus, tends to become hypertrophic and polypoid. In rare cases the mucous membrane atrophies instead.

The respiratory system functions as a whole, although for descriptive purposes it is generally divided into upper and lower parts. Therefore, what affects the nose and sinuses is also likely to affect the lower respiratory tract. Expressions of the same disease might occur in both areas such as in Woakes syndrome (nasal polyposis and bronchial asthma). Alternatively, infectious sinusitis as a primary problem can cause secondary contamination of the lungs.

Bacterial Infections

The more common bacterial rhinosinusitis is discussed in Chapter 11. There are, however, a few uncommon bacterial infections of the nasal mucosa that are important.

DIPHTHERIA. Diphtheria is an infection that is caused by a virulent strain of Corynebacterium diphtheriae. Although diphtheritic rhinitis is comparatively rare in developed nations, it can occur as the primary point of infection. The child with diphtheria becomes febrile and quickly develops a membranous rhinitis, with ulceration of the nasal mucosa and a blood-stained, purulent discharge. The ulcers are covered by a gray, adherent membrane. Diagnosis is made easily by Gram stain of a smear and by the appropriate cultures on Löffler's medium. Treatment is with diphtheria antitoxin and penicillin given parenterally and nasal irrigations with warm saline solution.

TUBERCULOSIS. Nasal tuberculosis presents as an indolent, painful ulcer of the cartilaginous septum. Initially, painful, small nodules are present on the mucosa, which coalesce and disintegrate to form an ulcer that eventually involves the cartilage. Dissolution of the cartilage causes a septal perforation. Nasal tuberculosis is usually secondary to advanced pulmonary disease and is treated with antituberculous medications such as isoniazid and ethambutol.

SYPHILIS. Syphilis is caused by infection with Treponoma pallidum, which might affect the nose in both its acquired and congenital forms.

ACQUIRED SYPHILIS. Primary chancres of

the nose are rare in acquired syphilis. Secondary syphilis presents with "mucous patches," which are superficial ulcers that may involve all mucosal surfaces. Diagnosis depends on clinical awareness and is confirmed by dark-field examination of a smear of mucus and by serologic tests. Treatment is with large doses of penicillin (2 million units) by intramuscular injection. Tertiary syphilis of the nose presents as gummatous lesions, which are areas of necrosis that usually involve the bony nasal septum. Disintegration of the septum and collapse of the nasal bridge causes saddling of the nose. Treatment is by local debridement and large dose of penicillin given parenterally.

CONGENITAL SYPHILIS. Congenital syphilis has all the stigmata of the secondary and tertiary forms of acquired disease. The nasal alae of the infant are crusted and fissured. Profuse rhinorrhea (snuffles) is present. The nose might be saddled. Diagnosis and treatment are the same as for the acquired form. Early therapy will control most of the features of congenital syphilis.

YAWS. Yaws is a treponemal disease that is endemic to parts of equatorial Africa. The features and course of yaws disease might be clinically indistinguishable from those of syphilis.

RHINOSCLEROMA. Rhinoscleroma is an unusual, potentially fatal inflammatory disease of the nose, which is endemic among members of the lower socioeconomic strata of Central America, parts of Africa, and South America. Rhinoscleroma might present as a tumescence of any part of the nose, which expands and eventually ulcerates. Rhinoscleroma is probably caused by Klebsiella rhinoscleromatis, an organism that has not been identified in every case. The histologic picture is dominated by large, foamy macrophages. Early lesions might respond to vigorous treatment with streptomycin or tetracycline. If the patient survives, the lesions regress, leaving an atrophic rhinitis.

Fungal Infections of the Nose and Paranasal Sinuses

Two groups of fungi cause severe infections in the nose and sinuses: Phycomycetes and Aspergillus.

PHYCOMYCETES (MUCORMYCOSIS). Phycomycetes have septated hyphae and tend to infect the paranasal sinuses of middle-aged and elderly diabetics. The organism spreads rapidly, invading blood vessels, causing arterial and venous thromboses, and, therefore, sharply defined areas of infarction and extensive necrosis. The patient presents with high fever, chills, headache, bloodstained nasal discharge, rapidly increasing swelling of the eyelids and cheek, proptosis, and paralysis of the extraocular muscles. The patient quickly becomes severely ill and can even become comatose, with signs of cavernous sinus thrombophlebitis. The middle turbinate and other parts of the nose become gray-black and necrotic early in the course of the disease (Figure 10.7). Roentgenograms show opacification of the ethmoid, maxillary, frontal, and, sometimes, sphenoid sinuses. Diagnosis is confirmed by microscopic examination of a wet preparation of tissue from the middle turbinate. If this test is negative, special

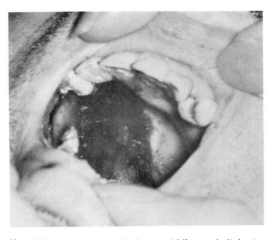

Fig. 10.7. Mucormycosis in a middle-aged diabetic. Necrosis of the maxilla caused by intravascular thrombosis is sharply demarcated.

stains of paraffin sections are necessary. Cultures take too long to be of use in diagnosis. Treatment must be based on a clinical diagnosis and must be prompt and extremely vigorous. Surgical debridement is performed early, with removal of all necrotic tissue. The infected tissue is usually avascular and should be excised until bleeding bone and soft tissue are encountered. Antifungal agents are administered intravenously. Amphotericin B is currently the drug of choice. Significant mortality results from the disease.

ASPERGILLUS. Infection of the nose and paranasal sinuses by Aspergillus species is uncommon but can occur at any age. Aspergillus infections might present as an acute or chronic problem and are more prevalent in immunologically compromised patients. No specific symptoms and signs are diagnostic of Aspergillus infection, except for the lack of response of a rapidly advancing rhinosinusitis to antibiotic therapy. Diagnosis is usually made by surgical exploration and biopsy. Treatment is by wide drainage and the administration of the appropriate antifungal agents.

RHINOSPORIDIOSIS. Rhinosporidiosis is infection caused by Rhinosporidium seeberi, which is a yeast-like fungus with an affinity for warm, moist surfaces. The disease is endemic in parts of India and Central and South America. The patient, usually a young child or young adult, presents with finger-like polypoid masses growing from the nasal mucosa. These are pale, tan-colored, and bleed readily. Diagnosis is made by histologic examination of the polyp, in which clusters of fungal sporangia can be recognized easily. Treatment is by surgical removal of all abnormal tissue and vigorous use of systemic antifungal agents.

BLASTOMYCOSIS. Blastomycoses is a group of yeast-like fungi that are endemic to Central and South America. Blastomycosis presents as chronic ulcerations in the upper aerodigestive tract, particularly the tongue and larynx, but might also involve the nose and paranasal sinuses. Treatment is by intravenous antifungal medications such as amphotericin B.

Allergic Rhinitis

Allergy plays a most important basic role in many nasal problems. It is, therefore, important to obtain a history of allergy in every patient with nasal symptoms. For instance, a well-documented relationship exists between nasal allergy and bronchospasm; these conditions should be considered to be merely expressions of the same allergic diathesis. Acute allergic rhinitis presents with a classic triad of symptoms: nasal obstruction, watery rhinorrhea, and episodic sneezing. However, wide variation exists in presentation, and it is possible for chronic allergy to be expressed by only two of the three symptoms. Long-standing allergic rhinitis might cause formation of nasal polyps.

ALLERGENS. Inhalants are the most frequent nasal allergens. Food allergens might also be important but are difficult to trace. Aspirin is a common ingested allergen. In the sensitive patient aspirin will cause chronic rhinitis, polypoid changes in the mucosa, and chronic nasal obstruction. Inhalant allergens are ubiquitous. Probably, every individual will react adversely to something in his or her environment. The commonest agents are pollens, animal dander, fungal spores, house dust, feathers, and detergents. House dust is a particularly active inhalant, which really consists of many substances such as spores, dander, fabric dust, and so on. Allergy to house dust causes perennial symptoms, whereas allergy to pollens is seasonal.

EXAMINATION. The mucosa, particularly on the inferior turbinate, is characteristically swollen, boggy, pale, and wet, and might completely obstruct the nasal passage. There is profuse, clear, watery secretion. On posterior rhinoscopy the posterior ends of the inferior turbinates are violaceous and swollen, and, in the chronic state, might have a mulberry-like appearance. In addition, in the chronic case polypoid changes might occur in the middle meatus.

INVESTIGATION. HISTORY. A detailed personal and family history is essential for diagnosis. Occasionally, the evidence for allergy might be more tenuous (e.g., when the only personal or family expression of allergy is eczema). Frequently, a careful history is all that is necessary but might entail detailed detective work on the part of the patient. Skin tests are performed if the history is not definitive.

BLOOD TESTS. The differential eosinophil count is significant but can be nearly normal with chronic allergy. It is now accepted that IgE is the prime carrier of reaginic hypersensitivity in humans, but the level of IgE in the serum of allergic patients is only sometimes elevated, especially during the acute phases. The radioallergosorbent test (RAST) measures antigen-specific IgE and is currently widely used for both diagnosis and as a guide for immunotherapy.

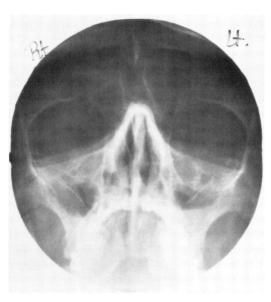

Fig. 10.8. Radiologic study of a young woman with allergic rhinosinusitis. There is generalized haziness of the sinuses, caused by thickening of the mucosa, and fluid levels in both maxillary sinuses.

RADIOLOGY. During an acute episode of allergic rhinitis, radiologic examination will show diffuse involvement of all paranasal sinuses and even collections of fluid in the sinuses (Figure 10.8). The maximum changes occur in the maxillary and ethmoid sinuses.

SKIN TESTS. Skin tests are done either by scratches or by injection. The scratch method is less reliable but is still the method of choice in children. Most allergists use predetermined dilutions of extracts of allergen. Small quantities of extracts of different substances are injected intracutaneously on the forearm, arm, or back. A red wheal indicates a positive reaction to a given allergen. An alternative method was described by Hansel (1953) in which the patient is tested with serial dilutions that are carefully titrated to an end point of minimal reaction.

NASAL SMEARS. Examining specially stained smears of nasal secretions for the presence of eosinophil and mast cells might be useful diagnostically.

TREATMENT. If one or a number of allergens are identified, treatment can be by one of three methods: avoidance or elimination of the allergen, medications (antihistamines and corticosteroids), or immunotherapy.

The first-line treatment of allergic rhinitis is a combination of antihistamine-decongestant medication that is taken orally. Many commercial preparations are available. Patients may respond satisfactorily to one preparation but not to another, and, therefore, a period of trial and error might be necessary until the right combination is found. Even this trial-and-error stage might be temporarily effective. Antihistamine-decongestants are most useful for control of the temporary symptoms of seasonal allergy. Corticosteroids are used only for severe cases and for quick results. They may be given orally (e.g., prednisone or betamethasone in sliding doses) or, alternatively, may be used topically (e.g., beclomethasone as a spray).

Avoidance or elimination of allergens is not always practical. House dust can be substantially reduced by daily cleaning, oiling the floors, and so on, and the use of an electric dust extractor. Pets can be banished from the indoors, but animal danders persist on furniture and fabric for a long time.

Immunotherapy is the only available specific treatment for allergic disorders. Basically, immunotherapy is the administration, by injection, of small, but increasing, doses of an allergen, with the goal of stimulating the body's defensive mechanism. Of course, the allergens must first be identified. Generally effective immunotherapy requires high doses of allergens, and this is usually achieved only after a long time and many injections. The process, although scientifically rational, is tedious, time-consuming, and expensive but can be effective in properly selected cases.

A number of other therapeutic maneuvers are sometimes temporarily effective in the treatment of allergic rhinitis. The more common of these are cautery of the inferior turbinates and injection of corticosteroids into the inferior turbinates.

Chronic Nonallergic Rhinitis

Chronic nonallergic rhinitis is a state of perennial nasal engorgement and rhinorrhea that is not really an inflammation of the mucosa. There are a number of causative factors in chronic nonallergic rhinitis such as autonomic dysregulation, hypothyroidism, environmental irritants, such as cold air, the menstrual cycle, pregnancy, antihypertensive medications (e.g., Rauwolfia serpentina), alcohol, tobacco, and cannabis.

VASOMOTOR RHINITIS. Vasomotor rhinitis is a form of chronic nonallergic rhinitis that is supposedly caused by dysfunction of the autonomic regulation of the nasal mucosa. The patient complains of nasal obstruction and profuse rhinorrhea with clear, watery mucus. There is no, or only occasional, sneezing and no watering of the eyes. The nasal obstruction can vary from complete obstruction to subtle stuffiness. The rhinorrhea can be an almost constant flow of clear, watery fluid requiring the use of many handkerchiefs each day. The nasal mucosa is pale, violaceous, soft, boggy, and watery. It responds to manipulation by shrinking but quickly rebounds. The inferior turbinate and anterior septum are the areas that are most affected. No tenderness develops over the sinuses. Strangely, patients with this condition are not prone to upper respiratory tract infections or sinusitis. Roentgenograms show clear sinuses.

TREATMENT. The treatment consists of controlling the causative factors if they are identifiable. Autonomic dysfunction is more difficult to treat. Anticholinergic medicines are useful, but the side-effects are usually intolerable. Cautery of the inferior turbinates might help for a few months. Interrupting the autonomic parasympathetic supply by cutting the vidian nerve was a popular therapeutic modality but gives only temporary relief.

Cerebrospinal Rhinorrhea

Leakage of cerebrospinal fluid into the nose occurs when a defect is present in the dura and bone of the roof of the nose (cribriform plate), roof of the ethmoid sinuses (fovea ethmoidalis), roof of the sphenoid sinus, or even in the temporal bone. The defect might be secondary to fractures of the floor of the anterior or middle cranial fossae, iatrogenic after surgery of the sinuses or nose, or can be spontaneous, probably as a result of a congenital dehiscence in the bone.

The patient may complain of a profuse, unilateral, watery rhinorrhea on bending forward or on lying down. Alternatively, the presenting problem can be recurrent meningitis, and the leakage of fluid might not be obvious to the patient or examiner. The mucosa looks wet and boggy, and, if the patient bends forward with his head well down, a few drops of clear, watery fluid drips from the nose. The fluid should be tested for glucose; cerebrospinal fluid gives a positive result. Radioactive technetium, fluorescein dye, or metrizamide injected into the subarachnoid space might identify the point of leakage. Computed tomography might demonstrate fractures or herniation of intracranial contents.

Although some patients have intermittent cerebrospinal fluid rhinorrhea for many years, the condition is potentially dangerous because of the risk of meningitis. The leak should, therefore, be stopped via a transnasal or intracranial surgical technique.

Nasal Polyps

Nasal polyps are usually bilateral, gray, smooth, shiny, rounded, grape-like masses of swollen mucosa that develop in the ethmoid sinuses and present in the middle meatus (Figure 10.9). Polyps are caused either by allergy or infection, but allergy is, by far, the more frequent factor. Large polyps cause obstruction to nasal breathing and anosmia. Histologically, polyps consist of a loose, edematous, myxoid stroma covered by respiratory epithelium. The mucosa over older polyps might change to squamous epithelium.

Allergic polyps are usually bilateral, and, therefore, all unilateral lesions of the nose that resemble polyps should be carefully investigated before a biopsy or surgical removal is performed. A unilateral, polypoid, nasal mass might be a meningoencephalocele, neoplasm, hemangioma, or an antrochoanal polyp (see below).

TREATMENT. Large obstructing polyps require surgical excision. This is usually done with local anesthesia, using snares and punch forceps. Remove as much polypoid material as possible. Vigorously treat the underlying allergy or infection because polyps tend to regrow. Their rate of growth can be reduced by the administration of topical or systemic corticosteroids. If recurrence is difficult to control, an ethmoidectomy might be necessary (see Chapter 22).

Antrochoanal Polyps

An antrochoanal polyp is a large, single, usually unilateral polyp that extends from the maxillary sinus into the posterior nasal passage, through the posterior choana into the nasopharynx, and might present as a pendulous mass in the oropharynx. Patients complain of unilateral nasal obstruction or of a mass in the throat. There

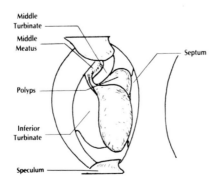

Middle Turbinate

Middle Meatus

Septum

Polyps

Inferior Turbinate

Speculum

Fig. 10.9.   Diagram of a nasal polyp. Most polyps present in the middle meatus, are bilateral, and are caused by allergy.

Frontal View

is no pain. Antrochoanal polyps probably originate in the maxillary sinus or adjacent ethmoid sinus. Removal of an antrochoanal polyp must include excision of both maxillary and nasal components.

Foreign Bodies

It is not unusual for otherwise normal children to insert various types of foreign bodies into their noses. Materials usually encountered are bits of paper, erasers, beads, seeds, stones, plastic toys, and so on.

The patient presents with unilateral nasal obstruction and a foul-smelling discharge. The symptoms may persist for a long time, possibly for years, and there is no pain. The child will almost always deny placing a foreign body in his nose. On examination, a thick, purulent, foul-smelling discharge is usually present in one nasal passage. The mucosa is pink, granular, and swollen, and might obscure the foreign body, which is usually lodged between the middle turbinate and the septum. Foreign bodies must be removed from the nose, otherwise, a rhinolith forms from the deposition of calcium salts around the foreign material.

Children usually require general anesthesia. Intubate the child to prevent the possible aspiration of the foreign body, and place a gauze pack in the nasopharynx and oropharynx. Extract the foreign body with a curved instrument, which is passed behind the foreign material and then drawn forward and out through the vestibule. Bleeding is usually minimal.

The Nose and Systemic Granulomatous Diseases

SARCOIDOSIS. Sarcoidosis is an idiopathic, systemic, granulomatous disease that is most prevalent in young black females; however, Caucasians and males are also affected. Sarcoidosis may present as nasal obstruction, cough, hoarseness, and lymphadenopathy in the neck, parotid area, or hilar nodes. The nasal mucosa becomes swollen and granular but no rhinorrhea is present. The erythrocyte sedimentation rate may be elevated.

Sarcoidosis may cause a characteristic hilar lymphadenopathy that can be seen on a chest roentgenogram. Diagnosis is made by biopsy of a lymph node, if one is available, or biopsy of the nasal, laryngeal, or tracheal mucosa. Histologically, noncaseating granulomas occur, with multinucleated giant cells.

There is no specific treatment for sarcoidosis. Corticosteroids can control the acute phases. Plasmaquin might control the early stages of the disease.

WEGENER'S GRANULOMATOSIS. Wegener's granulomatosis is really a form of necrotizing vasculitis. The disease tends to involve the respiratory tract, kidneys, skin, and other organs. Wegener's granulomatosis might present with nasal, otologic, pulmonary, or renal symptoms, even as recurrent sinusitis or otitis media. The nasal mucosa ulcerates, crusts, and bleeds

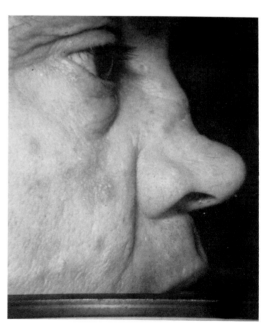

Fig. 10.10.   Saddling of the nose in a 43-year-old man with Wegener's granulomatosis. The cartilage of the septum has dissolved, and the corresponding dorsum has settled.

easily. The cartilaginous skeleton of the septum is lost, resulting in saddling of the nose (Figure 10.10). Roentgenograms of the chest may identify granulomas even as cavitated lesions. Renal involvement causes microscopic hematuria or proteinuria. Wegener's granulomatosis is diagnosed by biopsy of available tissue. Histologically, granulomas are present, with giant cells and occlusion of vessels, whose walls are indistinct because of the loss of elastic tissue. Wegener's granulomatosis is treated with corticosteroids and cyclophosphamide and is now considered to be a curable disease.

MIDLINE LETHAL GRANULOMA. Midline lethal granuloma is a rapidly progressive, ulcerative lesion of the midline structures of the face and mouth. The condition is uncommon and usually afflicts adults.

The histologic picture is frequently confusing, but increasing evidence exists to suggest that most cases of midline lethal granuloma are really highly undifferentiated malignant lymphomas. Nevertheless, differentiation between midline lethal granuloma and Wegener's granulomatosis is sometimes extremely difficult. Midline lethal granuloma is usually treated with radiation therapy and chemotherapy.

BIBLIOGRAPHY

Anggard, A.: Capillary and shunt blood flow in the nasal mucosa of the cat. Acta Otolaryngol. (Stockh), 78:418, 1974.
Bray, D.A.: Head and neck skin cancer: Preplanned pathologically controlled excision and reconstruction. Laryngoscope, 92:783–794, 1982.
Ishizaka, K., and Ishizaka, T.: Identification of gamma E antibodies as a carrier of reaginic activity. J. Immunol., 99:1187, 1967.
Kornblut, A.D., et al.: Wegener's granulomatosis. Laryngoscope, 90:1453–1465, 1980.
Malcomson, K.G.: The vasomotor activities of the nasal mucous membranes. J. Laryngol., 73:73, 1959.
Mygind, N.: Nasal Allergy, Part III. Oxford, Alden Press, 1979.
Pillsbury, H.C., and Fischer, N.D.: Rhinocerebral mucormycosis. Arch. Otolaryngol., 103:600–602, 1977.
Stoksted, P.: The physiologic cycle of the nose under normal and pathologic conditions. Acta Otolaryngol. (Stockh), 42:175–179, 1952.
Wide, L., Bennich, H., and Johannson, S.G.O.: Diagnosis of allergy by an in vitro test for allergen antibodies. Lancet, 2:1105, 1967.

Chapter 11

SINUSITIS AND NEOPLASMS OF THE NOSE

ACUTE SINUSITIS

"Sinusitis" is a much-abused diagnosis. Inflammation of the paranasal sinuses is comparatively common and is usually associated with viral upper respiratory tract infections or allergic reactions. Acute sinusitis, however, is not the cause of every spurious headache and certainly does not occur every day year in and year out in the same patient. A diagnosis of sinusitis should be made only after taking a careful history and performing a thorough examination.

Symptoms

A history of antecedent upper respiratory tract infection with rhinorrhea, nasal obstruction, sneezing, mild fever, and so on is usually present. Initially, the rhinorrhea is watery and profuse, but as bacterial infection supervenes, the discharge becomes thicker, more purulent, and, sometimes, bloodstained. One or more parts of the face become painful: the cheek and upper teeth in maxillary sinusitis; the ipsilateral forehead in frontal sinusitis; retro-orbital discomfort in ethmoiditis; and vague retro-orbital, vault, or temporal headache in sphenoid sinusitis. Pain is exaggerated by bending forward. Swelling and redness of the cheek, forehead, and/or upper eyelid occur occasionally, but not always. Fever and malaise increase.

Examination

Palpate carefully the areas over the representative sinuses, as detailed in Chapter 1. The nasal mucosa is reddened, edematous, and moist, particularly over the turbinates, which might be sufficiently swollen to occlude the nasal passages. Therefore, it might be necessary to shrink the mucosa with a topical vasoconstrictor to enable a more thorough examination. Mucopurulent material is present on the floor of the nose and usually in the middle meatus. Alternatively, discharge might be seen only with posterior rhinoscopy. Posterior rhinoscopy might also identify the flow of material above the middle turbinate, which indicates infection of the posterior ethmoid or sphenoid sinuses. A sample of the nasal secretions is taken under direct vision from the middle meatus for Gram stain, culture, and sensitivity studies. The organisms that are most frequently isolated are Streptococcus pneumoniae, Hemophilus influenzae, and (less frequently) Staphylococcus aureus.

Radiology

Standard routine roentgenograms are obtained. These will show opacification from mucosal swelling and/or air-fluid levels in the involved sinuses (Figure 11.1). Tomography is used only if more details are necessary.

119

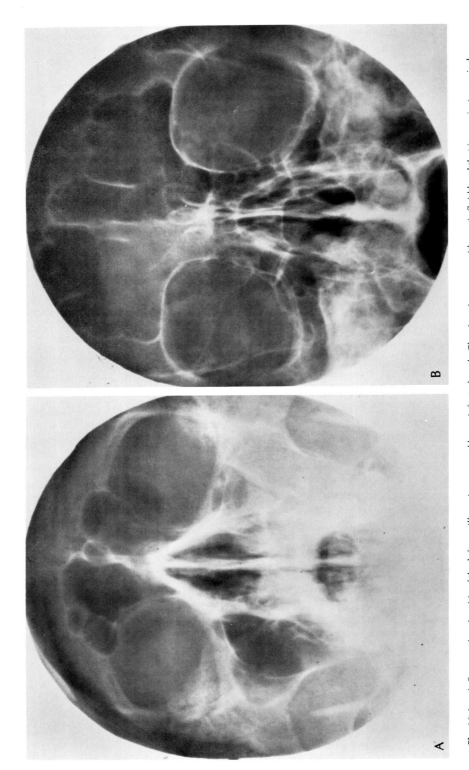

Fig. 11.1. *A.* Suppurative sinusitis of the left maxillary sinus caused by an infected tooth. The sinus is opaque with an air-fluid level that is seen just superiorly. The other sinuses are clear. *B.* Acute right frontal sinusitis in a different patient. An air-fluid level is present in the frontal sinus, and the ethmoid sinus is opaque.

Predisposing Factors

Any condition that compromises the natural drainage of the sinuses will predispose to sinusitis. The commonest factors are chronic allergy, severe deviation of the nasal septum, neoplasms (e.g., osteoma), and traumatic deformity of the nasofrontal duct. Dental infection might spread directly to the maxillary sinus.

Treatment

Draining the sinuses is essential and is best accomplished by reducing the swelling of the nasal mucosa, particularly around the ostia of the sinuses. Use topical vasoconstrictors liberally (e.g., oxymetazoline 4 times daily) to reduce edema and open the ostia. An oral antihistamine-decongestant preparation, such as chlorpheniramine maleate-phenylephrine, is helpful. Antibiotics should be begun only after sampling for the presence of bacteria. Most cases of sinusitis will respond to oral penicillin or one of its synthetic derivatives (e.g., ampicillin, 250 to 500 mg orally four times daily).

MAXILLARY SINUSITIS OF DENTAL ORIGIN. Only a comparatively thin plate of bone usually separates the cavity of the sinus from the apices of the posterior maxillary teeth, and even these plates might be absent. Apical infection of the teeth spreads easily through this flimsy barrier. The resulting sinusitis occurs spontaneously, without the usual antecedent upper respiratory tract infection and sometimes without clinical symptoms. The nasal secretions are profuse, thick, yellow, and foul smelling. The cheek is tender and the offending tooth is usually, but not always, tender on percussion. The sinusitis is treated with antibiotics and might require surgical drainage; the tooth is either extracted or a root canal performed.

CHRONIC SINUSITIS

Symptoms

Sinusitis becomes chronic when factors are present that keep the infection active. The usual predisposing factors have already been listed, but probably the most frequent cause is chronic allergy. Chronic sinusitis is not a common problem. The patient complains of constant, perennial, purulent nasal discharge, postnasal drip, and stuffiness of the head. Intermittent frontal and facial pain occurs from the frontal and maxillary sinuses, respectively, or the patient complains of retroorbital pain or temporal or vault headache from the ethmoid and sphenoid sinuses.

Frequently, a nocturnal cough develops because of drainage of nasal secretions into the larynx in the recumbent position. With superimposed acute episodes there is fever, pain, swelling and redness over the forehead or orbit and increase in rhinorrhea.

Examination

In chronic sinusitis moderate tenderness occurs over the forehead or cheeks. The nasal mucosa is red, loses its luster, and has a velvety appearance. Small, yellow, adherent crusts of dried secretions and purulent exudate develop in the middle meatus if the maxillary or frontal sinuses are involved or in the superior meatus if the posterior ethmoid or sphenoid sinuses are involved. Strands of thick, yellow, mucopurulent secretions are present on the posterior and lateral walls of the nasopharynx.

Radiology

Roentgenograms show opacification from mucoperiosteal thickening of and, possibly, air-fluid levels in the involved sinuses. Acute or chronic sinusitis might involve all the sinuses on one side, might be totally bilateral, or might be confined to a single sinus. The walls of the sinuses may lose their sharp definition because of chronic inflammation.

Treatment

The organisms involved are usually Streptococci, Hemophilus influenzae,

Staphylococci, and Klebsiella species. The appropriate antibiotics are taken orally for a prolonged period of time if they seem to be effective. Topical vasoconstrictors are not of much help. All predisposing factors must be corrected. If, despite these measures, chronic sinusitis continues, surgical ablative maneuvers become necessary. Before surgery is considered, the maxillary sinus is lavaged three times by the technique that is described in Chapter 22. For the maxillary sinus, a radical sinusectomy is performed via a Caldwell-Luc approach (see Chapter 22). All the mucosa is removed, and an opening is made in the inferior meatus (nasoantral window) for better drainage into the nose. For ethmoid sinusitis, the ethmoid labyrinth is exenterated by an intranasal or external approach. The frontal sinus requires an osteoplastic flap and obliteration of the sinus or a Lynch-type procedure (see Chapter 22).

COMPLICATIONS OF SINUSITIS

Acute Sinusitis

Fortunately, most episodes of acute sinusitis resolve without residium. Many complications, however, are possible, and the same complications occur with acute and chronic sinusitis. Infection might spread beyond the sinus but remain extracranial, or might spread intracranially and cause meningitis or an intracranial abscess. Bacteremia or septic shock might develop.

Early diagnosis of a complication of sinusitis depends on clinical suspicion and protracted illness despite the appropriate treatment of the primary problem. Computed tomography has become an invaluable tool for investigating the complications of sinusitis and should be used earlier rather than later.

Maxillary Sinusitis

Complications secondary to maxillary sinusitis are uncommon. The commonest is probably chronicity of the sinusitis. In rare cases a true osteomyelitis of the maxilla occurs in infants, but this is much rarer in adults and develops only when a predisposing factor is present such as the spread of a dental infection.

Ethmoiditis and Frontal Sinusitis

The ethmoid and frontal sinuses should be considered as a single complex. The following is a list of the complications that are possible after ethmoiditis and frontal sinusitis:

Extracranial
—orbital cellulitis
—orbital abscess
—Blindness
—osteomyelitis of the frontal bone

Intracranial
—extradural abscess
—subdural abscess
Meningitis
Cerebral abscess
Cavernous sinus thrombophlebitis

ORBITAL CELLULITIS AND ORBITAL ABSCESS. The ethmoid sinuses are separated from the orbit by the paper-thin lamina papyracea. Infection penetrates this plate easily. Therefore, the commonest complication of ethmoiditis is the spread of infection to the orbit, which initially presents as a cellulitis of the orbit and later as an orbital abscess. The upper eyelid becomes swollen, red, hot, and the eye is painful (see Figure 11.3). The globe is usually displaced inferiorly and laterally. Swelling might spread to the forehead and close the eye. If an abscess forms, the eyelid becomes tense, shiny, and fluctuant. Blindness might occur from excessive edema of the orbital tissues and secondary compression of the orbital veins. Computed tomography in the axial plane will demonstrate opacification of the ethmoid sinus and edema of the adjacent orbital tissues (Figure 11.2). Ultrasonography is also useful for investigating the contents of the orbit.

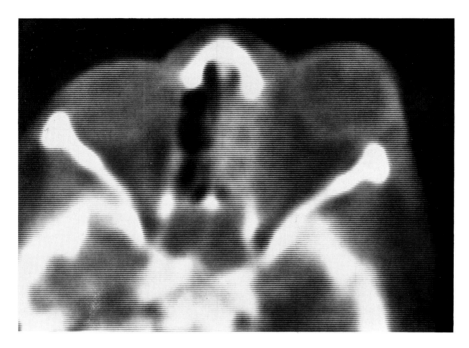

Fig. 11.2.   Computed tomography in a 4-year-old with orbital cellulitis secondary to ethmoiditis. Clouding of the ethmoid sinus extending into the orbit can be seen. The globe is displaced forward.

Treatment is with large doses of antibiotics given intravenously (e.g., ampicillin, 500 mg every 4 hours), topical vasoconstrictors (e.g., oxymetazoline), or 2% cocaine applied with a cotton tampon inserted into the middle meatus every 6 hours. If swelling progresses rapidly, corticosteroids are sometimes necessary. If antibiotics fail to control the infection, the ethmoid sinuses must be surgically exenterated and the orbital abscesses drained.

CONJUNCTIVITIS AND PSEUDOTUMORS. Orbital cellulitis must be differentiated from acute conjunctivitis and orbital pseudotumors. Conjunctivitis can cause substantial swelling and redness of the eyelids and chemosis. There is, however, purulent exudate in the conjunctival sac, which is not seen in orbital cellulitis secondary to sinusitis.

Pseudotumor of the orbit is an acute, idiopathic, granulomatous inflammation of the extraocular tissues. The eyelids become red, swollen, and painful, and paresis or paralysis of one or more extraocular muscles might occur. Fever, leukocytosis, and clinical or radiologic evidence of sinusitis are absent. The erythrocyte sedimentation rate is moderately elevated.

Computed tomography in the axial plane shows diffuse, patchy thickening of orbital tissues, characteristic swelling of the adjacent extraocular muscle, and a normal ethmoid sinus. The radiologic picture is almost diagnostic.

Pseudotumor is a clinical diagnosis. Before considering a biopsy a bolus of Hydrocortisone, 100 mg should be given intravenously. Most cases of pseudotumor will resolve rapidly over 6 to 12 hours after the administration of intravenous corticosteroids.

OSTEOMYELITIS OF THE FRONTAL BONE. Infection might spread from the frontal sinus to the diploë of the frontal bone and then progress rapidly. The pa-

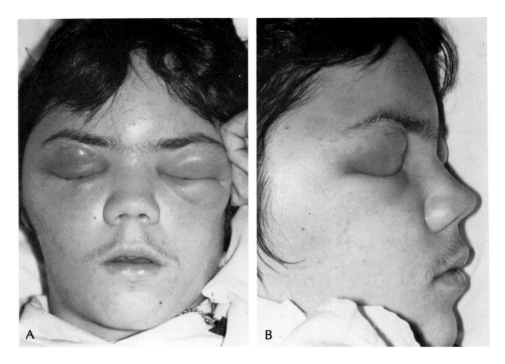

Fig. 11.3. Frontal (Fig. 11.3A) and lateral (Fig. 11.3B) roentgenograms of a 17-year-old patient with frontal osteomyelitis secondary to sinusitis. A smooth, doughy swelling of the forehead and edema of the eyelids are present.

tient quickly becomes extremely ill. The eyelids, forehead, and scalp are grossly edematous (Pott's puffy tumor) (Figure 11.3). Early diagnosis must be made on a clinical basis because radiologic changes, although characteristic, take 10 to 14 days to develop. The earliest roentgenographic changes are expansion of the diploic venous spaces, followed later by mottling of the bone (Figure 11.4). Some therapeutic guidance is possible from a Gram stain of a smear and from culture of nasal secretions. The more common causative organisms are Streptococcus pyogenes or Staphylococcus aureus. Osteomyelitis of the frontal bone is a dangerous problem that demands prompt, vigorous treatment with massive doses of intravenous antibiotics. The drugs of choice are clindamycin, lincomycin hydrochloride (Lincocin), and cefazolin sodium (Kefzol). Bony sequestra are removed surgically

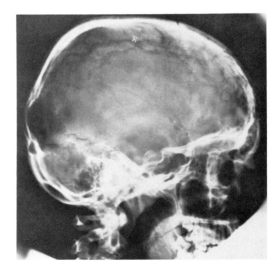

Fig. 11.4. Skull roentgenogram of patient in Figure 11.3. There is patchy erosion of the frontal bone and widening of the diploic veins.

when the acute phase has subsided. The frontal sinuses must be drained early in the course of the disease. If the condition is not controlled by antibiotics, infected bone must be removed surgically.

Sphenoiditis

The major complications of sphenoiditis are thrombophlebitis of the cavernous sinus, meningitis, and cerebral abscess.

THROMBOPHLEBITIS OF THE CAVERNOUS SINUS. This is always a potential problem in paranasal sinusitis but particularly so with sphenoiditis. The patient quickly becomes ill, toxic, has a fever, and is lethargic. The ipsilateral eyelids swell rapidly. Proptosis, chemosis, and partial or total external ophthalmoplegia are present (Figure 11.5). Papilledema, engorgement of the retinal veins, and rapid depression of visual acuity occur. Thrombophlebitis of the cavernous sinus is potentially fatal. Immediate antibiotic therapy should be started on the basis of a Gram stain of a nasal smear. Penicillin G, chloramphenicol, oxacillin, cefazolin sodium (Kefzol), and Meticillin in various combinations are useful. The use of anticoagulants is controversial and should be considered only if there is evidence of uncontrolled progression after initiation of antibiotic therapy. Corticosteroids might

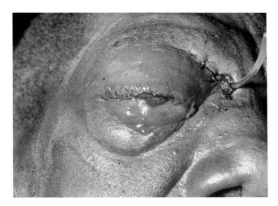

Fig. 11.5. Cavernous sinus thrombophlebitis in a 50-year-old man. Massive edema of the orbit and conjunctiva and a marked proptosis are present.

be valuable in reducing edema and preventing blindness. The involved sinus must be drained as soon as the patient's condition allows.

Intracranial Complications of Sinusitis

Meningitis, extradural abscess, cerebral abscess, and cortical thrombophlebitis are all possible complications of sinusitis. The symptoms and signs of meningitis are well known. The patient complains of severe headache. He is febrile, toxic, lethargic, and becomes comatosed. The neck is stiff, and Kernig's sign is positive. The diagnosis is confirmed by lumbar puncture. Treatment must be vigorous, with intravenous antibiotics. The involved sinus must be drained as soon as possible.

Extradural abscesses are difficult to diagnose unless gas forming organisms are present. Computed tomography of the head will, however, show extradural collections.

An abscess of the frontal lobe secondary to sinusitis can be silent initially. The only indicator might be a change in the patient's affect or behavior. Cerebral abscesses are diagnosed early only if the clinician is highly suspicious. Ancillary diagnostic maneuvers, such as computed tomography, radioisotope brain scans, and angiograms, should be obtained sooner rather then later. Glial cellulitis might respond to antibiotics, but if an abscess forms, it must be drained immediately.

Thrombophlebitis of the cortical veins is, fortunately, a rare occurrence. Focal neurologic signs are present, and the patient quickly becomes comatosed. Diagnosis is primarily based on clinical suspicion. Treatment must be prompt and maximal with antibiotics, drainage of the involved sinus, and, possibly, corticosteroids to reduce the cerebral edema.

CYSTS OF THE PARANASAL SINUSES

Three types of cysts are found in the paranasal sinuses: retention cysts, muco-celes, and cysts of dental origin. Cysts of dental origin are discussed in Chapter 14 (see the section entitled "Cysts of the Jaw").

Retention Cysts

Retention cysts are probably caused by blockage of the ducts of mucous or serous glands and are common in the maxillary sinus. They are asymptomatic and are discovered incidentally on roentgenography. Retention cysts appear as smooth, rounded, slightly opaque masses on the floor and medial or lateral wall but seldom on the roof of the sinus. If, however, these cysts expand to fill the sinus, they cause facial pain or headache.

Small retention cysts require no treatment. Larger, asymptomatic cysts can be decompressed by aspiration or by opening the sinus through a Caldwell-Luc approach.

Mucoceles

Mucoceles are slowly expanding, cystic masses that are supposedly caused by obstruction of the ostium of the sinus, which might be secondary to trauma or chronic infection or might be idiopathic. They are more common in the ethmoid and frontal sinuses. Mucoceles have fibrous walls, contain thick mucoid material, and grow slowly. Initially, they expand, and later they erode the walls of the sinuses.

Roentgenographically, the contour of the frontal sinus becomes rounded and the usual scalloped appearance is lost. The ethmoid expands and loses its intercellular septa. Eventually, mucoceles erode through bone. Mucoceles of the frontal and ethmoid sinuses usually expand into the orbit, causing slow inferolateral displacement of the globe. This benign course produces a cosmetic problem but seldom diplopia. Occasionally, a mucocele becomes infected and forms a mucopyocele, with all the symptoms and clinical findings of acute orbital cellulitis (Figure 11.6). The mucocele might then require immediate drainage to relieve the pressure.

Mucoceles are treated by surgical excision. Adequate exposure is necessary, and the wall of the mucocele must be completely removed.

Mucoceles of the sphenoid sinuses (which are rare) expand into the cavernous sinuses, causing vault headache and involvement of the third, fourth, and sixth cranial nerves.

NEOPLASMS OF THE NOSE AND PARANASAL SINUSES

Neoplasms of the nose and paranasal sinuses are neither common nor rare. Most of the true neoplams of the paranasal sinuses are malignant.

Benign Neoplasms

Benign neoplasms are a variety of papillomas, osteomas, and fibromas. Benign neoplasms cause symptoms by obstruction of a nasal passage when they block the outflow of a sinus, resulting in a secondary sinusitis. A benign neoplasm may also cause a cosmetic deformity. Most osteomas occur in the frontal and ethmoid sinuses. The inverted nasal papilloma is a locally invasive, histologically benign lesion that has a small, but definite, tendency to malignant metaplasia.

Malignant Neoplasms*

Squamous cell carcinoma is the most frequent type of malignancy of the paranasal sinuses, and adenocarcinoma is a distant second. Other malignancies, such as malignant melanomas, lymphomas, and esthesioneuroblastomas, do occur but much less frequently. The maxillary and ethmoid sinuses are the usual sites of malignancies in the nasal cavity. Carcinoma of the nose and paranasal sinuses is common in certain geographic area and is more frequent among workers in the nickel and furniture industries. Early lesions are rel-

---

*For more general information on head and neck cancer, including malignant neoplasms of the nose and paranasal sinuses, see Chapter 20.

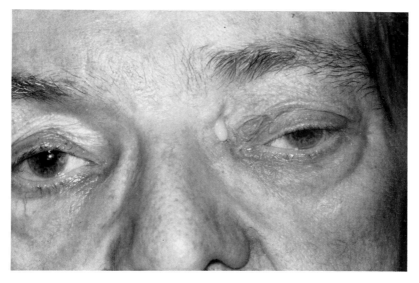

Fig. 11.6. Infected mucocele of the ethmoid sinus that has ruptured spontaneously. A fistula is present above the medial canthus. Note the displacement of the globe downward and outward.

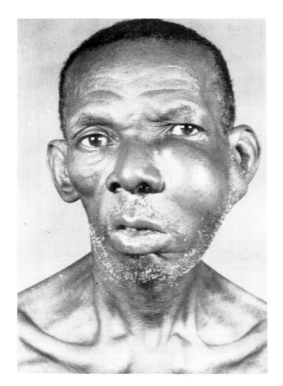

Fig. 11.7. Advanced carcinoma of the left maxilla. The left cheek is substantially swollen, and the left eye is displaced superiorly. The tumor has metastasized to the preauricular lymph node.

atively asymptomatic; therefore, diagnosis is usually late. The patient might complain of one or more of the following symptoms: unilateral, bloodstained rhinorrhea, nasal obstruction, pain and loosening of the teeth, swelling of the cheek, gums, or palate, or displacement of the eye with diplopia (Figure 11.7). Diagnosis is established by biopsy, and the extent of the tumor is determined by careful physical examination and by radiologic study, including computed tomography and radioactive bone scans. The typical roentgenographic picture is opacification of a single sinus, with expansiion and erosion of the bony walls (Figure 11.8). Treatment is with surgery, radiation therapy, or a combination of both modalities.

OTHER NASAL PROBLEMS

Epistaxis

Spontaneous epistaxis (bleeding from the nose) is a common problem, particularly in children up to the age of 7 to 8 years. The incidence falls among teenagers and young adults and then rises again among the elderly. Most cases of epistaxis

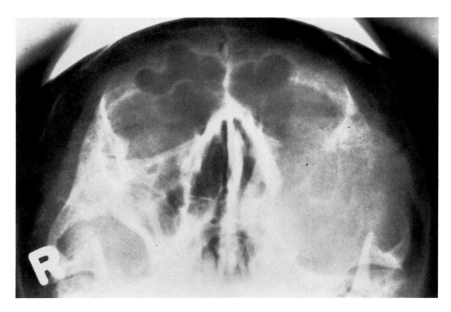

Fig. 11.8. Water's position roentgenogram of a patient with advanced carcinoma of the left maxilla. There is opacification of the maxillary sinus and erosion of the roof and lateral and medial walls.

are self-limiting, with loss of only a few milliliters of blood. In the elderly adult, however, epistaxis is a potentially life-threatening problem. Epistaxis can be the herald of or secondary to systemic disorders such as thrombocytopenic purpura and leukemia.

The most common site of bleeding is Little's area (Kiesselbach's plexus) (see Figure 10.5). Epistaxis is more frequent at night and usually occurs and stops spontaneously. Bleeding is easily controlled by pinching the nose and by inducing reflex vasoconstriction with ice packs on the face. More severe or recurrent bleeding requires cauterization of Keisselbach's plexus or nasal packing.

CAUTERY. First, anesthetize the anterior septum by a pledget of cotton that has been soaked with topical anesthetic (4% xylocaine or 4% cocaine). When the mucosa is anesthetized, carefully cauterize the area with one of the following: a silver nitrate stick, a bead of chromic acid, a 25% solution of trichloracetic acid, a hot-tipped electric cautery, or uni- or bipolar electric

cautery. Be careful to avoid burning too deeply.

In the older patient the bleeding point might be high anteriorly from the anterior ethmoid artery, far posteriorly from the sphenopalatine artery (a terminal branch of the internal maxillary artery). In these cases brisk arterial bleeding is handled by cautery, if possible, or by packing. Packing can be either anterior or posterior.

PACKING OF THE NOSE. Good lighting, a nasal speculum, bayonet forceps, packing material, and a topical anesthetic (4% lidocaine with 0.5% phenylephrine) are necessary for packing the nose (see Figure 11.11).

TECHNIQUE OF ANTERIOR PACKING. If at all possible, first anesthetize the mucosa. Four percent lidocaine and 0.5% phenylephrine, either sprayed or applied with a tampon, usually gives adequate anesthesia and might even provide temporary hemostasis. Packing material can be either ribbon gauze, 0.5 to 1 in. in width (plain or impregnated with iodoform) or gauze impregnated with petroleum jelly (0.5 to 1.0

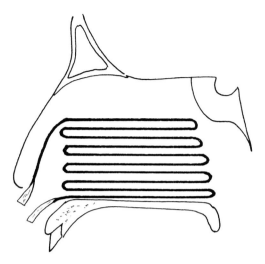

Fig. 11.9. Anterior nasal packing is done under direct vision with good lighting and bayonet forceps. Packing is begun on the floor of the nose and is built upward, each layer being pressed firmly into place.

in. wide strips 36 in. long). Place the packing in layers, beginning on the floor of the nose and building upward layer by layer, pressing each layer firmly downward until the passage is filled (Figure 11.9). Cut off excess material at the level of the anterior nares. For better hemostasis, the packing material can be soaked with a vasoconstrictor (e.g., 2% cocaine or 1% phenylephrine hydrochloride [Neo-synephrine]). When the packing is in place, tape a gauze sponge across the anterior nares.

For brisk posterior epistaxis, anterior packing is insufficient, and a posterior pack might be necessary. A posterior pack is a large mass of material, usually gauze, that fills the posterior choana, against which a more effective hemostatic anterior pack can be placed (Figure 11.10).

TECHNIQUE OF POSTERIOR PACKING. Good light, a nasal speculum, a posterior nasal pack (usually a 4 × 4 gauze sponge tied firmly into a tight roll, with two or three free-hanging 8 in. lengths of string), rubber catheters (10 to 14 French), material for anterior packing, bayonet forceps, and topical anesthesia are necessary for posterior packing of the nose.

If time allows, anesthetize the nose and throat. Pass one end of a catheter through the nasal passage, retrieve it from the oropharynx, and deliver it through the mouth. Tie two of the loose strings of the pack to this catheter (Figure 11.11). Pull the catheter back to deliver the strings through the anterior nares. Put a clamp (hemostat) on the catheter or string. Pull the string and catheter gently, but firmly and swiftly, simultaneously guiding the pack with the index finger of the other hand behind the soft palate into the nasopharynx and into the choana. That is, the pack should not pass into the nasal passage. The nasal string is pulled taut while the anterior pack is placed very firmly and far posteriorly against the posterior pack. The nasal strings are anchored around a gauze or dental roll to prevent slippage, and the third string is brought out through the corner of the mouth and taped to the cheek. Alternatively, one string is passed into each nasal passage and they are tied together around the columella and a protective dental roll.

There are alternative methods of tamponading the nose. A variety of balloons have been designed, and even Foley catheters have been used. In cases of severe epistaxis the packing is usually left in place for 3 to 5 days and is then gently removed. Nasal packing is uncomfortable. Most of these patients are admitted to the hospital, particularly if posterior packing is necessary. They should be given adequate analgesics but must not be heavily sedated. Hypertension, anemia, and other associated problems must be concurrently treated.

If bleeding is not controlled by packing, the offending artery or its main trunk must be ligated. The anterior and posterior ethmoid arteries are ligated as they penetrate the medial wall of the orbit, and the internal maxillary artery in the pterygomaxillary space is ligated by a transantral approach.

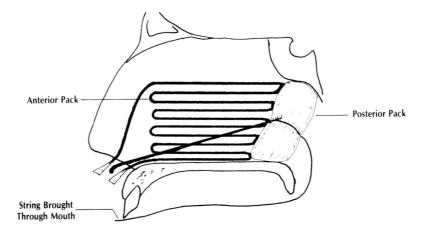

Fig. 11.10.   The principle of a posterior nasal pack. The pack is a bolster for a firmer, more efficient anterior pack.

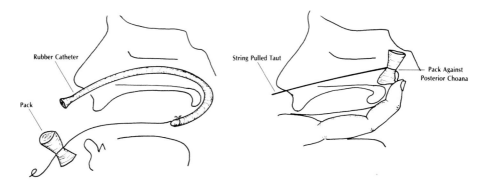

Fig. 11.11.   Placing a posterior pack (see text).

Nasal Obstruction and Stuffiness

Nasal obstructions and stuffiness are common complaints and should be regarded as symptoms and not as diagnoses.

ORGANIC CAUSES. Nasal obstruction can be caused by a problem at the anterior nares, nasal passage, posterior choana, or in the nasopharynx. The following is a list of the organic causes of nasal obstruction:

1. Congenital—choanal atresia, meningoencephaloceles, and hemangioma.
2. Traumatic—deviation of the nasal septum (see the section on this topic later in this chapter), hematoma of the nasal septum, adhesions, cicatricial stenosis, and stenosis of the nasopharynx.
3. Inflammatory—allergic rhinitis with or without polyps, antrochoanal polyp, infective rhinitis (acute viral or bacterial chronic sinusitis).
4. Neoplastic—usually unilateral, benign, or malignant. Neoplasm of the nasopharynx.
5. Pressure from spectacles.
6. Adenoid hypertrophy in children.
7. Foreign body in the nose—usually unilateral.
8. Miscellaneous—collapse of the alar cartilages in the elderly and in cases of facial nerve dysfunction, medication rhinitis, and atrophic rhinitis.

ATROPHIC RHINITIS. This is a most distressing problem. The nasal mucosa becomes thin and atrophic and loses most of

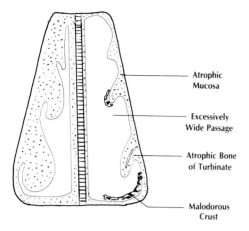

Fig. 11.12. Diagrammatic representation of atrophic rhinitis. The mucosa is thin, and the bones of the turbinates have been partially absorbed. Large, malodorous crusts are present.

its cilia and mucous glands. The tunica propria, bone of the turbinates, and the olfactory epithelium also atrophy. The nasal passages widen considerably and what little mucus is produced dries into foul-smelling crusts, which the patient cannot smell (Figure 11.12). The patient becomes a social outcast. He complains of nasal obstruction, even when the nose is clean, because the flow of air is no longer smooth and lamellar but is interrupted by numerous eddy currents.

The nasal mucosa and underlying turbinates might atrophy secondarily from a variety of factors such as mechanical or chemical trauma, chronic sinusitis, syphilis, rhinoscleroma, and gross deviation of the nasal septum. Most of the patients, however, have idiopathic atrophic rhinitis. In previous generations a particular type of atrophic rhinitis known as "ozena" was common, but better living conditions and nutrition have reduced its incidence in the developed nations. Ozena remains a problem in the underdeveloped countries.

Treatment of atrophic rhinitis is difficult. Etiologic factors must be defined and treated appropriately. Irrigate the nose with saline three or four times daily, and paint the mucosa with glycerine or a light oil containing eucalyptus and menthol. Spraying with estrogens (e.g., Premarin dissolved in peanut oil) is sometimes effective. Numerous surgical procedures have been tried, primarily submucosal implants. A more successful maneuver is to close the nasal passage by suturing together flaps of skin from the vestibule. These flaps are reopened 1 year later.

RHINITIS MEDICAMENTOSA. All topical vasoconstrictors cause rebound vasodilation 3 to 4 hours after application, which might, in turn, result in the recurrence of nasal obstruction (necessitating the reuse of the vasoconstrictor). In this way patients become "addicted" to the use of nasal drops and sprays, In a few weeks the nasal mucosa becomes characteristically pink, velvety, and slightly thickened. Medication rhinitis can persist for many years and is treated by withdrawing all nose drops and sprays. Withdrawal can be extremely difficult for the patient because of rebound nasal obstruction, and oral decongestants or corticosteroids might be needed until the nasal mucosa adjusts.

DEVIATION OF THE NASAL SEPTUM. Deviation of the nasal septum from the midline might be devlopmental or secondary to trauma. The Caucasian nasal septum is comparatively long vertically for the rest of the nose. The septum, therefore, tends to buckle during growth and deviates to one side, forming ridges, spurs, and concavities (Figure 11.13). This deformity causes varying degrees of obstruction.

All components of the septum might be involved. The septal cartilage is buckled, distorted, duplicated, or dislocated to one side of the free edge of the maxillary crest with which it usually articulates. Ridges and spurs form at the junction of the perpendicular plate of the ethmoid and vomer. If the obstructiion warrants, deviation of the nasal septum is corrected by a septoplasty (see Chapter 22). These are surgical procedures designed to correct the skeletal

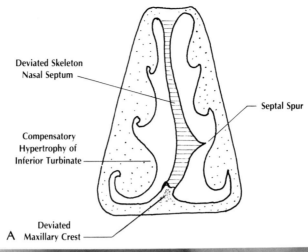

Deviated Skeleton
Nasal Septum

Septal Spur

Compensatory
Hypertrophy of
Inferior Turbinate

Deviated
A   Maxillary Crest

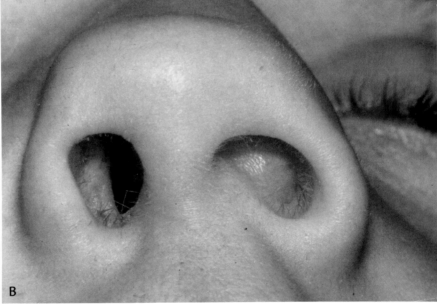

B

Fig. 11.13   *A. Diagrammatic representation of deviation of the nasal septum with a septal spur. The spur is a sharp bony excrescence that is usually formed at one of the articulations of the septum. B. Photograph of gross deviation of the cartilaginous septum.*

malalignment and return the septum to a more median position.

IDIOPATHIC NASAL STUFFINESS. It is not unusual for patients to complain of nasal stuffiness and for a thorough physical examination to be negative. These patients migh have transient "allergic" reactions or they may be fixated on their noses. They are constantly sniffling and hawking. Treatment should be minimal because these patients quickly become addicted to nose drops and sprays.

DISORDERS OF OLFACTION

Disorders of the olfactory system are much more prevalent than is supposed and can be classified as hyposmia, anosmia, cacosmia (malodor), and parosmia.

Hyposmia

Hyposmia is a common complaint and is frequently familial. Many people have an inherent difficulty in either recognizing the presence of or identifying odors.

Anosmia

Anosmia might be a genetic disorder, as in Kallmann's syndrome, which is anosmia and hypogonadism in females. Anosmia is possible after fractures of the anterior cranial fossa and by contrecoup injuries of the occiput. Viral infections of the upper respiratory tract sometimes cause temporary or permanent damage to the olfactory tract. Nasal obstruction secondary to polyps or neoplasms also causes anosmia, which can sometimes be reversed by relieving the obstruction. Atrophic rhinitis is accompanied by anosmia.

A reliable therapy for hyposmia and anosmia has not yet been developed. Zinc sulphate given orally supposedly helps and should be tried.

Cacosmia

Cacosmia is the perception of a real malodor, which is usually caused by chronic sinusitis. Treatment of the cause eliminates the problem.

Parosmia

Parosmia is the sensation of altered olfaction in the absence of an adequate environmental explanation. Parosmia is sometimes caused by lesions, such as neoplasms, along the olfactory tract.

Psychosomatic

Psychosomatic disorders of the olfactory system are common. The more bizarre symptoms are frequently associated with mental disorders.

BIBLIOGRAPHY

Batsakis, J.G.: Tumors of the Head and Neck. Chapter 7. Baltimore, Williams and Wilkins Company, 1974.

Evans, F.O., et al.: Sinusitis of the maxillary antrum. N. Engl. J. Med., 293:735, 1975.

Fairbanks, D.N.F., Vanderveen, T.S., and Bordley, C.: Intracranial complications of sinusitis. In Otolaryngology. Edited by G. English. Hagerstown, Maryland, Harper and Row Publishing, Inc., 1980.

Goodwin, J.W., et al.: The role of high-resolution computerized tomography and standardized ultrasound in the evaluation of orbital cellulitis. Laryngoscope, 92:728–732, 1982.

Gray, L.P.: Deviated nasal septum. Ann. Otol. Rhinol. Laryngol., 87(Suppl. 50):1978.

Montgomery, W.W.: Surgery of the Upper Respiratory System. 2nd Ed.. Vol. 1. Philadelphia, Lea & Febiger, 1979.

Park, R.K.: Olfaction. Otol. Clin. North Am., 6:636, 1973.

Ritter, F.N.: The Paranasal Sinuses. St. Louis, C.V. Mosby C., 1973.

Schramm, V.L., Curtin, H.D., and Kennerdell, J.S.: Evaluation of orbital cellulitis and results of treatment. Laryngoscope, 92:732–738, 1982.

Yarinton, C.T.: Cavernous sinus thrombosis revisited. Proc. Roy. Soc. Med., 70:456–459, 1977.

Chapter 12

MAXILLOFACIAL TRAUMA

MANAGEMENT

Trauma of the soft tissues and bony skeleton of the face is collectively known as maxillofacial trauma. In most medical centers the management of these cases is undertaken by a team that consists of an otolaryngologist, oral surgeon, neurosurgeon, and, sometimes, a plastic surgeon. Trauma to the face is a frequent by-product of automobile accidents, and every physician should be able to assess these injuries and make intelligent plans for their management. Basic guidelines for management have been established that must be adhered to. All patients with moderate to severe facial trauma should be assessed for concomitant injury to the brain and cervical spine. A thorough physical examination and the appropriate roentgenograms are needed to rule out abdominal and thoracic injuries.

History

Before a history is taken, examine the patient to assess the cerebral function and the patency of the airway. Inquire about and note the mechanism of injury, the volume of blood that has been lost, and the level of consciousness immediately after injury. If possible, obtain a history of previous facial injuries and surgery and details of the pertinent past medical history.

Physical Examination

First, check cerebral function, patency of the airway, pulse rate, blood pressure, and rate of respiration. This is most important. Physical examination should be performed promptly before any swelling obscures the landmarks, and all findings, including negative test results, should be recorded. Note carefully any deformity of the forehead, eyelids, globes, nose, cheeks, and lower jaw. Palpate the nasal bones and cartilaginous nose and note areas of tenderness, bony crepitus, or subcutaneous emphysema. Palpate in this order (Figure 12.1): the forehead, supraorbital rims, medial canthal areas, infraorbital rims, cheeks, mandible, and alveolar ridges. Hold the teeth and alveolar ridges between the thumb and index finger and check for mobility. Assess and carefully record the function of all cranial nerves, particularly the reaction of the pupils, visual acuity, and the function of the trigeminal and facial nerves. Check for diplopia. Examine the nasal and oral cavities and check the alignment (occlusion) of the teeth. Perform indirect laryngoscopy. Examine the neck carefully for lacerations, bruises, tenderness, swelling, and subcutaneous emphysema. Record the circumference of the neck. Palpate the larynx, noting

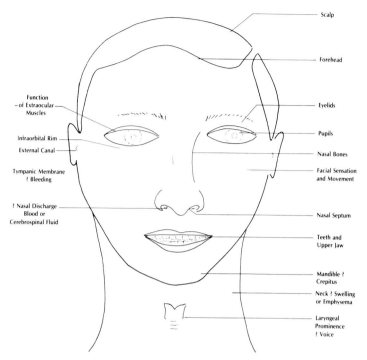

Scalp

Forehead

Eyelids

Function
— of Extraocular—
Muscles

Pupils

Infraorbital Rim

Nasal Bones

External Canal

Facial Sensation
and Movement

Tympanic Membrane
? Bleeding

? Nasal Discharge
Blood or
Cerebrospinal Fluid

Nasal Septum

Teeth and
Upper Jaw

Mandible ?
Crepitus

Neck ? Swelling
or Emphysema

Laryngeal
Prominence
? Voice

Fig. 12.1. Important points in assessment of a patient with facial trauma.

whether the thyroid cartilage is normal or flattened.

Examine the chest and abdomen. Perform a thorough neurologic examination and carefully record all positive and negative clinical findings, particularly of the cranial nerves and especially vision and function of the facial nerve. Cranial neuropathy from edema might develop many hours and even as much as 1 or 2 days after the injury. Early documentation of function is, therefore, extremely valuable as a guide to therapy. For instance, immediate facial paralysis suggests direct trauma to the facial nerve and is an indication for exploration and repair. Late-onset facial paralysis, however, is attributed to edema and is treated expectantly.

Radiographic Examination

Radiographic examination is important in the investigation and management of maxillofacial trauma. Obtain routine roentgenograms of the nasal and facial bones. For the nasal bones, lateral and occlusal positions are best. A Water's position is useful for the maxilla. Oblique positions and the panorex are most helpful for studying the mandible. Tomograms are useful in identifying fracture lines. They are particularly valuable in trauma around the orbit and for assessing blow-out fractures.

Important Points in General Management

Maxillofacial injuries are repaired to restore function and for cosmesis. There are well-defined priorities in the management of these patients, as follows:

1. Establish an airway.
2. Stop all obvious bleeding and establish intravenous lines for control of blood volume.
3. Stabilize the neck. A fracture of the cervical spine must be assumed until proven otherwise.

4. Assess all trauma to the brain. These injuries have first priority.

5. Check for abdominal injuries.

6. Radiologic studies should be obtained only when the patient's general condition is satisfactory and has been stabilized. Do not send the patient to a distant radiologic facility if acute obstruction of the airway or further profuse bleeding is possible.

7. Clean and suture all soft-tissue lacerations.

8. If cerebral or abdominal injuries require surgery, suture facial lacerations at the same time.

9. Manipulate and fix fractures of the facial bones. This can be done up to 10 days later.

FRACTURES OF THE NOSE. Fractures usually cause deviation or depression of the nose (Figure 12.2). Fractures might be simple linear or comminuted, and both the bony and cartilaginous skeletons might be involved. A frontal blow fractures both nasal bones and possibly the bony and cartilaginous septum, causing flattening of the nose. A blow from the side usually fractures both nasal bones, causing deviation of the nose to the opposite side. Displace-

ment is best determined by examining from above, viewing the nose from the forehead. Fractures are frequently, but not always, accompanied by epistaxis. Swelling, obvious deviation or flattening of the nose, tenderness, malalignment of fragments, and, sometimes, crepitus are present. The nasal septum might be deviated, lacerated, or swollen. Roentgenograms confirm but are not essential for the diagnosis (Figure 12.3).

TREATMENT OF NASAL FRACTURES. *Instruments.* Bayonet forceps, wire applicators, cotton, Walsham's forceps, Asche forceps, scalpel handle, Gillies' elevator, and topical anesthetic (4% cocaine solution or 4% lidocaine), 1% lidocaine with 1:100,000 epinephrine for injection, are required to treat a nasal fracture.

Technique. Nasal fractures can be manipulated with local anesthesia. Using Walsham's forceps, the bony fragments are elevated and maneuvered back to their pretrauma positions. Asche forceps are used to manipulate the nasal septum, which is replaced in the midline. Mild de-

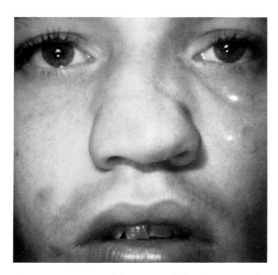

Fig. 12.2. Fracture of the nose with displacement. The bridge of the nose is splayed and deviated to the right.

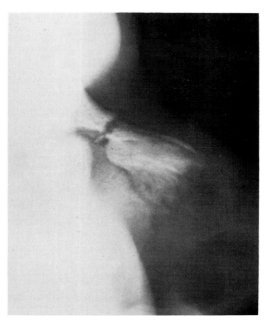

Fig. 12.3. Roentgenogram of the nasal bones with a wide fracture.

viations, if seen acutely, can be handled without anesthesia by pressure applied swiftly with the examiner's thumb. After manipulation, the nose is splinted with an external splint, and, at times, internal packing is required. A simple external splint can be made with plaster of paris cut into a T shape, molded on the forehead and nose, and kept in position with strips of tape. Alternatively, a prefabricated splint made of sponge rubber with metal backing can be used. If the fragments are unstable, it might be necessary to keep them in place with external metal splints anchored with through-and-through stainless steel wires.

Because cosmesis is a most important factor, it is sometimes best to wait a few days until swelling subsides before manipulating nasal fractures to obtain the best cosmetic results.

Compound fractures should be handled immediately. Soft-tissue lacerations must be cleaned and sutured and fractures manipulated and fixed.

SEPTAL HEMATOMA. Injury to the septum might cause a subperichondrial hematoma. One or both sides of the septum swells and obstructs the nasal passage. If the hematoma is not evacuated, the septal cartilage might die and the dorsum of the nose collapse ("saddle nose"). The hematoma must be relieved by a wide incision in the mucosa, and, at the same time, the septal fragments are repositioned and kept in place by intranasal packing for 5 to 6 days.

BLOW-OUT FRACTURES. By definition, a blow-out fracture is exclusively a fracture of one of the walls of the orbit, usually the floor, without involvement of the orbital rims or other facial bones. Blow-out fractures occur if a sudden increase in intraorbital pressure occurs from a blow (such as with a ball or fist), which causes the thinner walls to give way. The danger of a blow-out fracture is the possibility of entrapment of one of the extraocular muscles, usually the inferior rectus, and dis-

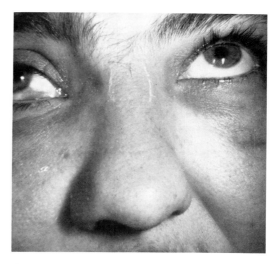

Fig. 12.4. Limitation of upward gaze in a patient with fracture of the floor of the right orbit. The inferior rectus muscle is trapped in the fracture, preventing upward rotation of the globe.

placement of orbital contents into the maxillary sinus, which causes enophthalmos and diplopia. The eyelids swell immediately, and the patient might complain of diplopia; however, visual acuity is not usually impaired. If the nose is blown forcefully, subcutaneous emphysema develops immediately. With a fracture of the floor of the orbit, voluntary movement of the globe on upward gaze might be limited (Figure 12.4). Diagnosis is further enhanced by testing the mobility of the inferior rectus muscle with traction on the tendon after anesthetizing the conjunctiva. Fixation indicates entrapment in a fracture.

Routine roentgenograms of the paranasal sinuses and orbit and tomograms are obtained. These will identify a soft-tissue mass in the roof of the maxillary sinus or in the ethmoid sinus and the position of the displaced fragments of bone (Figure 12.5).

The management of blow-out fractures depends on the severity of the injury. Mild forms, without trapping of muscle, require no treatment. If the inferior or lateral rectus muscles are trapped, the fracture

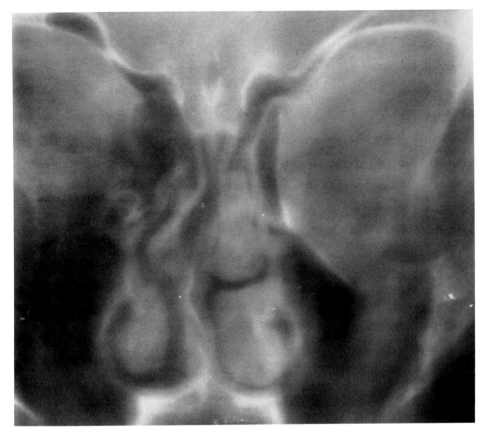

Fig. 12.5. Blow-out fracture of the orbit caused by a blow with a fist. A soft-tissue density is present in the roof of the maxillary sinus and the medial segment of the orbital floor is displaced inferiorly.

should be explored through an appropriate external incision. The floor of the orbit is exposed and soft tissue is reduced and kept in place with a supporting plate of alloplastic material, cartilage, or bone.

FRACTURES OF THE MAXILLARY-ZYGOMATIC COMPLEX. Fractures of the middle third of the face can be either bilateral (i.e., involving both sides across the midline) or unilateral.

BILATERAL FRACTURES. Bilateral fractures were studied by Le Fort (1901), who found that these fractures follow well-defined patterns and offered the following classification (Figure 12.6).*

---
*It should be noted that the pterygoid plates are also always fractured.

Le Fort I (Guérin fracture)
—the fracture separates the entire teeth-bearing areas of the maxilla from the rest of the facial skeleton. The inferior half of the maxilla, hard palate, and the base of the nasal septum become mobile and might be displaced, with secondary malocclusion of the teeth.

Le Fort II (pyramidal fracture)
—the median block of the middle third of the face separates from the rest of the facial skeleton and skull. Fracture lines pass across the roof of the nose into the medial floor of the orbit, the infraorbital foramen, across the zygomaticomaxillary

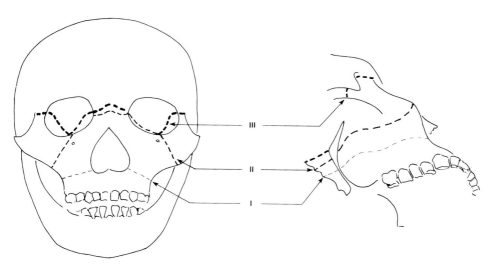

Fig. 12.6. Le Fort lines. These are the lines of bilateral fractures across the midline of facial bones (see text). The nasal septum is also always fractured.

junction, then posteriorly across the middle of the pterygoid plates. Therefore, the whole complex of the nose, both maxillae, and the hard palate become mobile as a single block. Considerable epistaxis results.

Le Fort III (craniofacial disjunction)
—all the facial bones are separated from the skull. Fracture lines pass through the roof of the nose and the ethmoid sinuses into the superior orbital fissure, across the frontozygomatic suture and zygomatic arch, and through the base of the pterygoid process. The facial skeleton is displaced downward and tilts backward so that the face looks longer and more concave. The lower eyelids and cheeks flatten ("dish face"). There is usually massive epistaxis and even cerebrospinal fluid rhinorrhea. Facial swelling develops rapidly and might hide the changes in contour.

In all of these fractures the relationship between maxilla and mandible changes so that the posterior upper molars are too low,

preventing complete closure of the mouth (malocclusion with an open bite).

Treatment. Major displaced fractures of the facial bones are treated by realignment of maxilla to mandible and facial skeleton

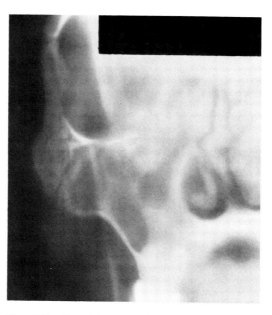

Fig. 12.7. Tripod fracture. There are fractures in the infraorbital rim and maxilla, frontozygomatic suture, and the zygomatic arch. The free segment might rotate around a horizontal or vertical axis.

to the base of the skull. The fragments are held in place by a variety of methods: intermaxillary fixation (anchoring maxilla to mandible), interfragment wiring, fixating fragments to the skull, or attaching fragments to an external apparatus, which is usually worn on the head (halo or skullcap). With careful attention to detail the cosmetic result can be most satisfactory.

UNILATERAL FRACTURES. The most common lateral fracture is the "tripod" fracture of the zygomaticomaxillary complex. This is caused by a lateral blow to the side of the face. There are three fracture lines: one on the zygomatic arch, which is usually depressed, one that starts at the frontozygomatic suture and runs along the lateral wall of the orbit, and one in the floor of the orbit, which passes through the infraorbital canal and the anterior and lateral walls of the maxilla (Figure 12.7). These fractures essentially isolate the zygomatic bone, which is then free to rotate around vertical or horizontal axes. The zygomatic arch is depressed, and the body of the zygoma might be impacted. On palpation,

fractures of the zygomatic arch feel like depressions and those in the infraorbital rim feel like step deformities. The eminence of the cheek is flattened, and the cheek is hyperesthetic if the infraorbital nerve is involved. Both of these conditions become permanent if the fractures remain untreated. In rare cases fractures of the zygomaticomaxillary complex might involve the contents of the superior orbital fissure. Dysfunction of the third, fourth, and sixth cranial nerves occurs, with external ophthalmoplegia, ptosis of the upper eylids, proptosis, a fixed dilated pupil, and pain over the distribution of the ophthalmic division of the trigeminal nerve. Treatment is by manipulation, which usually requires disimpaction and wiring of the fragments to the more stable, adjacent frontal and maxillary bones.

FRACTURES OF THE ZYGOMATIC ARCH (FIGURE 12.8). Isolated fractures of the zygomatic arch can occur from direct blows. There are two or more fracture lines and the central segment is depressed. This causes flattening of the arch, which is cos-

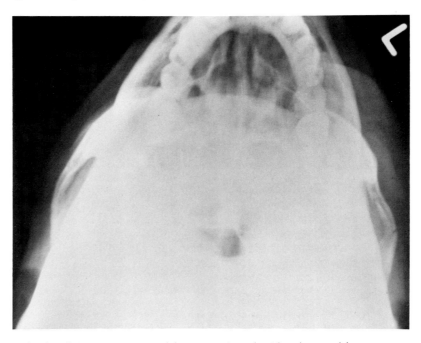

Fig. 12.8. "Bucket handle" roentgenogram of the zygomatic arch with a depressed fracture.

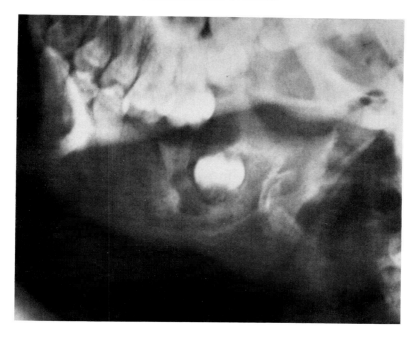

Fig. 12.9. Osteomyelitis of the mandible secondary to an infected tooth. Note the tooth remnant, the lucency around the root of the tooth, and a tract that extends inferiorly. This patient presented with a chronic fistula on the skin of the submandibular area.

metically unacceptable and which might also compromise opening of the mouth because of limitation of motion of the coronoid process. Most fractures of the zygomatic arch can be treated by simple elevation via the Gillies' approach. In this approach an incision is made over the temporalis muscle. The temporalis fascia is incised, and a blunt, flat elevator is passed between fascia and muscle deep to the arch, which is elevated by leverage.

Trauma to the Mandible

TOOTH EXTRACTIONS. Dental caries is the most prevalent "disease" that afflicts mankind. It is ubiquitous and affects all age groups. Extraction of teeth is, therefore, the most frequently inflicted trauma to the jaws. Extraction sockets usually heal swiftly and cleanly. Complications are, however, possible. The most frequent complications of extractions are infection, a dry socket, or development of a reparative granuloma.

POSTEXTRACTION INFECTION. Fortunately, infection occurs infrequently after tooth extraction, but it can be a substantial problem. Infection can be either in the soft tissues or in bone. Soft-tissue infection might spread rapidly into the fascial spaces of the floor of the mouth to produce Ludwig's angina (see Chapter 19). With osteomyelitis of the mandible, the clinical picture evolves more slowly. Postextraction, a doughy swelling, erythema, and tenderness on sustained pressure develop over the mandible. Roentgenograms are not helpful initially because changes in bone may take 10 to 14 days to become identifiable radiologically (Figure 12.9). Culturing material from the tooth socket might yield a specific organism.

Osteomyelitis is treated with large doses of intravenous antibiotics. Clindamycin is currently the agent of choice for osteomyelitis, and intravenous therapy is continued for a minimum of 4 weeks.

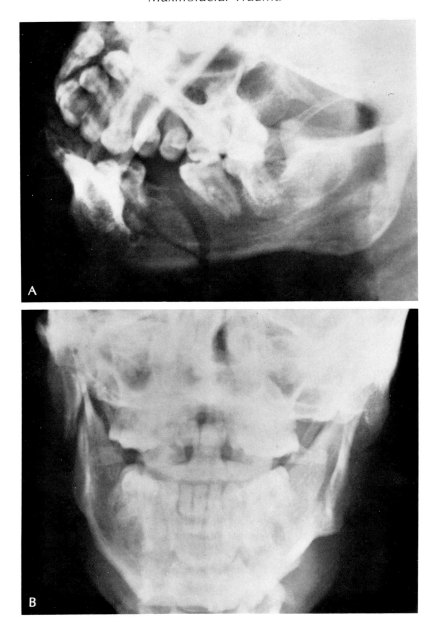

Fig. 12.10. *A.* Comminuted fracture of the body of the mandible. *B.* Fracture of the neck and ramus of the mandible with displacement of fragments.

TRAUMA TO THE TEETH. A blow to the tooth might cause pulpal hemorrhage, fracture, or loosening of the tooth. Hemorrhage into the pulp is not apparent until a few weeks later. The tooth becomes, and remains, discolored (brown, purple, or black) but stays in place. Fractured teeth are common in maxillofacial trauma. Teeth may be fractured horizontally or vertically. Horizontal fractures usually result in a nonviable crown segment, which must be discarded. A vertically split tooth, how-

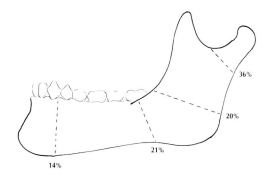

Fig. 12.11. Diagrammatic representation of the more frequent fractures of the mandible.

ever, can sometimes be salvaged by banding and fixation to adjacent teeth.

FRACTURES OF THE MANDIBLE. Fractures of the mandible are caused by direct trauma and are the second commonest facial fractures. Trauma is usually followed immediately by bleeding from the mouth and pain on opening the mouth. Swelling and tenderness of the jaw develop rapidly. Deformity might be obvious, and crepitus can sometimes be elicited. The teeth may be loosened or in malocclusion, and deep tears of the mucosa might occur, which bleed profusely. The diagnosis is confirmed by roentgenograms (Figure 12.10). With fractures of the condyles, the maximum swelling might be in the preauricular areas and can be mistaken for masses in the parotid glands.

Most of the fractures of the mandible occur in one of three areas: base of the neck (36%), the angle (20%), and along the body (21%). The area of the chin accounts for 14% of fractures (Figure 12.11). Midline fractures of the mandible are rare. In addition to a fracture of the mandible, a blow on the point of the chin might fracture and posteriorly displace the posterior wall of the glenoid fossa, which is the anterior wall of the external auditory canal.

Mobile fragments of the mandible are displaced out of alignment by the unbalanced contraction of attached muscles. For instance, central segments are pulled downward and posteriorly by the geniohyoid muscles. The ramus, however, rotates medially from contraction of the masseter and pterygoid muscles.

Fractures of the mandible are treated by reduction, splinting, and fixation. Splinting and fixation are accomplished in a number of ways (Figure 12.12). Briefly, they are as follows:

1. Direct wiring of fragments to each other.
2. Intermaxillary fixation with arch bars, wire loops, or rubber bands.
3. External splints.
4. Internal splints (e.g., Gunning splints).
5. Circumferential wires.

Fixation is continued for a minimum of 6 weeks. Intraoral hygiene is mandatory and is best accomplished by jets of water from a Water Pik or similar device. Diet is restricted to liquids taken through a straw. Antibiotics (e.g., Kefzol and clindamycin)

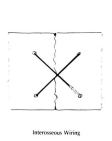

Interosseous Wiring

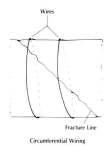

Circumferential Wiring

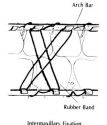

Intermaxillary Fixation

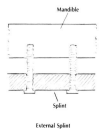

External Splint

Fig. 12.12. Methods of fixation and stabilization of mandibular fractures.

should be prescribed in the appropriate doses with all compound fractures.

Fractures of the condyle of the mandible are usually not amenable to manipulation. Most of these patients, however, retain satisfactory mobility of the jaw and should be encouraged to move the jaw soon after injury. Occasionally, it is necessary to remove the neck and condyle to prevent ankylosis of the temporomandibular joint.

BIBLIOGRAPHY

Bernstein, L., and McClurg, F.L.: Mandibular fractures: A review of 156 consecutive cases. Laryngoscope, 87:957–961, 1977.

Dingman, R.O., and Natvig, P.: Surgery of Facial Fractures. Philadelphia, W.B. Saunders Co., 1964.

Kane, N.P., and Kane, L.A.: Open reduction of nasal fractures. J. Otolaryngol., 7:183–186, 1978.

Knight, J.S., and North, J.F.: The classification of malar fractures. An analysis of displacement as a guide to treatment. Br. J. Plast. Surg., 13:325, 1961.

Levine, P.A., and Goode, R.L.: Treatment of fractures of the edentulous mandible. Arch. Otolaryngol., 108:167–173, 1982.

McCoy, F.J., et al.: An analysis of facial fractures and their complications. Plast. Reconstr. Surg., 29:381, 1962.

Murray, J.A.M., and Moran, A.G.D.: The treatment of nasal injuries by manipulation. J. Laryngol. Otol., 94:1405–1410, 1980.

Rowe, N.L., and Killey, H.C.: Fractures of the Facial Skeleton. 2nd Ed. Edinburgh, E.S. Livingstone, 1968.

Smith, B., and Regan, W.F.: Blow-out fracture of the orbit. Am. J. Ophthalmol., 44:733, 1957.

Chapter 13

THE ORAL CAVITY

ANATOMY AND PHYSIOLOGY

Anatomy of the Oral Cavity

The anatomic limits of the oral cavity are the lips anteriorly and the anterior pillars of the tonsils posteriorly (Figure 13.1). The oral cavity, which is enclosed by walls of soft tissue and bone, contains the tongue, teeth, gums, and openings of the ducts of the salivary glands. The anterior wall is the mucosal surfaces of the lips. The lateral walls are the buccal surfaces of the cheeks. The roof is formed by the hard palate and the teeth-bearing alveolar ridges of the maxilla. The floor is formed by the soft tissue between the tongue and lower alveolus and contains the ducts of the submandibular salivary glands and the lingual and hypoglossal nerves. The floor of the mouth is bounded inferiorly by the mylohyoid muscle (the oral diaphragm). The mandible is the skeletal framework of the floor of the mouth and articulates with the temporal bone in the glenoid fossa. The temporomandibular joint is the only mobile articulation in the head. The oral mucosa, which is lined by thick, stratified squamous epithelium, contains innumerable mucous and minor salivary glands and taste buds. The mucosa might be deeply pigmented in the dark-skinned races. Saliva is also produced by the major salivary glands. The tongue is a muscular organ covered by a thick mucosa that contains filiform and fungiform papillae and taste buds.

For the sake of consistency in reporting, the different parts of the oral cavity have been clearly defined. The following is a list of the more pertinent areas:

1. Vestibule—the space between the teeth and lips.
2. Alveolar ridges—the teeth-bearing areas of the mandible and maxilla.
3. Anterior floor of mouth—the area between the posterior surface of the symphysis menti and the anterior tongue, which contains the papillae of Wharton's ducts.
4. Posterior floor of mouth—the area between the body of the mandible and the lateral root of the tongue.
5. Retromolar trigone—the triangular area of gum and soft tissue immediately posterior to the lower molar teeth.
6. Buccal mucosa—the mucous membrane of the cheeks.
7. Papilla of the parotid duct—found opposite to the second upper molar.
8. Fordyce spots—clinically visible pores of ectopic sebaceous glands on the posterior buccal mucosa.

BLOOD VESSELS AND NERVES. The oral cavity is richly supplied by the pal-

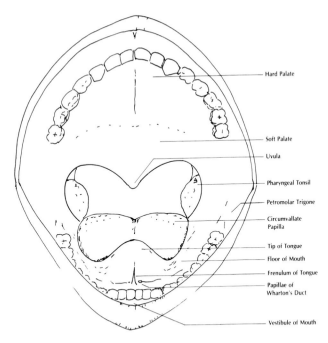

Fig. 13.1. Stylized diagram of the oral cavity showing the important areas to be noted on routine examination.

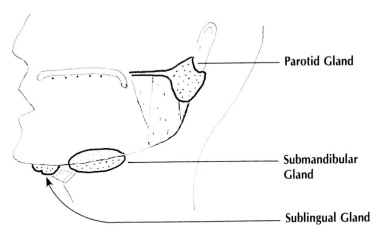

Fig. 13.2. The major salivary glands. The parotid, submandibular, and sublingual glands are shown. The minor glands on the palate are also shown.

atine and lingual arteries and branches of the facial and long sphenopalatine arteries. The nerve supply consists of viscerosensory, somatosensory, visceromotor, and somatomotor nerves. The somatosensory nerves are the lingual nerves to the tongue, the mandibular nerves to the floor of the mouth and buccal mucosa, and the greater and lesser palatine nerves to the palate. The viscerosensory nerve supply to the palate is through the petrosal nerves via the sphenopalatine ganglion and the palatine nerves. The viscerosensory nerve (taste) and the visceromotor nerve to the floor of the mouth, tongue, and submandibular salivary gland is the chorda tympani nerve. The somatomotor nerves are the hypoglossal nerves to the tongue and the mandibular nerve to the muscles of mastication and the mylohyoid muscle. The lymphatic vessels of the oral cavity drain into the upper and midjugular lymph nodes. Some cross-drainage occurs from the midtongue to the contralateral juguloomohyoid nodes.

THE SALIVARY GLANDS. There are three named groups of major salivary glands on each side of the oral cavity: the parotid, submandibular, and sublingual glands (Figure 13.2). In addition, thousands of minor glands are present in the mucosa of the oral cavity, pharynx, and epiglottis.

THE PAROTID GLAND. The parotid gland, the largest salivary gland, is almond-shaped and situated in the infra-auricular area between the ramus of the mandible and the mastoid process. It is incompletely split by the branches of the facial nerve into superficial and deep lobes. The gland is divided into segments, from each of which a duct drains into a larger collecting system. The main duct exits from the anterior border of the gland, runs horizontally just inferior to the arch of the zygoma on the lateral surface of the masseter muscle, then turns medially to enter the oral cavity opposite to the second upper molar tooth. The parotid glands secrete a large volume of watery saliva with minimal enzyme content. Parotid secretion is controlled by Jacobson's branch of the ninth cranial nerve through the tympanic plexus, the otic ganglion, and auriculotemporal nerves.

THE SUBMANDIBULAR GLAND. The submandibular salivary gland is tucked underneath the body of the mandible. The gland becomes more obvious in elderly people. It is a soft, slightly rubbery mass that is covered by a thin fascia. The gland rests on the lateral surface of the mylohyoid muscle but dips deep to the posterior edge of this muscle to lie on the hyoglossus muscle. Here, it is superficial to the hypoglossal and lingual nerves. The submandibular ganglion, in which secretomotor nerves from the chorda tympani synapse, is suspended from the lingual nerve. Section of the chorda tympani nerve stops secretion in the ipsilateral submandibular salivary gland. The main duct (Wharton's duct) leaves the anterior edge of the deeper part of the gland and passes upward and medially toward a papilla on the anterior floor of the mouth. The submandibular glands secrete saliva with a high enzyme content.

Physiology of the Oral Cavity

The oral cavity, jaws, teeth, and salivary glands function synergistically to hold, pulverize, moisten, lubricate, and partially digest food. The tongue initiates the act of swallowing by propelling the bolus of food backward into the oropharynx. If the lips, nasopharynx, and/or larynx remain open, food will escape into these portals rather than pass into the esophagus. These areas, therefore, have sphincteric mechanisms that close during the act of swallowing. The oral cavity is the portal of entry for all the food that we eat and a significant amount of the air that we breathe. Therefore, the mucosa is subject to much trauma and must be both resilient and tough. Consequently, the oral mucosa is covered by a thick squamous epithelium that has an extraordinary capacity for regeneration.

DISORDERS OF THE ORAL CAVITY

Congenital

Clefting of the lip and palate are common congenital anomalies of the face and oral cavity, with an incidence of around 1:1000 live births. Clefting can be either partial or complete (i.e., affecting only a small part of the lip or palate or involving the entire length of the palate) (Figure

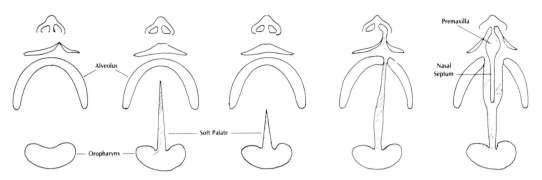

Fig. 13.3. Types of clefting of the lip and palate. These are the more usual defects. Clefting of the lip and palate can occur in any combination.

13.3). A cleft of the palate might also be entirely submucosal. Cleft palate is also a feature of many inherited syndromes of the head and neck.

CLEFT LIP. Clefting of the lip can be either unilateral or bilateral. A cleft occurs at the site of the philtrum (Figure 13.3) and involves the full thickness of the lip. Depression of the ipsilateral nasal ala is associated with a cleft lip. A cleft lip causes some difficulty with feeding and should be repaired early. Many repair techniques are available. Most are designed to restore continuity of the lip, lengthen the vertical height of the lip, restore the vermilion border and the Cupid's bow, and prevent notching. The technique described by Millard (1958) is probably the most widely used.

CLEFT PALATE. Clefting of the palate might involve both the hard and soft palates or only the soft palate and might be unilateral or bilateral around the premaxilla (Figure 13.3). With a bilateral cleft, the premaxilla is usually rotated forward out of alignment with the rest of the jaw.

A cleft palate creates an oronasal fistula because the palate normally forms the floor of the nose. Most children, however, eventually master the technique of swallowing and survive. Few require feeding by gavage.

Cleft palates are repaired within 2 years of birth, usually when the child is between

the age of 1 and 2 years. After repair, the alveolar ridges may collapse medially. This is prevented by fitting the child with arch expanders. The soft palate (velum) is usually shortened and scarred and seldom functions normally, causing significant incompetence of the velopharyngeal sphincter. The speech is usually hypernasal, and many patients require corrective surgical procedures such as pharyngeal flaps. Ninety percent of children with cleft palates have serous otitis media because of malfunctioning of the tensor veli palatini muscles.

SUBMUCOUS CLEFT OF THE PALATE. A submucous cleft is a clefting of only the middle layer aponeurosis of the soft palate. Instead of fusing in the midline, the palatal muscles course anteriorly to insert on the posterior edge of the hard palate. The two layers of mucosa on the oral and nasal surfaces are intact and together form a blue line down the middle of the palate. (Figure 13.4). A diagnostic notch is palpable in the median posterior edge of the hard palate. A submucous cleft of the palate might cause either mild or severe hypernasality. Submucous clefts are contraindications to tonsillectomy and adenoidectomy and should be looked for in all patients before these procedures are performed.

MACROGLOSSIA. The tongue is large in cretinism and Down's syndrome. The tongue might be grossly enlarged from an-

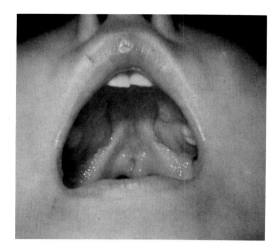

Fig. 13.4. Submucosal clefting of the palate in a 3-year-old patient. The bifid uvula is just visible. The thick lateral bands of the soft palate are the anteriorly directed palatal muscles.

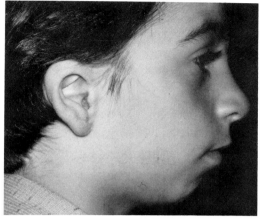

Fig. 13.5. Micrognathia in a 7-year-old boy. The mandible has been small and retrused since birth.

giomatous or lymphangiomatous malformation. In cretinism and hemangiomas the tongue might protrude between the lips at birth.

ANKYLOGLOSSIA ("tongue-tie"—congenital shortening of the lingual frenulum). The tip of the tongue is somewhat blunted and might even be grooved. The restricted mobility of the tongue causes a characteristic tongue-tied speech. If necessary, the frenulum is lengthened by incising horizontally and suturing vertically.

FISSURED TONGUE (scrotal tongue). This is a developmental anomaly in which the tongue is deeply fissured by transverse grooves. Frequently, a family history of the disorder is present. The condition has no clinical or pathologic significance and is usually asymptomatic, except for occasional mild inflammation caused by trapped food particles.

MICROGNATHIA. By definition, micrognathia means a small jaw. Hypoplasia of the mandible might be either unilateral or bilateral. Bilateral hypoplasia causes a micrognathia that is a feature of many syndromes (e.g., Pierre Robin syndrome). The chin is small and retrused, and the lower lip is far posterior to the upper lip (Figure 13.5). The volume of the oral cavity is reduced and is filled by the tongue, which is displaced posteriorly. Breathing and feeding are difficult and might require endotracheal intubation or a tracheostomy. Fortunately, in most cases the mandible grows to a reasonable size so that cosmesis and function become adequate.

Unilateral hypoplasia of the mandible occurs in association with maldevelopment of other derivatives of the first branchial arch apparatus such as deformities of the pinna, external auditory canal, and middle ear (hemifacial microsomia). The lower face is grossly lopsided, and the chin is displaced off the midline. Reconstructive surgery is possible when the child is older.

Trauma of the Soft Tissues of the Oral Cavity

Most traumatic lesions of the oral cavity are secondary to minor factors such as broken teeth, dentures, hard food, and so forth. The lesions are superficial, but painful, ulcers with yellow, fibrinous bases. If the aggravating factors are removed, the pain ceases within 3 or 4 days, and the ulcers heal spontaneously in 7 to 10 days. Application of a protective covering (e.g., Orabase) is helpful.

Penetrating wounds of the oral cavity

are not uncommon and occur in children who fall while holding sticks, pencils, and so on in their mouth. Deep, wide lacerations require suturing, but most of the more superficial wounds will heal spontaneously and do not usually become infected. Lacerations of the tongue bleed profusely, and sutures might be necessary for hemostasis.

Chemical burns of the oral cavity occur as a result of ingestion of concentrated acids or alkalies. The lips, tongue, and palatal arches are the usual sites of injury. Chemical burns are discussed in Chapter 18.

NICOTINE STOMATITIS. Smoking causes irritation of the oral mucosa and a very characteristic stomatitis. The mucosa is hyperemic, looks somewhat velvety, and has punctate pink spots, particularly on the hard and soft palates, which represent the orifices of the ducts of minor salivary glands. Cessation of smoking is the only method of treatment.

Inflammatory Disorders

Most inflammatory disorders of the oral cavity cause ulcerated lesions. Attention

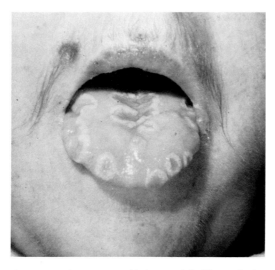

Fig. 13.6. Herpes stomatitis in an adult. The vesicular lesions have ulcerated. Note the lesions on the lips. Herpes stomatitis is common in immunologically suppressed patients.

must be paid to the color of the edge of the ulcer, which is an important differentiating feature. A red halo around the edge is characteristic of aphthous ulcers.

Infectious Diseases

VIRAL INFECTIONS. HERPES. The herpesvirus, particularly herpes simplex I, is the most frequent cause of viral stomatitis. Herpes angina is a highly contagious, sexually transmitted disease. Multiple small (less than 1 mm in diameter), painful ulcers develop, on the mucosa of the lips, alveolar ridges, palate, and even the pharynx and epiglottis (Figure 13.6). Ulceration is preceded by small vesicles without halos. These vesicles may coalesce to form larger lesions, and the regional lymph nodes might be enlarged and tender. A smear might show multinucleated giant cells or swollen, degenerating epithelial cells. The giant cells are diagnostic of viral infection. The herpesvirus can be grown from samples obtained by vigorously swabbing the ulcer.

Herpetic ulcers usually resolve in 7 to 14 days, but tend to be recurrent over the span of many years. Treatment is symptomatic (e.g., pasting the lesions with a bland covering, such as Orabase, is helpful, as is prescribing a soft, semiliquid diet). A recently described topical antiviral agent, Acyclovir, seems able to control and abort the early episodes of herpes labialis. Corticosteroids should not be used either locally or systemically. Herpetic lesions must be differentiated from aphthous ulcers.

APHTHOUS ULCERS. Aphthous ulcers are recurrent, painful lesions, 0.25 to 3.0 cm in diameter, which are usually found on the mobile mucosa of the lips, buccal mucosa, tongue, and soft palate. They are characteristically rimmed by a red halo and may occur singly or in groups, but they are usually present in fewer numbers than herpetic lesions (Figure 13.7). Infrequently, lymphadenopathy is associated

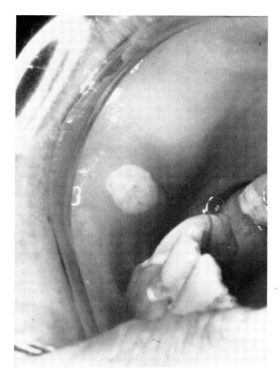

Fig. 13.7. Aphthous stomatitis. The small ulcerated lesions on the buccal mucosa are usually surrounded by a characteristic pink halo. The lesions are recurrent and painful. (Courtesy of C. Doku, D.M.D.)

with aphthous ulcers, but the white cell count is not elevated.

Differentiation between herpetic and aphthous ulcers is not easy and is based on the history, clinical examination, and microscopic examination of smears.

Like herpetic lesions, most aphthous ulcers resolve spontaneously in 7 to 14 days. Unfortunately, there is no definitive treatment for aphthous ulcers. Many different topical applications are recommended for the relief of pain, and each preparation has its staunch advocates. Silver nitrate, tannic acid, crystalline tetracycline, triamcinolone acetonide (Kenalog) are some of the remedies that are used. All might be helpful.

THE EXANTHEMA. Measles (morbilli) is characterized by a papular rash and the presence of Koplik's spots. Koplik's spots are tiny, grayish to white spots on a red base on the buccal mucosa opposite to the lower molars and sometimes also on the anterior buccal mucosa. They are the first truly diagnostic findings in measles. The skin rash appears 2 to 3 days later when Koplik's spots begin to fade. Treatment of measles is primarily supportive. Children should be vaccinated against measles early in life.

BACTERIAL INFECTION. ACUTE NECROTIZING GINGIVITIS (VINCENT'S ANGINA, TRENCH MOUTH). This is a highly contagious, rapidly progressive, acute, and painful gingivitis that occurs in young adults. The disorder is characterized by fever, fetid breath, bleeding ulcerated gums, and necrosis of the interdental papillae. The ulcers are covered by a dirty-gray, adherent pseudomembrane. A marked regional lymphadenopathy is present. The lesions are supposedly caused by synergism between a fusiform anaerobic bacterium and a spirochete (Borrelia vincentii). Treatment is by intensive local irrigations with warm saline solution and hydrogen peroxide and large doses of penicillin, 2 million units daily, preferably given systemically. Differential diagnosis includes secondary syphilis, sickle cell anemia, and candidiasis.

FUNGAL INFECTIONS. CANDIDIASIS. Candida albicans is the organism that is most frequently involved in fungal infections of the mouth. Candidiasis is fairly common in infants but usually affects only the immunologically compromised adult (e.g., diabetics and patients on chemotherapy). Candidiasis also occurs secondary to antibiotic therapy.

The patient complains of soreness of the mouth. Lily-white patches of fluffy, adherent pseudomembrane are found on the palate, buccal mucosa, and pharynx (Figure 13.8). Removal of the membrane leaves a raw, bleeding surface. Diagnosis is supported by the history and confirmed by identifying fungal hyphae on a smear stained with periodic acid-Schiff (PAS) and by culturing.

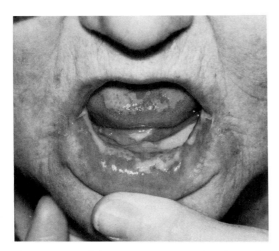

Fig. 13.8. Candidiasis in a woman undergoing radiation therapy. Candidiasis is a frequent occurrence in immunocompromised patients.

Early, mild lesions respond to gargling with nystatin suspension or painting with gentian violet. Severe, extensive infections require intravenous amphotericin B. Antibiotics must be avoided.

LICHEN PLANUS. Lichen planus is char-acterized by a delicate, white, lacelike pattern on the buccal mucosa (Figure 13.9). There are, however, three forms of lichen planus: reticular, ulcerative, and bullous. The reticular lesions, which may be asymptomatic or cause mild burning, are more common on the mucosa of the cheeks, gums, and undersurfaces of the tongue. Ulcerative and bullous lichen planus presents as a chronic, painful ulceration of the buccal mucosa, gingiva, tongue, palates, or lips, in that order. The ulcer is superficial, sometimes hemorrhagic, and is occasionally surrounded by the reticular pattern of the disease. Clinical diagnosis might be difficult, and biopsy is frequently necessary for confirmation. The lesions must be differentiated from pemphigus by a Tzanck smear and determination of antinuclear antibody levels, both of which are positive in pemphigus, from lupus erythematosus (L.E.) by an L.E. preparation of a blood smear, and from carcinoma by biopsy. Treatment is symptomatic, with topical anesthetic lozenges and topical corticosteroids such

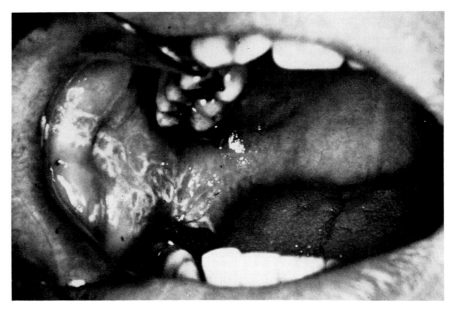

Fig. 13.9. Lichen planus. A white, lacelike pattern is present on the buccal mucosa. Lichen planus is usually asymptomatic but might become ulcerated and symptomatic. (Courtesy of C. Doku, D.M.D.)

as betamethasone or triamcinolone. Severe symptoms are controlled by injecting a mixture of 2 ml of 1% lidocaine and 1.2 mg of betamethasone into the base of the ulcer.

SYPHILIS. Syphilis can cause painful lesions in the mouth in all three of its stages: primary, secondary, and tertiary.

PRIMARY SYPHILIS (CHANCRE). A chancre is the characteristic ulcerative lesion of primary syphilis and develops at the site of initial infection. A crateriform ulcer develops, with a clean, shiny center that is surrounded by a firm induration. Regional lymph nodes are enlarged, hard, and shotlike. Chancres may persist for 2 weeks to 2 months and, as such, might be mistaken for a carcinoma. Therefore, any suspicious lesions, particularly among members of the younger age groups, must never be palpated with an ungloved finger, and scrapings should be examined by dark-field illumination before biopsy. In the oral cavity, however, dark-field examination requires much experience for correct interpretation. Serologic tests for syphilis might be negative or only weakly positive at this stage and should be repeated in 4 weeks.

SECONDARY SYPHILIS. The classic oral signs of secondary syphilis are painful, serpiginous, superficial ulcerations on the buccal mucosa, palate, and pharynx. Fever, lymphadenopathy, and a papular rash are associated with this stage.

TERTIARY SYPHILIS. The classic lesion of tertiary syphilis is the gumma, which is rarely seen today. A gumma is a localized area of necrosis that might involve the tongue, hard palate, pharynx, or epiglottis. A substantial loss of tissue occurs, which is followed by dense scarring.

Syphilitic Tongue. In the advanced stages of syphilis the tongue develops deep, longitudinal furrows that are irritated by trapped food particles. The patient complains of soreness of the tongue. The incidence of carcinoma of the tongue is increased in these patients.

Syphilis is treated with massive doses of penicillin, given either intravenously or intramuscularly. The standard dose is 2.5 million units as a single dose for primary lesions, 2.5 million units every 7 days for three doses for secondary and tertiary lesions, and 500,000 units per kilogram of body weight for congenital lesions.

The Oral Cavity in Systemic Diseases

Ulcerations of the oral cavity are frequently an expression of or part of a systemic disease such as pemphigus, erythema multiforme, and agranulocytosis. Both soft tissue and bone might be affected. The most common expression of systemic disease in the oral cavity is ulceration. Other forms of expression are ecchymosis (as in leukemia and thrombocytopenia purpura), pigmentation, as in the Peutz-Jeghers syndrome (freckle-like pigmentation and colonic polyps), and mucosal atrophy of the cheeks and tongue (e.g., in pernicious anemia).

PEMPHIGUS. Pemphigus is a rare, probably autoimmune disease of the middle-aged and elderly. Multiple, painful, shallow ulcers develop on different parts of the skin, lips, oral cavity, and gastrointes-

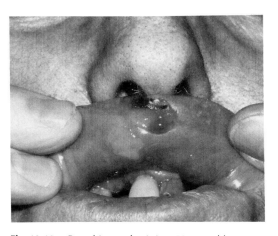

Fig. 13.10. Pemphigus vulgaris in a 70-year-old woman. The large, superficial ulcer on the lip was initially vesiculated. Lesions on the skin of the upper chest were also present.

tinal tract. Lesions begin as bullae that rupture and leave ulcers (Figure 13.10). Pemphigus is a debilitating disease of the elderly, and the gastrointestinal lesions might cause fatal hemorrhage. Lesions are controlled by moderate to high doses of corticosteroids.

ERYTHEMA MULTIFORME. In this condition extensive, painful, superficial ulcerations are present, which are confined to the anterior oral cavity. First there are large bullae, which quickly ulcerate. The lesions are virtually indistinguishable from those of pemphigus. Biopsy and immunofluorescent studies will distinguish erythema multiforme from herpetic infections, allergic stomatitis, and other ulcerative lesions. Erythema multiforme is self-limiting but can be treated with topical corticosteroids.

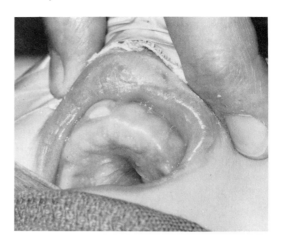

Fig. 13.12. Gingival hyperplasia in a 5-year-old patient on phenytoin since birth. Only one tooth is partially visible. The other teeth are present but are covered by the hypertrophied gum.

MIDLINE LETHAL GRANULOMAS. This condition begins as a deep ulceration of the midline structures of the oral cavity and/or face, which spreads rapidly. Histologic diagnosis might be exceedingly difficult, but midline lethal granuloma is now considered to be a virulent form of malignant lymphoma. Unchecked, the lesions erode the full thickness of the bony and soft palates and destroy the median structures of the face. Radiation therapy and, sometimes, chemotherapy is the treatment of choice. Corticosteroids and antibiotics might give temporary remission but are not curative.

Wegener's granulomatosis and periarteritis nodosa are other disorders of the autoimmune system that may cause persistent ulceration of the oral cavity.

Idiopathic Disorders

MEDIAN RHOMBOID GLOSSITIS. Median rhomboid glossitis is characterized by a rhomboid-shaped, dark pink, smooth, and usually depressed area devoid of papillae that is just anterior to or around the foramen cecum of the tongue. The condition is usually asymptomatic, and no treatment is required. Median romboid glossitis is now considered to be a developmental anomaly.

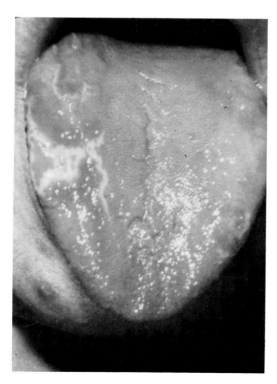

Fig. 13.11. Geographic tongue. The lesions are areas of denudation of the papillae of the tongue. The condition is asymptomatic.

GEOGRAPHIC TONGUE. The geographic tongue might or might not be mildly symptomatic. The disorder is characterized by the presence of constantly changing and migrating serpiginous areas of lingual epithelium that are smooth and shiny because of a lack of papillae. These areas are surrounded by a distinct white or cream-colored border that is caused by localized thickening of the epithelium (Figure 13.11). The shape of the involved area is constantly changing—advancing and receding. The cause of geographic tongue is unknown, and the condition requires no treatment.

RANULA ("frog-like"). A ranula is a thin-walled, translucent cyst in the floor of the mouth. Ranulas are supposed to be retention cysts of blocked minor salivary glands and may develop in childhood or early adulthood. A ranula can be extremely large, pushing the tongue upward, or it might invade deeply into the submental tissues. They are treated by excision or marsupialization.

GINGIVAL HYPERPLASIA. Patients who are medicated with phenytoin (Dilantin) may develop diffuse hyperplasia of the gingiva. The gums become grossly thickened and grow over, and perhaps completely cover, the teeth (Figure 13.12). The condition is asymptomatic and usually regresses when the medication is withdrawn. Gingival hyperplasia can be minimized by maintaining good oral hygiene.

BIBLIOGRAPHY

Chang, T.W.: Herpetic angina following orogenital exposure. J. Am. Vener. Dis. Assoc., 1:163–164, 1975.

Goldhalber, P.S., and Gliddon, D.P.: Present concepts concerning the etiology and treatment of acute necrotizing ulcerative gingivitis. Int. Dent., 14:468–496, 1964.

Gorlin, R.J., Pindborg, J.J., and Cohen, M.M.: Syndromes of the Head and Neck. 2nd Ed. New York, McGraw-Hill, 1976.

Gorlin, R.J., and Goldman, H.M. (eds.): Thomas's Oral Pathology. 6th Ed. St. Louis, C.V. Mosby Co., 1970.

Grabb, W.C., Rosenstein, S.W., and Bzoch, K.R. (eds.): Cleft Lip and Palate. Boston, Little, Brown, and Co., 1971.

McCarthy, F.P., and McCarthy, P.L.: Oral medicine. N. Engl. J. Med., 252:1079, 1955.

Michaels, L., and Gregory, M.M.: The pathology of non-healing midline granuloma. J. Clin. Pathol., 30:317–327, 1977.

Millard, R.D.: Columella lengthening by the forked flap. Plast. Reconstr. Surg., 22:454–457, 1958.

Mine, M.K.: Diseases of the tongue. Oral Surg., 9:619, 1956.

Shklar, G., and McCarthy, P.L.: Oral Manifestations of Systemic Diseases. Woburn, Massachusetts, Butterworth Publications, Inc., 1976.

Smith, R.J.H., Sessions, R.B., and Bean, S.F.: Benign mucous membrane pemphigoid. Ann. Otol. Rhinol. Laryngol., 91:142–144, 1982.

Chapter 14

NEOPLASMS OF THE ORAL CAVITY

NEOPLASMS OF THE SOFT TISSUES OF THE ORAL CAVITY

Benign Neoplasms

FIBROMAS. Fibromas are smooth, rounded, or papilliferous, painless masses of fibrous tissue that develop in the denture-bearing areas after prolonged use of dentures (Figure 14.1). They represent hyperplasia of the subepithelial stroma. Early lesions might subside with adjustment of the denture, but mature lesions require excision as well as adjustment of the dentures.

Isolated fibromas are sometimes found elsewhere in the oral cavity, particularly along the bite line of the buccal mucosa.

EPULIS. An epulis is any excrescence from the gum, which is more frequently a fibromatous mass secondary to chronic local trauma.

GIANT CELL GRANULOMA. This is a soft, painless, pink, brown, or bluish mass on the gum that is probably a reaction to trauma. Often, a localized, smooth, excavation of the adjacent cortical bone occurs. Histologically, numerous giant cells are present in an areolar stroma. The lesions tend to recur after removal. Hyperparathyroidism might cause similar tumors (e.g., brown tumors), and, therefore, the levels of serum alkaline phosphatase, parathy-roid hormones, and serum calcium should always be assayed.

PAPILLOMA. Papillomas are usually small, soft, pedunculated, irregular, cauliflower-like mucosal masses (Figure 14.2). The surface might be either white, from the buildup of keratin, or pink. Papillomas are asymptomatic and are found at any age, even at birth. The usual sites of occurrence are the free edge of the soft palate, the tongue, and lips. Histologically, finger-like cores of fibrous tissue are covered by thick squamous epithelium.

Diagnosis is made easily on clinical examination. If papillomas are clustered together, they must be differentiated from verrucous carcinoma or verruca vulgaris by biopsy. They are easily removed surgically. Neonatal and juvenile papillomas are more frequent in the children of women with condyloma acuminata.

PIGMENTED NEVUS. Pigmented nevi are flat, blue, asymptomatic nodules on the oral mucosa. Excision is indicated only if they cause symptoms.

AMALGAM TATTOO. An amalgam tattoo is a deep blue, patchy discoloration of the oral mucosa caused by amalgam, which is the substance usually used for dental fillings. They are common in the lower gums and buccal mucosa. Amalgam tat-

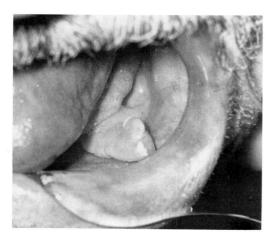

Fig. 14.1. A large denture fibroma on the left lower jaw. These excrescences are found under ill-fitting dentures and are usually asymptomatic.

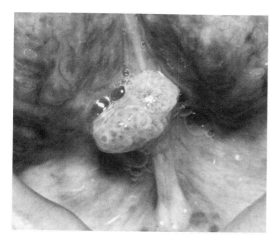

Fig. 14.2. Pedunculated squamous papilloma on the frenulum of the tongue.

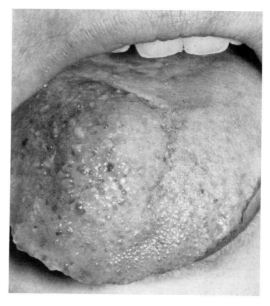

Fig. 14.3. Lymphangioma of the tongue in a 12-year-old girl. The tongue has almost been replaced by a mass of dilated lymph channels.

toos are not tumors but may be mistaken for melanomas. No treatment is necessary.

LYMPHANGIOMAS AND HEMANGIOMAS. Lymphangiomas and hemangiomas of the tongue and buccal mucosa might be congenital or might present later in life. Lymphangiomas present as firm, almost vesiculated, irregular swellings of the tongue or buccal mucosa; they are usually painless but might be painful if infected (Figure 14.3). A hemangioma presents as a mass of dilated, compressible blood vessels that blanches with pressure but refills rapidly with the release of pressure. Histologically, lymphangiomas and hemangiomas are frequently combined, and most lymphangiomas occurring in this area are really lymphangiohemangiomas. In the tongue they may grow to an enormous size and should be excised if they cause obstruction. Complete excision, however, can be most difficult because of the lack of clear demarcation between lymphangiomatous and normal tissue. Hemangiomas of the tongue are treated by wedge resection, with preservation of enough lingual tissue for reconstruction.

Malignant Neoplasms*

Ninety percent of the malignant neoplasms of the oral cavity are squamous cell carcinomas, and 90% of patients with squamous cell carcinomas are heavy consumers of alcohol and tobacco (in the form of cigarettes). Other causative factors are

---

*For more general information on cancer of the head and neck, including malignant neoplasms of the oral cavity, see Chapter 20.

a fissured tongue (e.g., from syphilis) and ill-fitting dentures. A particularly high incidence of cancer of the oral cavity occurs in western India and parts of Africa where the betel nut is chewed as a stimulant. A number of the malignant neoplasms of the oral cavity originate in the salivary glands, and these will be discussed in Chapter 15.

Squamous cell carcinoma occurs in every part of the oral cavity in the following order of frequency: lips, anterior floor of the mouth, mobile tongue, retromolar trigone, posterior floor of the mouth, alveolar ridges, palate, and base of the tongue. Carcinoma of the oral cavity might be surrounded by an area of leukoplakia or erythroplasia, both of which are premalignant lesions and must be considered in planning treatment. These neoplasms usually begin as firm, raised areas or as ulcerations. Eventually, all of these areas ulcerate (Figure 14.4). Ulcers are typically deep, with firm, rolled edges that are surrounded by a zone of induration. The tumors, however, might be exophytic or infiltrative beneath an intact mucosa. Some lesions are superficial, staying on the surface, and involve comparatively wide areas, while others are smaller but infil-

trate deeply. Lesions of the anterior floor of the mouth, anterior tongue, and base of the tongue metastasize comparatively early. Metastasis is first to the jugular chain of lymph nodes and later to more distant structures (Figure 14.5).

Malignancies of the oral cavity are seldom diagnosed in their early stages because they are asymptomatic, causing pain and paralysis only after achieving a substantial size. Patients may complain of pain, difficulty with dentures, bleeding, loosening of the teeth, or might seek medical assistance because of an expanding jugular lymph node, the primary lesion being asymptomatic. All lesions of the oral cavity may cause referred otalgia; that is, the patient complains of pain in his ear, which is clinically normal because the source of the pain is in his mouth. This is because the sensory innervation of both areas is by the same nerve (the fifth cranial nerve) (Figure 14.6).

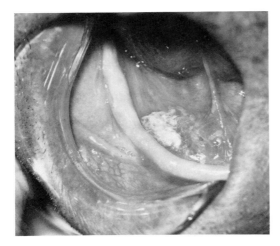

Fig. 14.4. Squamous cell carcinoma of the anterior floor of the mouth. A raised, ulcerated lesion is present between the tongue and alveolus.

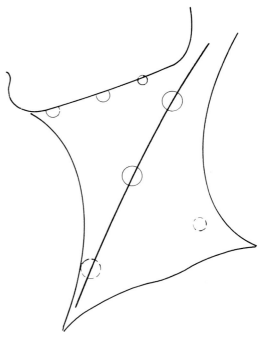

Fig. 14.5. Common sites of nodal metastases from lesions of the oral cavity. Small submandibular nodes are difficult to palpate.

Cancer of the mouth is a potentially multifocal problem, and a thorough search must be made for a second primary in the oral cavity, pharynx, and larynx. There is a 6 to 10% incidence of a secondary primary malignancy developing in the esophagus.

PREMALIGNANT LESIONS. LEUKOPLAKIA AND ERYTHROPLASIA. The word leukoplakia refers to a white plaque, and erythroplasia refers to a red patch on a mucosal surface. Both are descriptive terms and are not diagnostic. Leukoplakia might be caused by epithelial dysplasia, lichen planus, or candidiasis. Leukoplakia from epithelial dysplasia occurs on any part of the oral mucosa and represents a thickening of the keratin layer of the epithelium (Figure 14.7). This form of leukoplakia must be considered to be premalignant and should be extensively biopsied. Intravital staining with 1% toluidine blue helps to identify suspicious areas. Dysplastic leukoplakia should be excised, but extensive raw areas may need skin grafts.

Erythroplasia might also represent a superficial malignant change in the surface epithelium. Erythroplasia is frequently found around established infiltrative malignancies.

SPECIFIC SITES OF MALIGNANCIES IN THE MOUTH. ANTERIOR FLOOR OF THE MOUTH. The patient complains of a painful ulceration under the anterior tongue. Usually, one or both ducts of the submandibular salivary glands are involved, and secondary swelling of the salivary gland might occur from ductal obstruction. The tumor might spread to the anterior mandible. Therefore, the mandible should always be studied radiologically.

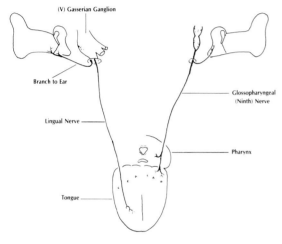

Fig. 14.6. Anatomy of referred otalgia. The ear is innervated by four sensory nerves, with the major contribution from the fifth and ninth cranial nerves.

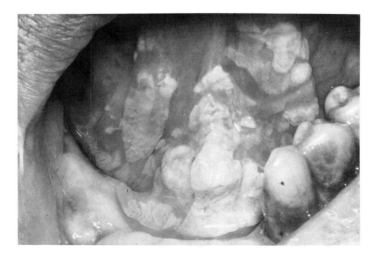

Fig. 14.7. Extensive leukoplakia in a heavy smoker. Patches have the appearance of "white paint."

POSTERIOR FLOOR OF THE MOUTH. This is a hidden area that is frequently missed on routine examination. The primary complaint is pain because these lesions are never small when the patient presents. The tumors spread in all directions to involve the adjacent gum, undersurface of the tongue, and infiltrate into the underlying submandibular salivary gland.

Lesions of the anterior and posterior floor of the mouth are treated according to their stage. Early lesions are treated with primary surgery, while moderate-sized and larger lesions are treated with radiation therapy or a composite resection (commando-type) of the tumor and adjacent mandible in continuity with a radical neck dissection (see Chapter 22).

PALATE (ROOF OF THE MOUTH). Squamous cell carcinoma of the hard palate is uncommon. Most of the malignancies of the hard palate are from the minor salivary glands. The soft palate, however, is a more common site of carcinoma and should be considered along with the tonsils and tonsillar pillars as a single unit. The lesions are frequently preceded by patches of erythroplasia.

A submucosal mass that displaces the soft palate and tonsil anteriorly and me-dially is likely to be a neoplasm from the deep lobe of the parotid gland.

MOBILE TONGUE. Most of these lesions begin on the lateral border or tip of the tongue (Figure 14.8). They account for over 60% of all cancers of the tongue and infiltrate deeply, causing fixation of the tongue. Careful bidigital palpation is necessary to assess whether the tumor approaches or crosses the midline.

Treatment is by surgery or radiation therapy or a combination of the two. Smaller lesions should be excised with a comfortable (1.0 to 1.5 cm) margin of normal tissue. Larger lesions require a hemiglossectomy, hemimandibulectomy, and radical neck dissection. Total glossectomy is sometimes necessary.

BASE OF THE TONGUE. Malignancy of the base of the tongue is seldom seen as an early lesion. These tumors metastasize early and have a poor prognosis. The patient's primary complaint might be constant pain in the throat, otalgia, odynophagia, dysphagia, or aspiration, or he may present because of metastatic cervical lymphadenopathy. Mirror examination of the base of the tongue and larynx and digital palpation are mandatory. Palpation may be the only way of detecting a sub-

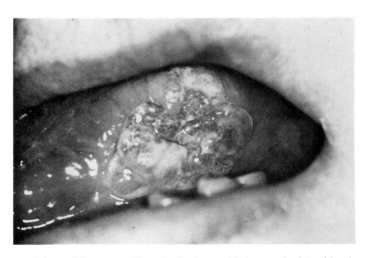

Fig. 14.8. Carcinoma of the mobile tongue. The raised, ulcerated lesion on the lateral border of the tongue was most painful.

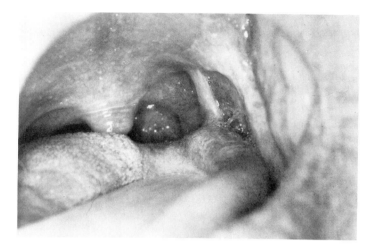

Fig. 14.9. Carcinoma of the retromolar trigone presenting as a deep infiltrating ulcer with rolled edges.

mucosal lesion. Lesions are better assessed with direct laryngoscopy or by radiologic study, and computed tomography is particularly helpful. These lesions tend to infiltrate the substance of the tongue, spreading into the root of the tongue toward the hyoid bone and epiglottis.

Carcinoma of the base of the tongue is treated by radiation therapy; surgery is seldom feasible.

GUMS AND RETROMOLAR TRIGONE (Figure 14.9). Carcinoma of the gums is more common in patients with poor dental hygiene and those with ill-fitting dentures. Patients complain of painful ulcerations and loose teeth, which are sometimes mistaken for chronic dental abscesses. These tumors infiltrate down to and through the periosteum to involve the mandible. Lesions on the retromolar trigone extend posteriorly to the medial pterygoid and masseter muscles and may cause trismus. Carcinoma of the gums and retromolar trigone are best treated by radiation therapy (to 5000 rads) followed by a wide excision that includes part of the mandible and a radical neck dissection in continuity (composite resection, commando). With vigorous therapy, there is a 50% five-year survival rate.

BUCCAL MUCOSA. Carcinoma of the buccal mucosa is common in western India because of the habit of chewing the betel nut. A high incidence of carcinoma of the buccal mucosa also occurs in parts of East Africa, where tobacco is chewed. Patients present with a substantial, painful ulcer that bleeds easily and which is surrounded by a zone of leukoplakia or erythroplasia (Figure 14.10). Tumors infiltrate into the buccal fat pad and buccinator muscle.

Radiation therapy of malignancies of the

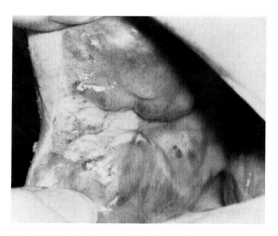

Fig. 14.10. Carcinoma of the buccal mucosa in a 55-year-old man who was a heavy smoker and drinker.

oral cavity and tongue is delivered by external radiation using a cobalt or electron beam or by a combination of external radiation and implant techniques, with radium or iridium needles or radon seeds. The node-bearing areas of the neck are included in the portals.

MELANOMA. Melanomas do occur in the oral cavity but are rare. They present as rapidly expanding, pigmented lesions on the buccal mucosa, palate, or lip. Treatment is by wide surgical excision with a neck dissection and chemotherapy. The prognosis is poor. Malignant tumors of the salivary glands will be discussed in Chapter 15.

NEOPLASMS OF THE BONY JAWS

Tumors of the bony jaws may be derived from the bone of the mandible, maxilla, or, more commonly, from tooth-forming tissues (odontomas). Only the more common neoplasms will be discussed in this Chapter.

Benign Neoplasms

FIBROUS DYSPLASIA. Fibrous dysplasia is a disorder of tissue regulation and is really similar to a hamartoma. In fibrous dysplasia all the tissue components of bone are present but their ratio is altered. Usually, a preponderance of fibrous tissues exists, with varying amounts of bone. Fibrous dysplasia might be monostotic or polyostotic. Most of the monostotic forms occur in the facial bones. Their rates of growth vary considerably, but, with time, a large number become sclerotic. About 15% of the lesions become malignant.

Patients present early in life with progressive, smooth, painless, diffuse, hard swelling of one side of the face, usually involving the maxilla or mandible. The forehead and zygoma are less affected. Roentgenograms might show a typical "ground glass" appearance of the bone, or, alternatively, an erosive process can be simulated. Histologically, wide areas of fibrous tissue with spicules of bone are present.

Treatment is by sculpturing the bone back to normal, cosmetically acceptable, contours. Recurrences are common. Malignant metaplasia is indicated by rapid increase in the rate of growth. A biopsy must be performed and consideration given to wide excision. Radiation therapy of the benign form predisposes to malignant change.

TORUS PALATINUS. A torus palatinus is a hard, bony excrescence in the midline of the posterior hard palate, usually found in adults. The surface is grooved into four rounded quadrants (Figure 14.11). A torus palatinus may grow to substantial size and be a problem with the fitting of dentures, in which case consideration can be given to removal. It may also become infected secondary to erosion of the overlying mucosa. The sequestrum and the remainder of the torus must then be removed surgically.

OSTEOMA (Torus Mandibularis). Osteomas of the mandible are common. They are usually multiple, asymptomatic, hard, round, smooth, white excrescences on the lingual surface close to the midline (Figure 14.12). They may cause problems with dentures but seldom require removal.

CYSTS OF THE JAWS. Cysts of the jaws might be either single or multiple. A simple classification of cysts of the jaws is listed below, but one should remember that cysts of the jaws (particularly of the mandible) are pathologically complex entities. Multiple cysts of the jaws may be associated with multiple cutaneous "nevoid" basal cell carcinomas and skeletal anomalies. The classification is as follows:

1. Odontogenic—radicular
                 —dentigerous
                 —odontoma
2. Solitary bone cysts
3. Neoplastic—ameloblastoma

RADICULAR CYSTS. A radicular cyst is the most common cystic lesion of the jaws.

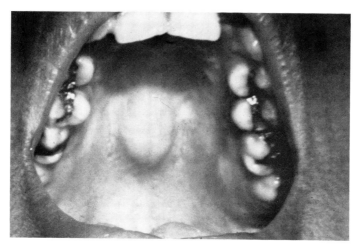

Fig. 14.11. Torus palatinus. This is a smooth, bony excrescence in the midline of the posterior hard palate. (Courtesy of C. Doku, D.M.D.)

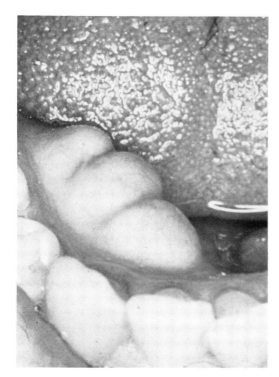

Fig. 14.12. Exostoses of the mandible. These are asymptomatic, round, smooth, white masses of bone on the lingual surface of the mandible. (Courtesy of C. Doku, D.M.D.)

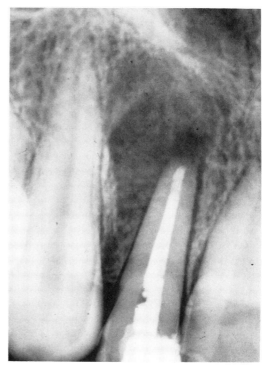

Fig. 14.13. Radicular cyst of the mandible. A large defect is present in the bone at the apex of a previously infected tooth. (Courtesy of C. Doku, D.M.D.)

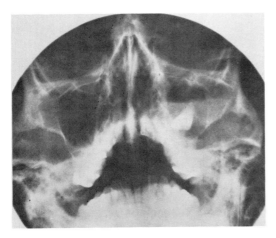

Fig. 14.14. Infected dentigerous cyst of the maxilla. An ectopic tooth is present in the wall of a cyst, which occupies most of the maxillary sinus. The horizontally demarcated opacification is caused by purulent exudate.

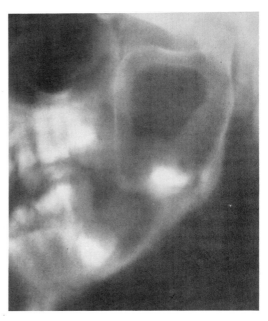

Fig. 14.16. Tomogram of an ameloblastoma of the mandible. A large, cystic lesion has expanded the ramus. The involved part of the mandible was excised.

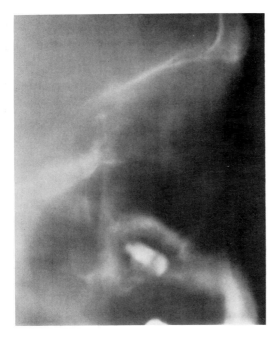

Fig. 14.15. Tomographic roentgenogram of a composite odontoma. This is a dense mass that originates in tooth-forming tissue.

Radicular cysts develop secondary to apical infection and are always at the apices of diseased teeth (Figure 14.13). The cyst might present as an expansion of the mandible or might be relatively asymptomatic, being discovered on routine radiologic examination. Radicular cysts are lined with a flat, almost squamoid, epithelium. They are treated by extraction of the tooth and removal of the lining of the cyst. The cavity fills spontaneously with fibrous tissue.

DENTIGEROUS CYSTS. A dentigerous cyst is associated with an unerupted tooth. The cyst is formed by the continued expansion of the tooth capsule. The unerupted tooth remains in the wall of the cyst and is the characteristic feature of a dentigerous cyst (Figure 14.14). Dentigerous cysts are found in the maxilla or mandible, can be large, and may become infected. They are treated by excision.

SOLITARY BONE CYSTS. Solitary bone cysts are individual cystic spaces in the jaws that are lined by a layer of fibrous tissue. They may expand to occupy a substantial part of the bone.

BENIGN NEOPLASMS FROM TOOTH DERIVATIVES. ODONTOMAS. An odontoma is a benign tumor that is derived from the tooth-forming tissues. It consists of the basic elements of the teeth compounded into one mass. Radiologically, odontomas present as a cystic or solid mass without a surrounding halo (Figure 14.15). Treatment is by surgical removal.

CEMENTOMA. A cementoma is a benign tumor that is derived from the periodontal lamina. Well-formed teeth are enclosed in a membrane that resembles a halo on roentgenography. Treatment is by surgical removal.

AMELOBLASTOMA. Ameloblastoma (adamantinoma) is a benign, cystic neoplasm that is common in the mandible but uncommon in the maxilla. It is derived from the enamel-producing layer of the teeth and presents as a slowly progressive, painless expansion of one side of the jaw. Roentgenograms show a cystic honeycombed or multichambered, expanded area in the mandible within a thin, eggshell-like layer of cortical bone (Figure 14.16).

Ameloblastomas are treated by segmental excision of the mandible and reconstruction with a bone graft or by extensive curettage and filling of the cavity with bone chips. Ameloblastomas tend to recur and a few become malignant.

MALIGNANT NEOPLASMS

OSTEOSARCOMA. Osteogenic sarcoma sometimes occurs in the mandible and more rarely in the maxilla and presents as a rapidly expanding, painful mass that ulcerates into the gums. Roentgenograms show a lytic lesion in the bone. These lesions may metastasize to the lungs. Treatment is by wide excision followed by combination chemotherapy.

MALIGNANT NEOPLASMS OF THE TOOTH-FORMING TISSUES. In rare cases ameloblastomas undergo malignant change to become an ameloblastic sarcoma or carcinoma. Myxomas are fibromatous, nonmetastasizing, locally invasive tumors that probably arise from the tooth pulp. The are treated by radical excision.

BIBLIOGRAPHY

Batsakis, J.G.: Tumors of the Head and Neck. 2nd Ed. Baltimore, Williams and Wilkins, 1979.

Bhaskar, S.N.: Bone lesions of endodontic origin. Dent. Clin. North Am., November, 1967, 421.

Bhaskar, S.N., and Dubit, J.: Central and peripheral hemangioma. Oral Surg., 23:385, 1967.

Dinerman, W.S., and Myers, E.N.: Lymphangiomatous macroglossia. Laryngoscope, 86:391, 1976.

Gardner, D.G.: Peripheral ameloblastoma. Cancer, 39:1625, 1977.

Krause, C.J., et al.: Carcinoma of the oral cavity. A comparison of therapeutic modalities. Arch. Otolaryngol., 97:353–358, 1973.

MacComb, W.S., and Fletcher, G.H.: Cancer of the Head and Neck. Baltimore, Williams and Wilkins, 1967.

Quint, J.H., Lehrman, M., and Loveman, C.E.: Reparative giant cell granuloma. Oral Surg., 17:142, 1964.

Robinson, H.B.G.: Ameloblastoma, a survey of 379 cases from the literature. Arch. Pathol., 23:831, 1937.

Smith, H.W.: Cystic lesions of the maxilla, I. Arch. Otolaryngol., 88:315, 1968.

Spiro, R.N., and Strong, E.W.: Epidermal carcinoma of the oral cavity and oropharynx. Arch. Surg., 107:381–384, 1973.

Chapter 15

DISORDERS OF THE SALIVARY GLANDS

THE SALIVARY GLANDS

Saliva

Saliva is produced by the major salivary glands and by the innumerable minor glands that are located in the mouth and pharynx. About 1 L of saliva is produced daily in a normal adult, mostly by the parotid glands, which are primarily serous glands. The submandibular glands have both serous and mucous cells. The secretion of saliva is controlled by the parasympathetic system. The secretomotor nerves to the parotid gland are from the inferior salivary nucleus via the glossopharyngeal nerve and through the tympanic plexus and otic ganglion. The secretomotor nerves of the submandibular gland originate in the superior salivary nucleus, run in the facial nerve, and exit into the middle ear in the chorda tympani, which joins the lingual nerve and enters the submandibular gland after synapsing in the submandibular ganglion. Parasympathetic stimulation increases salivary flow, while sympathetic activity decreases the flow of saliva. Saliva is mostly water but also contains traces of sodium, potassium, and calcium salts, ptyalin (α-amylase), maltase, lysozymes, immunoglobulins, and mucus. Saliva moistens, lubricates, and partially digests food.

DISORDERS OF THE SALIVARY GLANDS

Congenital Disorders

CONGENITAL SIALECTASIA OF THE PAROTID GLAND. Sialectasia of the parotid gland resembles bronchiectasia in that the peripheral acini are dilated and retain puddles of saliva, making the gland prone to recurrent, usually staphylococcal, infection. The problem presents in the young child when the gland becomes swollen and tender, and the overlying skin might be reddened. The papilla of the parotid duct (Stensen's duct) might be swollen and pink. With gentle massage of the gland and duct, a bead of pus can be expressed from the papilla. This finding is diagnostic, and the pus can also be used for bacteriologic study. Without a thorough examination, mumps is usually diagnosed at the first episode, but the second episode of swelling tells the true story. Each episode is treated with the appropriate antistaphylococcal antibiotics, such as dicloxacillin, and fluids, taken liberally by mouth. Sialography is performed when the infection subsides and demonstrates the characteristic punctate globular expansion of the acini, which confirms the diagnosis. The condition becomes less problematic as the child grows older.

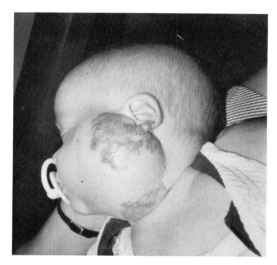

Fig. 15.1.　Hemangioma of the parotid gland.

DUPLICATION ANOMALIES OF THE EXTERNAL AUDITORY CANAL (see Chapter 5). Duplication anomalies of the external auditory canal might present as an acute infection in the region of the parotid gland. Differential diagnosis from suppurative parotitis is aided by identifying the mouth of a tract on the floor of the external canal and by the presence of normal saliva.

HEMANGIOMA OF THE PAROTID GLANDS. Congenital hemangioma of the parotid gland presents in the neonate or infant as a soft, compressible, painless swelling in the pre- and infra-auricular areas. The overlying skin might be obviously involved (Figure 15.1), in which case the diagnosis is self-evident, or the skin might contain only a few dilated, venous channels. Occasionally, a bruit is audible with a stethoscope. Diagnosis is enhanced by computed tomography with intravenous contrast, in which the vascular mass is well demonstrated. An open biopsy is occasionally necessary.

The behavior of congenital hemangiomas varies considerably. Most show increased growth soon after birth, which is followed either by a slower, but continuous, rate of growth or by spontaneous regression. Therefore, active therapy is considered only after a period of waiting for spontaneous remission to occur. Continued growth might be slowed by a course of corticosteroids (prednisone). Surgical excision of a hemangioma of the parotid gland has a high risk or permanently injuring the facial nerve and is unlikely to achieve complete removal.

Inflammatory Disorders

Inflammatory disease of the salivary glands might be viral or bacterial, might be confined to a single gland, or might affect many glands simultaneously. A significant decrease in the salivary flow might occur, or salivary flow might be unaffected. Sudden inflammation of a single gland in an otherwise healthy person usually indicates ductal obstruction by calculi or neoplasms. Many glands are simultaneously and chronically involved in autoimmune diseases, such as Sjogren's disease, and in iatrogenic disorders (e.g., iodism).

Viral Infections

MUMPS. Mumps is a highly contagious, systemic, viral infection that usually presents with fever and swelling of the salivary glands, particularly the parotid glands. In addition, the gonads, brain, and pancreas are afflicted to variable degrees. A low total white cell count and a relative lymphocytosis occur, and the serum amylase might be elevated. Diagnosis is confirmed by determination of rising antibody titers in acute and convalescent serum.

Other viral infections cause acute swelling of the salivary glands, particularly the cytomegaloinclusion virus and coxsackievirus.

Bacterial Infections

ACUTE SUPPURATIVE PAROTITIS. Acute suppurative parotitis is usually a staphylococcal infection that is secondary to general debility or poor oral hygiene. The gland becomes acutely swollen, and exquisitely tender, with erythema of the

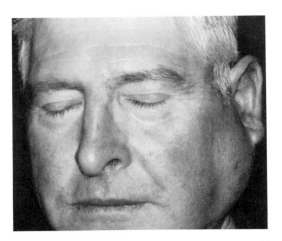

Fig. 15.2.   Acute suppurative parotitis in a 60-year-old man. The parotid gland is grossly swollen, tense, and tender. The overlying skin is red, and the patient is toxic.

overlying skin (Figure 15.2). The patient quickly shows signs of systemic toxicity. Diagnosis is confirmed by expressing pus from Stensen's duct. Untreated, an abscess forms deep to the tense parotid fascia. Treatment is by rehydration and the administration of the appropriate antibiotics, such as oxacillin administered intravenously. Abscesses are drained via horizontal incisions in the fascia parallel to the direction of branches of the facial nerve.

Acute suppuration of the submandibular salivary gland is usually secondary to obstruction by a calculus or to general debility. Acute, tender, painful swelling of the submandibular area develops. The overlying skin becomes pink, and pain is aggravated by eating. Gentle massage of the gland might force a bead of pus through the ductal papilla. Mixed bacterial flora are present, with Staphylococci and Streptococci predominating. Treatment is with antistaphylococcal antibiotics. When the infection has settled, the calculi are removed (see the section on salivary gland calculi in this chapter).

CHRONIC SIALOADENITIS. Chronic sialoadenitis is a questionable entity. Diffuse enlargement and intermittent pain

develop in the salivary glands, particularly the parotid glands. Sialography demonstrates persistent, irregular dilatation of the peripheral ducts and varying degrees of sialectasia. Treatment is by sialogogues, such as potassium iodide, gentle frequent massage of the gland, and irrigation of the ductal system with a mild antiseptic solution. If the severity of the problem warrants, parotid secretion can be reduced by tympanic neurectomy, in which the secretomotor fibers are sectioned on the promontory of the middle ear where they are part of the tympanic plexus.

Salivary Gland Calculi

Calculi are calcified bodies that form in the ductal systems of the salivary glands. Calculi are common in the submandibular glands and rare in the parotid and sublingual glands. They consist of calcium salts, which are probably deposited around a microscopic foreign body. Calculi may be very small, even less than 2 mm in diameter. They cause symptoms by obstruction of salivary flow. The smaller calculi get washed into the main duct and impact in the ductal papillae. Larger calculi stay within the gland close to the hilum. Obstruction occurs suddenly during a meal,

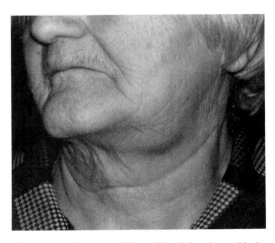

Fig. 15.3.   Chronic swelling of the left submandibular salivary gland in a 70-year-old woman. The condition is secondary to the calculus that is shown in Figure 15.4B.

the gland swells and becomes tense and painful within a few minutes. The patient stops eating, and over the ensuing 1 or 2 hours the swelling subsides. If true impaction occurs, the swelling persists, and the pain subsides only to be exacerbated by the next meal (Figure 15.3). Alternatively, intermittent obstruction might occur over a long period of time. Calculi in Wharton's duct are frequently palpable. Most, but not all, calculi are radiopaque and are easily demonstrated by roentgenography. The best positions for submandibular calculi are tilted oblique roentgenograms of the mandible and occlusal roentgenograms to show the floor of the mouth (Figure 15.4). Sialography is seldom necessary.

Small calculi, impacted in Wharton's duct, are easily removed by infiltrating the overlying mucosa with a small quantity of local anesthesia (1% lidocaine) and cutting down on the calculus with a pointed scalpel. Larger stones in the substance of the gland require excision of the whole gland.

The Salivary Glands in Systemic Disorders

The salivary glands are frequently involved in systemic diseases. These systemic diseases may specifically and almost always involve the salivary glands, or the glands might be more peripherally affected.

Specific Disorders

SJOGREN'S SYNDROME. Sjogren's syndrome is a multiorgan systemic disorder that is characterized by atrophy of the salivary glands and the secretory glands of the eyes, nose, larynx, trachea, and bronchi. The joints, lymph nodes, and other organs are also affected. Patients complain of dryness of the mouth and eyes, nasal crusting, and mild or severe respiratory symptoms. Inflammatory arthritis might be present. The salivary glands, particularly the parotid glands, may enlarge considerably (Figure 15.5), with superadded,

acute inflammatory episodes, or the salivary glands may become smaller and indurated. Xerophthalmia causes keratoconjunctivitis and corneal ulcers, and xerostomia results in discoloration and carious disintegration of the teeth. All symptoms may be present in varying degrees.

Sjogren's syndrome is probably an autoimmune disorder. The characteristic histopathologic finding is dense infiltration of the glandular acini by small lymphocytes, which is confirmed easily by taking a deep biopsy from the mucosal surface of the lower lip. Malignant lymphoma develops in a significant percentage of patients with Sjogren's syndrome.

Presently, no curative treatment exists for Sjogren's syndrome. Replacement of tears and saliva by artificial solutions and stimulation of bronchial secretions by expectorants, such as potassium iodide, are useful. Prognosis varies depending on the rapidity of the progression of the disease. Some patients survive for decades and others die from pulmonary infections.

MIKULICZ'S DISEASE (BENIGN LYMPHOEPITHELIOMATOUS HYPERPLASIA). The only difference between Sjogren's syndrome and Mikulicz's disease is that Mikulicz's disease is confined to salivary and lacrimal glands. The histopathologic patterns are identical, and the methods of management are the same.

Nonspecific Disorders

Nonspecific enlargement of the salivary glands, particularly of the parotid glands, occur in a number of unrelated systemic disorders.

SARCOIDOSIS (UVEOPAROTID DISEASE). In the head and neck, sarcoidosis may present as discrete nodular swellings of the parotid glands, nasal obstruction, or cervical lymphadenopathy and, rarely, facial paralysis. Sarcoidosis should be considered in the differential diagnosis of any diffuse swelling of the salivary glands. A chest roentgenogram might demonstrate

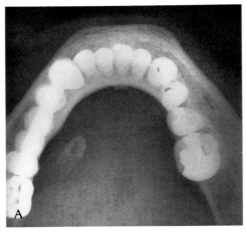

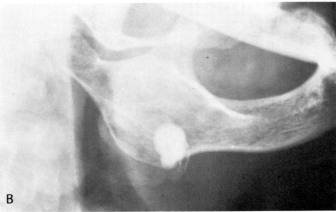

Fig. 15.4. Calculi of the submandibular salivary gland. *A.* Medium-size calculus in Wharton's duct. *B.* Large intraglandular calculus. The calculus is better seen by more tilt, which angles it away from the mandible.

mediastinal lymphadenopathy and parenchymal granulomas or scarring. Diagnosis is made by biopsy of an obvious lesion (e.g., nasal mucosa, parotid gland, and mediastinal lymph node), or by finding sarcoid nodules in the retina.

RHEUMATOID ARTHRITIS. In severe rheumatoid arthritis there might be xerostomia and dryness of the nose because of atrophy of the salivary and nasal mucous glands. The salivary glands do not enlarge but may feel slightly thickened.

DIFFUSE FATTY INFILTRATION OF THE PAROTID GLANDS. Diffuse fatty infiltration of the parenchyma of the parotid glands occurs in alcoholism, chronic di-

abetes, protein-calorie malnutrition, and iodism. Sialograms are normal. Treatment is directed at correction of the cause.

Neoplasms of the Salivary Glands

Tumors of the salivary glands are common. By far, the majority of tumors of the salivary glands are of epithelial rather than stromal origin. One third of the tumors are malignant, and the majority occur in the parotid glands. The most frequent tumor of all of the salivary glands at every age is a pleomorphic adenoma (96% of which are benign). Generally, tumors of the major salivary glands are likely to be benign,

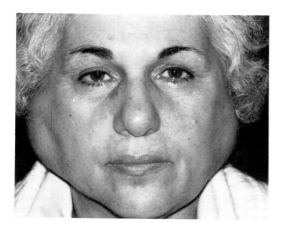

Fig. 15.5. Sjogren's disease. Gross enlargement of the parotid glands has occurred. The patient also complained of dryness of the eyes and mouth.

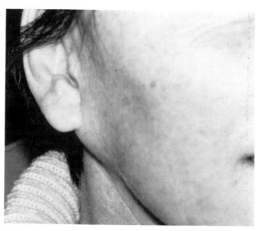

Fig. 15.6. Pleomorphic adenoma (mixed tumor) of the parotid gland in a 42-year-old woman. A firm, rounded mass is immediately posterior to the angle of the mandible.

while those of the minor glands are more likely to be malignant.

Histologic interpretation of tumors of the salivary glands can be most difficult, and electron microscopy is now a common adjunct.

Benign tumors of the parotid glands do not cause facial paralysis. Therefore, any tumor that causes facial paralysis must be assumed to be malignant. Most tumors of the salivary glands are asymptomatic in their early stages. Benign tumors may grow to huge dimensions and remain asymptomatic, but malignant neoplasms eventually cause pain.

Malignant neoplasms of the salivary glands metastasize by the lymphatic vessels to the regional lymph nodes or by hematogenous spread to the lungs and bones.

Benign Tumors

PLEOMOPHIC ADENOMA. The commonest neoplasm of all the salivary glands in every age group is the pleomorphic adenoma (mixed tumor), so-called because it seems to contain many different tissue types: epithelium, cartilage-like tissue, and glandular tissue. The tumor, however, is probably derived from only one cell type

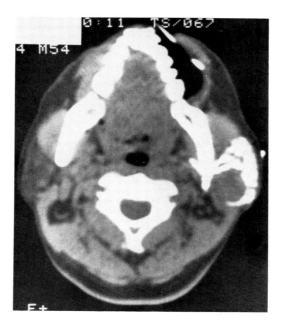

Fig. 15.7. Computed tomography with sialogram demonstrates a round, intraglandular, pleomorphic adenoma.

(myoepithelial cells). Most pleomorphic adenomas are benign, but 2 to 5% are malignant.

A pleomorphic adenoma presents as a painless, firm to hard, smooth, rounded mass that occurs most frequently in the superficial segment of the parotid gland, usually in the tail of the gland just posterior to the angle of the mandible (Figure 15.6). Pleomorphic adenomas may grow to enormous size without causing dysfunction of the facial nerve. Tumors may also occur in the deep lobe of the parotid gland, presenting as a pharyngeal mass and displacing the tonsil and adjacent soft palate downward and forward. Radiographically, pleomorphic adenomas can be nicely demonstrated by combining sialography and computed tomography (Figure 15.7). Pleomorphic adenoma of the parotid gland is managed by performing a superficial lobectomy, which is an en bloc excision of all glandular tissue superficial to the branches of the facial nerve. Pleomorphic adenoma of the deep lobe is handled by first excising the superficial lobe and then carefully removing the deep lobe, preserving the facial nerve.

Pleomorphic adenomas of the submandibular gland require total resection of the gland. Adenomas of the minor salivary gland are excised with a generous rim of normal tissue.

WARTHIN'S TUMOR (CYSTADENOMA LYMPHOMATOSUM). This tumor is a fluid-filled, cystic mass that presents in the region of the tail of the parotid gland. The mass is asymptomatic, and patients usually complain about cosmesis rather than pain. The facial nerve is never involved. Histologically, a Warthin's tumor consists of a thin capsule with papilliferous projections of endothelium-lined tissue in which numerous lymphocytes are present. Warthin's tumor might be multicentric, with more than one lesion in one parotid gland. These tumors are easily excised.

ONCOCYTOMA. Oncocytomas are firm, rounded masses in the parotid gland. They are rare tumors and are clinically indistinguishable from other benign tumors. Histologically, they are composed almost exclusively of oncocytes with pink, granular

cytoplasm. Treatment is by excision via a superficial parotid lobectomy.

Malignant Tumors

ADENOID CYSTIC CARCINOMA (CYLINDROMA). Adenoid cystic carcinoma, the most frequent malignant tumor of the salivary glands, is a disease mostly of young adults but can occur at any age. It is an insidious tumor that causes no symptoms in its early stages, except occasionally in the parotid gland, where a deep, dull ache might develop. The histologic pattern is one of multiple, discrete, solid masses of small, darkly staining cells. In the center of many of these masses are small cystic spaces with eosinophilic material, which gives a pattern resembling Swiss cheese (Figure 15.8). The tumor tends to spread along the perineural spaces and the circulatory system so that regional and distant pulmonary metastases occur early. Adenoid cystic carcinomas grow slowly, however, and can persist for 10 to 15 years without significantly affecting the patient. Similarly, metastases might persist for many years without causing symptoms or morbidity. Adenoid cystic carcinoma is treated by total surgical excision of the involved gland with a wide margin of normal tissue, followed by radiation therapy.

MUCOEPIDERMOID CARCINOMA. Mucoepidermoid carcinoma is a comparatively recently recognized form of malignant tumor of the salivary glands. The tumor presents as a firm, ill-defined mass in one of the salivary glands. Histologically, there is a mixture of malignant glandular and epidermoid tissue. Mucoepidermoid carcinoma seems to occur in two forms: a slow-growing, indolent tumor and a more aggressive, rapidly expanding tumor that metastasizes early.

Mucoepidermoid tumors are treated by excision of the primary tumor with a generous margin of normal tissue. For the more aggressive tumors, a concomitant radical neck dissection is recommended. Radia-

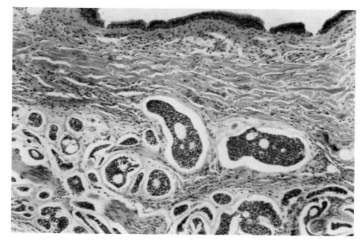

Fig. 15.8. Histopathology of adenoid cystic carcinoma of the submandibular salivary gland. Cores of cells with central mucin-containing cystic spaces are present. A nerve bundle is visible in the lower left quadrant of the field. The lesions spread along the perineural spaces.

tion therapy is given if surgery is considered unlikely to control the disease.

Trauma to the Salivary Glands

The only important injury to the salivary glands is sharp incisional trauma to the parotid gland, which frequently damages the facial nerve and Stensen's duct. The facial nerve and parotid duct should be reapproximated with fine sutures. The duct is repaired over a polyethylene tube, which is left in place for 2 weeks. Occasionally, incisive trauma to a salivary gland might result in a salivary-cutaneous fistula. This is treated by either a pressure dressing or open repair, and might even necessitate total excision of the salivary gland. Alternatively, salivation can be suppressed by radiation therapy or by section of the appropriate secretomotor pathway.

Drooling

Drooling is caused by excessive salivation or from an inability to control swallowing, as occurs often in mental retardation. The parotid glands produce the largest volume of saliva, and parotid secretion is controlled by Jacobson's nerve,

which is a branch of the ninth cranial nerve. Jacobson's nerve is the major contributor to the tympanic plexus, which lies on the promontory of the middle ear. It is possible, by way of a transcanal approach, to interrupt the tympanic plexus (tympanic neurectomy) in the middle ear and thereby reduce the volume of parotid secretions. This is significantly beneficial to many patients with excessive drooling.

Xerostomia (Dryness of the Mouth)

Xerostomia is caused by external drying factors, such as mouth breathing, or by the reduction of salivation. Salivation is reduced by either intrinsic or extrinsic factors.

INTRINSIC FACTORS. CONGENITAL. Congenital xerostomia is rare but does occur.

INFLAMMATORY. Most febrile illnesses cause dryness of the mouth.

IDIOPATHIC. The sicca syndrome and Sjogren's disease.

EXTRINSIC FACTORS. Atropine-based medications and radiation therapy cause dryness of the mouth.

Long-standing xerostomia causes the buildup of plaque, which is an erosive layer of bacteria on the surface of the teeth. The enamel disintegrates, and the teeth rapidly become carious.

Xerostomia is treated by elimination of the causative factors. If this is not possible, the liberal use of artificial saliva is recommended.

BIBLIOGRAPHY

Bailey, H.: Congenital parotid sialectasis. J. Int. Coll. Surg., 8:109, 1945.

Eby, L.S., Johnson, D.S., and Baker, H.W.: Adenoid cystic carcinoma of the head and neck. Cancer, 29:1160–1168, 1972.

Eneroth, C.M., and Hamberger, C.A.: Principles of treatment of different types of parotid tumors. Laryngoscope, 84:1732, 1974.

Grey, J.M., Hendrix, R.C., and French, A.J.: Mucoepidermoid tumors of salivary glands. Cancer, 16:183, 1963.

Harril, J.A., King, J.S., and Boyce, W.H.: Structure and composition of salivary gland calculi. Laryngoscope, 69:481, 1959.

Nussbaum, M., Tans, S., and Som, M.L.: Hemangiomas of the salivary glands. Laryngoscope, 86:1015, 1976.

Rankow, R.M., and Polayes, I.M.: Diseases of the Salivary Glands. Philadelphia, W.B. Saunders Co., 1976.

Warthin, A.S.: Papillary cystadenoma lymphomatosis. J. Cancer Res., 13:116, 1929.

Work, W.P., and Hecht, D.W.: Inflammatory diseases of the major salivary glands. In Otolaryngology. 2nd Ed. Edited by M.M. Paparella and D. Shumrick. Philadelphia, W.B. Saunders Co., 1980. pp. 2235–2243.

Work, W.P.: New concepts of the first branchial cleft defects. Laryngoscope, 82:1581, 1972.

Chapter 16

THE PHARYNX

ANATOMY

The pharynx is derived from the ento-dermal surface and adjacent tissue of the branchial apparatus. It is an incomplete muscular tube, open anteriorly, that extends from the base of the skull to the inlet of the esophagus at the level of the sixth cervical vertebra. Traditionally, the pharynx is subdivided into three parts: the nasopharynx posterior to the nasal complex, the oropharynx posterior to the oral cavity, and the laryngopharynx posterior to the upper larynx (Figure 16.1). On each side the pharynx is composed of three thin, flat muscles, which are the superior, middle, and inferior constrictors. These are joined to those of the opposite side by a posterior median raphe. The muscles fit into each other like a stack of paper cups (Figure 16.2). The median raphe is attached superiorly to the pharyngeal tubercle on the inferior surface of the sphenoid bone and ends inferiorly at the inlet of the esophagus. From the median raphe the constrictors sweep downward and forward to insert into the stylohyoid ligament, the hyoid bone, and thyroid cartilages. Muscles are innervated by the pharyngeal plexus, whose primary motor component is supplied by the vagus nerve. The pharynx is lined internally by a thick mucosa covered by squamous ep-ithelium that contains discrete aggregates of lymphoid tissue.

The Nasopharynx

In the vault of the nasopharynx is the adenoid, which is a mass of lymphoid tissue with a central segment and two lateral bands. The surface of the adenoid is covered by a respiratory-type epithelium. The eustachian tubes open into the lateral walls of the nasopharynx. The adenoid is present at birth, but its size varies depending on age. The adenoid grows slowly to a maximum size around the age of 4 years and thereafter slowly regresses. In the adult

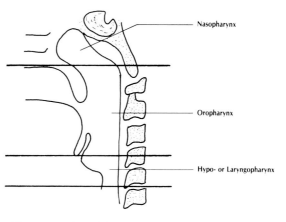

Fig. 16.1. The subdivisions of the pharynx. These are arbitrary divisions that are used for purposes of description.

175

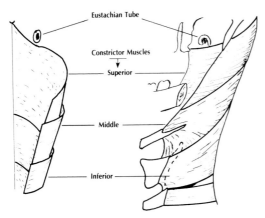

Fig. 16.2. The constrictor muscles. The thin muscles fit into each other and arise posteriorly from a central median raphe. There is a potentially weak area between the inferior constrictor and the cricopharyngeus muscle.

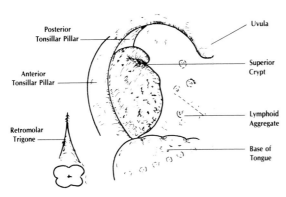

Fig. 16.3. The pharyngeal tonsils and associated structures. The tonsil is contained between the anterior and posterior pillars. Many aggregates of lymphoid tissue are present on the posterior pharyngeal wall.

the adenoid is usually only a comparatively small mass of tissue.

The Oropharynx

The oropharynx is bounded anteriorly by the oral cavity and the base of the tongue. The pharyngeal tonsils (faucial tonsils) are present in its lateral walls. The pharyngeal tonsils are large masses of lymphoid tissue, one on each side, which are contained in a fossa that is formed by the anterior and posterior tonsillar pillars (Figure 16.3). Their lateral surfaces are de-

marcated by a thin, white, glistening capsule. The tonsils (like the adenoid) are present at birth, grow to a maximum size around the age of 4 years and then regress slowly over many years. The size of the tonsils may vary considerably between individuals. The surface of the tonsil is covered by squamous epithelium and contains numerous crypts. Epithelial debris and saprophytic bacteria collect in these crypts and may present as small, yellow masses that should not be mistaken for pustules. The lingual tonsils are large aggregates of lymphoid tissue on the base of the tongue. They may be of considerable size. Other lymphoid aggregates are scattered throughout the posterior wall of the pharynx. The adenoid, pharyngeal tonsils, lingual tonsils, and lymphoid aggregates form a somewhat continuous circle of lymphoid tissue around the lumen of the pharynx that is known as Waldeyer's ring. The valleculae are two depressions between the epiglottis and the base of the tongue, which are separated from each other by a frenulum-like fold of mucosa.

The Laryngopharynx

The laryngopharynx is a small but important area that is bounded anteriorly by the larynx and posteriorly by the prevertebral fascia, and inferiorly by the inlet of the esophagus. Laterally, the laryngopharynx extends downward to two gutters (on each side of the larynx), which are the pyriform sinuses. Each wall of the pharynx contains innumerable minor salivary glands that keep the surface constantly moist. The important anatomic relationships of the pharynx are as follows (Figure 16.4): laterally, the common carotid and external and internal carotid arteries, vagus nerve, and contents of the neck; and posteriorly, the vertebral column with prevertebral muscles and fascia. The major vessels lie in a potential space that extends from the base of the skull to the thoracic inlet. This is known as the parapharyngeal space and contains the contents of the ca-

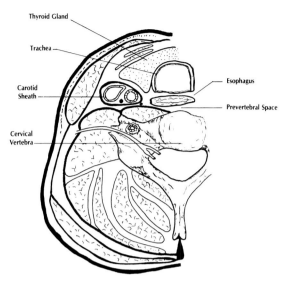

Fig. 16.4. Diagram of transverse section through the neck. Although the level is inferior to the pharynx, the relationships are the same.

rotid sheath and the jugular chain of lymph nodes.

PHYSIOLOGY

There are two primary functions of the pharynx: to serve as a conduit for air and food and as a propellor of food. The tube-like configuration of the pharynx allows air to pass from the nose to the larynx and food to pass from the mouth to the esophagus. Food, however, requires additional impetus and this is provided by the rhythmic contractions of the pharyngeal constrictors.

Deglutition

Food is pulverized, moistened, and partially digested during the act of chewing. The bolus of food is then passed by the tongue into the oropharynx. This initiates a well-coordinated sequential constriction of superior, middle, and inferior constrictor muscles, whereby the bolus is grasped by the pharynx and propelled inferiorly. A number of events take place simultaneously: the mouth is closed, the soft palate rises and closes off the nasopharynx,

the larynx rises and the epiglottis dips downward and posteriorly to close off the larynx, and the cricopharyngeus muscle, which is usually constricted, relaxes to open the inlet of the esophagus. Breathing ceases momentarily.

Secondary Functions

The pharynx has additional secondary functions. Evidence suggests that the tonsils and adenoid secrete immunoglobulins even early in utero, but this secretory activity peaks soon after birth. It has also been postulated that the cryptic surfaces of the tonsils allow for trapping of bacteria and, therefore, for immunologic surveillance so that natural antibodies are formed slowly. The pharynx is also part of the resonating chamber for speech.

DISORDERS OF THE PHARYNX

Congenital Disorders

Congenital anomalies of the pharynx are uncommon. Branchial pouches may persist as internal sinuses in the vicinity of the pharyngeal tonsils or they may extend to the skin of the neck as part of a fistula (see Chapter 19). An internal branchial sinus may cause recurrent unilateral tonsillitis.

THORNWALDT'S CYST. Thornwaldt's cyst is a smooth cystic structure that develops high in the vault of the nasopharynx in adults. Supposedly, these cysts are formed by closure of the mouth of a persistent pharyngeal bursa, which is a small embryonic evagination of pharyngeal epithelium. Patients complain of postnasal drip, an unpleasant taste, and, sometimes, otalgia. Thornwaldt's cysts are treated by wide marsupialization.

Traumatic Disorders

Traumatic injuries to the pharynx can be either mechanical or chemical.

MECHANICAL INJURIES. Penetrating injuries are comparatively rare but can occur from external or internal insult. Internal injury is more common in children who fall while holding sticks, pencils, and so forth in their mouths. All pharyngeal wounds are potentially dangerous because of the proximity of the large vessels of the neck and the possibility of infection of the parapharyngeal space. If injury to the great vessels is even suspected, the neck should be promptly explored through an external incision.

CHEMICAL INJURIES. Chemical trauma of the pharynx is caused by strong alkalies and acids and is more frequent among young children. Burns with sodium hydroxide (lye, Drano, and so on) are fairly common in many countries where these substances are still household items. Burns occur on the lips, oral mucosa, pharynx, esophagus, and even stomach, depending on the quantity ingested. The patient quickly develops severe pain in the mouth, throat, chest, and epigastrium and salivates profusely. The burnt areas are reddened initially but in a few hours are covered by a whitish, fibrinous deposit which makes them easier to identify. If seen early, the patient should be examined gently but carefully and supportive intravenous therapy begun. All patients should be examined endoscopically, preferably at least 6 hours after ingestion when the lesions are easier to recognize. Deep burns are treated with antibiotics and corticosteroids to prevent the formation of strictures. Superficial burns usually resolve spontaneously and only supportive measures are necessary.

Inflammatory Disorders

All inflammatory reactions of the pharynx cause soreness of the throat. Pharyngitis might be acute or chronic and infective or allergic.

INFECTIVE PHARYNGITIS. Infective pharyngitis is caused by viruses, bacteria, or fungi. Viruses are the commonest causative agents followed by β-hemolytic streptococci and Hemophilus influenzae (in children). Fungal infections are com-

paratively uncommon and tend to afflict infants (thrush, monilia) and immunologically compromised hosts.

VIRAL PHARYNGITIS. Viral pharyngitis is the commonest cause of infective pharyngitis and is frequently part of an upper respiratry tract infection. The usual agents are influenza, herpes simplex, adenoviruses, rhinoviruses, coxsackieviruses, and the Epstein-Barr virus.

The patient complains of severe pain in the throat, but the clinical findings are comparatively mild. Mild to moderate hyperemia and edema are present, particularly along the faucial pillars and lymphoid aggregates in the mucosa. Mild enlargement of the jugulodigastric nodes might occur. The leukocyte count is not elevated and might actually be depressed, and pharyngeal cultures grow only normal flora. Although this is the usual pattern, viral pharyngitis can be a severe problem, with high fever, mucosal ulcerations, extreme odynophagia, and cervical lymphadenopathy.

Treatment of viral pharyngitis is mainly symptomatic. Gargling with warm, diluted salt water is soothing (a half teaspoonful of salt in 8 oz of water). Analgesics can be used liberally (e.g., aspirin, 10 grains or acetaminophen, 360 mg three times daily) and are useful. Antibiotics are used only if a superinfection with bacteria develops. Lozenges containing a topical anesthetic give temporary relief. Soreness might persist for a long time after the physical signs have subsided.

Infectious Mononucleosis. Infectious mononucleosis is an infection caused by the Epstein-Barr virus (more frequent in young adults) that presents with acute sore throat, high fever, and mild to massive cervical lymphadenopathy. Frequently, the surfaces of the tonsils are ulcerated and covered by a shaggy, yellow exudate. The uvula is swollen, and fetor oris is present. Swelling of the tonsils and pharyngeal mucosa might cause respiratory obstruction. Hepatosplenomegaly and lymphadenopathy develop in other areas. Infectious mononucleosis can occur at any age but is usually a milder disease in children. Diagnosis is confirmed by serologic tests: a monospot test or heterophil antibody test, both of which depend on the agglutination of sheep red blood cells. Routine blood tests are usually not helpful. The white blood cells count is normal wih a relative lymphocytosis. Treatment is primarily supportive with warm saline solution irrigations, analgesics, and ample fluids by mouth. Ampicillin should not be used because it causes an unusually troublesome rash in these patients. Prolonged, severe dysphagia might necessitate the administration of intravenous fluids. The disease usually runs its course with spontaneous remission, but hepatic failure and encephalopathy are possible complications.

BACTERIAL PHARYNGITIS (ACUTE TONSILLITIS). The commonest infecting organisms in bacterial pharyngitis are β-hemolytic streptococci, Hemophilus influenzae, and Neisseria species. Hemophilus influenzae is more frequent in younger children. The pharyngeal tonsils, adenoid, and lingual tonsils are the most frequent sites of infection, in that order. Bacterial pharyngitis is usually an acute problem that presents with sore throat, frequently referred otalgia, fever, odynophagia, jugular lymphadenopathy, and polymorphonuclear leukocytosis. At first there is hyperemia of the pharyngeal mucosa, particularly the tonsillar pillars. Within a few hours the pharyngeal tonsils become red and swollen, and yellow patches appear on the crypts of the tonsils and sometimes on the pharyngeal lymphoid aggregates (Figure 16.5). All symptoms and physical findings may vary considerably. Punctate yellow spots may appear on the tonsils (follicular tonsillitis), the whole tonsillar surface might be involved (ulcerative tonsillitis), or the tonsil might be covered by a yellow-gray membrane (membranous tonsillitis).

Treatment. If possible, swab the pharynx for culture before treatment begins. Penicillin controls streptococci and Neisseria species. Hemophilus influenzae can be controlled by ampicillin or amoxicillin, which are, therefore, preferable in younger children. Oral antibiotics are useful if

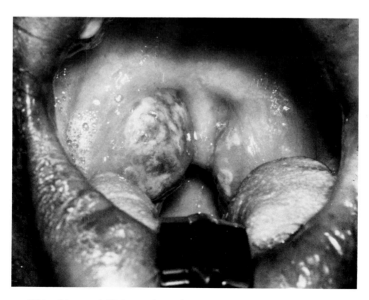

Fig. 16.5. Acute tonsillitis. Discrete follicles and membranous material are present on the surface of the tonsils. Large, tender jugulodigastric nodes were associated with the condition.

swallowing is still possible, but intramuscular or intravenous therapy might be necessary. Treatment is given for a minimum of 10 days.

More immediate symptomatic relief can be obtained with local treatment. Irrigations with a warm, diluted saline solution, gargles, and lozenges that contain a topical anesthetic are all soothing. Oral analgesics (e.g., aspirin, 10 grains, codeine, 30 mg, acetaminophen, 300 mg three times daily) give relief. Patients are encouraged to take fluids liberally by mouth.

Gonococcal Pharyngitis. Gonococcal pharyngitis is an acute, debilitating infection that is almost always secondary to orogenital sex, and its incidence is increasing. Ulceration of the pharyngeal tonsils and other lymphoid aggregates usually develops, which might be complicated by secondary septic arthritis. Diagnosis is made by a history of contact, Gram stain of a smear of the pharyngeal secretions, and by culture. Treatment is with single, large doses of penicillin (2 million units), given parenterally. Penicillin-resistant strains of gonococci, however, are becoming more frequent.

Diphtheria. Diphtheria is an infection by a virulent form of Corynebacterium diphtheriae and is still a potential problem because of the recent laxity in immunization programs. Diphtheria presents in children as an acute febrile illness, with soreness of the throat and substantial cervical lymphadenopathy. The oral cavity, soft palate, tonsils, and pharynx might be covered by an adherent, dirty-gray membrane that does not strip easily. The child rapidly becomes ill and might develop respiratory obstruction from involvement of the larynx. Toxic myocarditis might occur. Diagnosis is made on clinical presentation and confirmed by growth of the organism on MacConkey's medium. Treatment, which should begin immediately without waiting for the results of bacteriologic studies, is with diphtheria antitoxin and massive doses of penicillin (1 million units

of penicillin G every 4 hours), given intravenously. Diphtheria can either be fatal or leave a residual neuropathy. The disease can be prevented by immunization with a heat-killed vaccine such as DPT (diphtheria, pertussis, tetanus).

COMPLICATIONS OF BACTERIAL PHARYNGITIS. The more frequent complications of bacterial pharyngitis, in descending order of frequency, are cervical adenitis, which progresses to abscess formation, peritonsillar abscess, infection of the parapharyngeal space,* rheumatic fever, septic emboli, and acute glomerulonephritis. Respiratory obstruction is surprisingly rare.

Peritonsillar Abscess. Peritonsillar abscess results from infection of the potential space between the capsule of the tonsil and the superior constrictor muscle. These abscesses are usually unilateral and are more prevalent among younger adults. The principal symptoms are increasingly severe pain, mainly on one side of the throat and upper neck, severe odynophagia, trismus, and fever.

The soft palate is red, edematous, and bulges on one side. The area of maximal swelling is immediately superolateral to the upper pole of the tonsil. The tonsil is displaced downward, and medially pushing the edematous uvula across the midline (Figure 16.6). There is profuse salivation and tender enlargement of the ipsilateral jugulodigastric lymph node.

There are two methods of treating peritonsillar abscess: initial drainage and antibiotics and tonsillectomy a few weeks later, or, alternatively, initial intravenous antibiotics followed in 24 hours by tonsillectomy (tonsillectomy au chaud).

Drainage is accomplished with topical anesthesia by way of a small stab incision over the point of maximal swelling. A hemostat is passed through the incision into

---

*For a discussion of infection of the parapharyngeal space, see Chapter 19.

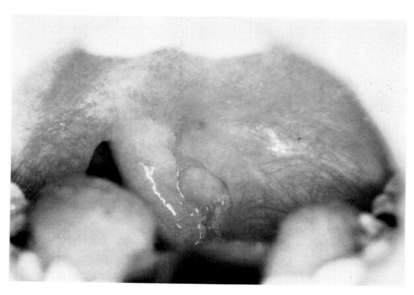

Fig. 16.6. Left peritonsillar abscess. The tonsil is displaced inferomedially, and the swollen uvula is draped over its surface. A large, smooth bulge is present above and just lateral to the superior pole.

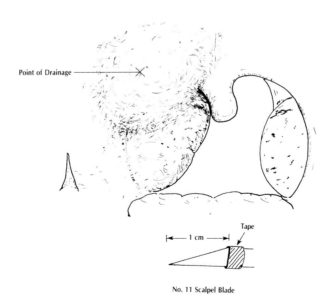

Point of Drainage

Tape

|← 1 cm →|

No. 11 Scalpel Blade

Fig. 16.7. Technique of draining a peritonsillar abscess. A blunt pointed instrument such as a hemostat is inserted into the incision and opened to facilitate drainage.

the abscess and its jaws are opened to increase drainage (Figure 16.7).

TONSILLECTOMY AND ADENOIDECTOMY. These two surgical procedures are frequently performed together. The indications for each, however, are different and should be considered separately, although the indications do sometimes overlap.

Tonsillectomy. The traditional indications for tonsillectomy are recurrent sore throat, recurrent bacterial pharyngitis, peritonsillar abscess, respiratory obstruction, dysphagia, and neoplasms. Pharyngitis is the most frequent indication. Two factors must be considered together: the frequency and severity of episodes. Six episodes per year is commonly accepted as an indication for surgery but five or seven might be equally acceptable. If the attacks are severe, fewer are needed for indicating surgery. Episodes of sore throat should be documented by competent examiners and not by parents, and patients must be assessed individually. The surgical technique of tonsillectomy is described in Chapter 22.

Adenoidectomy. The classic indications for adenoidectomy are respiratory obstruction, recurrent otitis media, and recurrent pharyngitis, but these indications are still loose and controversial. Respiratory obstruction is usually a local problem, with symptoms of nasal stuffiness and snoring. In rare cases, however, the obstruction might be sufficiently severe to cause cor pulmonale, in which case adenoidectomy and tonsillectomy are indicated even as an emergency. For many years partial compromise of the posterior nares was considered harmful. Supposedly, this caused secondary high arching of the palate, narrowing of the maxillary arch, and pectus cavum, although none of these have been conclusively proven.

The size of the adenoid mass can be assessed radiologically by a lateral roentgenogram of the nasopharynx. The role of the adenoid mass in the etiology of otitis media is currently being assessed. Adenoid-ectomy has been, and continues to be, an integral part of the treatment of recurrent otitis media, but no well-controlled prospective studies have been done that support or negate this practice.

Neoplasms of the Pharynx

BENIGN NEOPLASMS. Benign neoplasms of the pharynx are uncommon and are symptomatic only when they grow to a size that is large enough to cause the sensation of a lump in the throat, dysphagia, or obstruction of the airway. Papillomas, fibromas, lipomas, and pleomorphic adenomas of the salivary glands have all been described. Small papillomas are common but are asymptomatic. Benign neoplasms are treated by excision.

JUVENILE ANGIOFIBROMA OF THE NASOPHARYNX. Juvenile angiofibromas are hormone-related, adherent, fibrovascular tumors that occur on the vault of the nasopharynx in pubescent males (never in females). The tumor, which is firmly attached to the basisphenoid, consists of a mixture of fibrous tissue and large, thin-walled sinusoids without muscular walls. They expand in all directions: into the nasal cavity, pterygomaxillary space, and maxillary sinus (causing nasal obstruction and massive epistaxis), into the orbit (causing proptosis), and into the cranial cavity (causing neuropathies).

The primary blood supply to the tumor is the internal maxillary artery, but secondary contributions are acquired from adjacent tissue as the tumor expands, and both the external and internal carotid arterial systems might be involved.

The most frequent presenting symptoms are nasal obstruction and profuse, life-threatening epistaxis in an adolescent male. Angiofibromas are pink masses that are covered by a smooth mucosa and are sometimes visible on anterior and posterior rhinoscopy. The size and extent of the tumor, however, can only be assessed radiologically. Routine roentgenograms may show forward bowing of the posterior wall

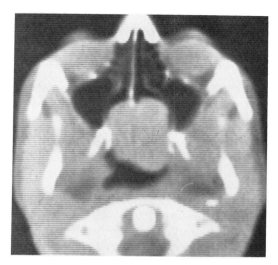

Fig. 16.8. Computed tomography with intravenous contrast in a 16-year-old boy demonstrates a large juvenile angiofibroma in the nasopharynx. The tumor fills the posterior nasal choanae. The presenting symptom was nasal obstruction.

of the maxillary sinus if the pterygomaxillary space is involved. Angiography and computed tomography with intravenous contrast are most helpful in determining the size and blood supply of the tumor (Figure 16.8).

The treatment of a juvenile angiofibroma depends on its size and accessibility. Surgery is the modality of choice but can be hazardous because of the blood loss. Evidence suggests that these tumors may regress partially with estrogen therapy. Therefore, preoperative preparation with estrogens or preoperative embolization of the accessible feeding vessels is advised. Small tumors are removed by a transpalatal approach, but larger tumors may require both transpalatal and transmaxillary sinus approaches. Radiation therapy might control these tumors but is usually reserved for unresectable lesions.

Juvenile angiofibromas supposedly involute spontaneously in early adulthood, but the overall mortality rate is around 3%, mainly from massive epistaxis.

MALIGNANT NEOPLASMS.* The most frequent malignant neoplasm of the pharynx is a squamous cell carcinoma. Lymphomas may originate in or secondarily involve Waldeyer's ring. Malignancies of the pharynx must be considered separately by anatomic area because tumors in each area cause different symptoms. Early lesions are usually asymptomatic. Larger lesions cause soreness of the throat, frequently referred otalgia, dysphagia, odynophagia, and hoarseness if the larynx is involved. Large lesions of the oropharynx and hypopharynx may present with respiratory obstruction. Malignancies of the pharynx metastasize early and may present initially because of an expanding metastatic cervical lymphadenopathy.

CARCINOMA OF THE NASOPHARYNX. Carcinoma of the nasopharynx is prevalent in Southern China, Southeast Asia, Hong Kong, and parts of East and North Africa and is related to infection with the Epstein-Barr virus. Patients with nasopharyngeal carcinoma have high levels of antibodies against the Epstein-Barr virus, but whether the relationship between the two is causal or incidental is still unknown.

Carcinoma of the nasopharynx spreads by infiltration of adjacent structures and metastasizes early. The common presenting symptoms are unilateral, serous otitis media caused by involvement of the eustachian tube, metastatic cervical lymphadenopathy (usually in the posterior triangle), nasal obstruction, and epistaxis. Alternatively, infiltration through the foramen lacerum, which is a common wall between the vault of the nasopharynx and the cavernous sinus, may compromise the fifth, sixth, third, or fourth cranial nerves. The presenting symptoms may then be anesthesia of the cheek and lower jaw, internal strabismus with diplopia, and external ophthalmoplegia, respectively. In-

---

*For a more general discussion of cancer of the head and neck, including malignant neoplasms of the pharynx, see Chapter 20.

filtration of the tumor posteriorly along the base of the skull toward the jugular foramen may cause a jugular foramen syndrome, which is concomitant involvement of the vagus, spinal accessory, and hypoglossal nerves. The presenting symptoms are, therefore, hoarseness, dysphagia, paralysis of the ipsilateral tongue, and paralysis of the sternocleidomastoid and trapezius muscles. The most frequent point of origin of carcinoma of the nasopharynx is the fossa of Rosenmüller, but the neoplasms are usually silent until they grow to substantial size or affect an adjacent structure. They are, however, capable of metastasizing while still only of microscopic size. There are two histologic types of carcinoma of the nasopharynx: squamous cell carcinoma and lymphoepithelioma, which is really an undifferentiated squamous carcinoma with a lymphocytic component. Carcinoma of the nasopharynx can be diagnosed early if the physician is especially suspicious because of the presenting symptoms such as persistent serous effusion in the middle ear of an adult. Definitive diagnosis is dependent on a biopsy, which is done transnasally or transorally. Random biopsies are taken to check for small lesions that are not visible. Any adult with a recent onset of serous otitis media that is unrelated to an upper respiratory tract infection or allergy should be considered to have a nasopharyngeal carcinoma until proven otherwise. Determination of Epstein-Barr virus antibody titers is helpful but not diagnostic. Evaluation of the extent of a nasopharyngeal lesion requires a thorough physical examination of the head and neck, including assessment of the cranial nerves and detailed radiologic study by routine skull roentgenograms and computed tomography (Figure 16.9). Nasopharyngeal carcinoma is treated by radiation therapy. Surgery is anatomically difficlt and usually impossible.

MALIGNANCIES OF THE OROPHARYNX. The tonsil is the most common site of carcinoma of the oropharynx. Other sites are the base of the tongue, faucial pillars, valleculae, and the posterior wall of the pharynx. Symptoms are soreness of the throat, odynophagia, referred otalgia, dysphagia, and cervical lymphadenopathy, usually of the midjugular nodes. Any of these might be the presenting symptom. Diagnosis is made by a thorough physical examination, including mirror examination and palpation. Lesions are firm, exophytic, and usually ulcerated. The tonsil is usually fixed at the time of diagnosis. Radiologic investigation with barium studies and computed tomography are useful to determine the extent of the lesions. All suspicious lesions must be biopsied for histologic study.

Malignancies of the oropharynx are treated by wide surgical excision, radiation therapy, or, more usually, a combination of both modalities.

MALIGNANCIES OF THE LARYNGOPHARYNX. Early malignancies of the laryngopharynx, particularly of the pyriform sinuses, are usually asymptomatic. Later, they may cause dysphagia, odynophagia, hoarseness, and referred otalgia. These le-

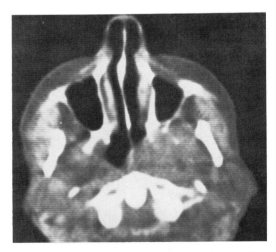

Fig. 16.9. Computed tomography scan of a nasopharyngeal cancer in a 60-year-old woman. A large mass is present in the posterior lateral wall of the nasopharynx, which obliterates the muscle planes in the infratemporal fossa. The pterygoid plates are eroded.

sions frequently present with asymptomatic, metastatic cervical lymphadenopathy. Carcinoma of the laryngopharynx is treated by surgery, radiation therapy, or a combination of both modalities. Malignancies of the posterior pharyngeal wall generally carry a poor prognosis.

Miscellaneous Disorders

PHARYNGEAL PARALYSIS. Unilateral paralysis of the pharyngeal musculature occurs with high lesions of the vagus nerve and lesions of the brainstem (e.g., pseudobulbar palsy, neoplasms of the posterior cranial fossa, stroke).

SYMPTOMS AND PHYSICAL FINDINGS. Four of the essential events for safe swallowing are affected: the ipsilateral soft palate is paralyzed and, therefore, does not ascend to close the velopharyngeal isthmus; the pharyngeal musculature is paralyzed and, therefore, cannot propel a bolus of food downward; the cricopharyngeus muscle fails to relax, which keeps the esophageal inlet closed; and, finally, the ipsilateral vocal cord is paralyzed in abduction and does not adduct to close the glottis. Dysfunction of the vagus nerve, therefore, may cause nasal regurgitation of food, dysphagia, aspiration, particularly of liquids, with the possibility of recurrent pneumonia, and hoarseness.

TREATMENT. Pharyngeal paralysis is most difficult to treat. There are no techniques available for reactivation of the musculature, and thus the treatment is primarily symptomatic. The two major problems are nutrition and aspiration, both of which can be handled by feeding via a nasogastric tube (a soft, weighted, silicone tube is preferred).

The voice can be improved by displacement of the paralyzed vocal cord medially with injection of Teflon paste into the substance of the cord. Occasionally, gastrojejunostomy and tracheostomy are necessary for the more difficult cases.

GLOSSOPHARYNGEAL NEURALGIA. Glossopharyngeal neuralgia is a rare, ill-defined condition that is characterized by unilateral, episodic, sharp, stabbing pain in the throat, which is usually centered around the tonsil. The full-blown syndrome suggests a pharyngeal equivalent of tic douloureux. Pain might be triggered by swallowing, talking, and so on. One possible causative factor is elongation of the styloid process and ossification of the stylohyoid ligament, which causes irritation of the adjacent glossopharyngeal nerve.

Treatment of glossopharyngeal neuralgia is generally unsatisfactory. An elongated styloid process can be shortened, or the rootlets of the glossopharyngeal nerve might be sectioned by an intracranial approach.

PHARYNGOESOPHAGEAL DIVERTICULUM (ZENKER'S DIVERTICULUM). A pharyngoesophageal diverticulum is a herniation of the pharyngeal mucosa in the posterior midline at the junction of the pharynx and esophagus. This is a pulsation diverticulum that occurs in Killian's dihiscence, which is a triangular-shaped

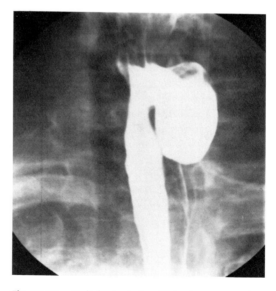

Fig. 16.10. Radiologic study with barium contrast in a 60-year-old man with a moderate-sized pharyngoesophageal diverticulum. The thickened cricopharyngeus muscle forms a common wall between the esophagus anteriorly and the diverticulum posteriorly.

area of potential weakness in the pharyngeal wall that is formed by the obliquely directed lower fibers of the inferior constrictor muscles and the transverse fibers of the cricopharyngeus muscle. Thickening and tightness of the cricopharyngeus muscle and dyskinesia of the esophagus are almost always associated with the disorder. Most diverticula expand posteriorly and to the left of the esophageal inlet, thereby distorting the cervical esophagus and increasing dysphagia.

Pharyngoesophageal diverticula are more frequent in the older age groups but can occur even in young adults. Patients complain initially of slight dysphagia. Later, the dysphagia increases, but regurgitation of food a few minutes or hours after ingestion also develops. Patients also notice a gurgling sensation on swallowing. Large divertiula might cause recurrent aspiration pneumonitis or cachexia from severe dysphagia.

Larger diverticula are sometimes palpable as a soft, compressible, crepitant mass in the lower left neck. Diagnosis is easily confirmed radiologically with a barium swallow (Figure 16.10).

Small diverticula are treated by stretching the cricopharyngeus muscle with esophageal dilators. Larger diverticula can be treated in one of three ways. The diverticulum can be excised via an external incision, while the cricopharyngeus muscle is simultaneously incised to relieve its constriction. Alternatively, the diverticulum can be rotated superiorly and sutured upside down (diverticulopexy) via an external incision. This is useful in older, debilitated patients. Lastly, an endoscopic technique can be used, which consists of using special instruments to excise part of the cricopharyngeus muscle that forms a common wall between the esophagus and the diverticulum. The results of all forms of treatment are generally satisfactory but recurrence is possible.

DISTENTION OF THE PHARYNX. In a few musicians who play wind instruments, particularly trumpet players, the pharynx distends considerably during the act of blowing but then subsides back to normal dimensions. This is primarily a cosmetic problem that requires no specific treatment. True lateral diverticula of the pharynx are rare.

BIBLIOGRAPHY

Bonding, P.: Tonsillectomy a chaud. J. Laryngol., 87:1171–1182, 1973.

Eagle, W.W.: Elongated styloid process: Further observations and new syndrome. Arch. Otolaryngol., 47:630–640, 1948.

Eisback, K.J., and Krause, C.J.: Carcinoma of the pyriform sinuses. A comparison of treatment modalities. Laryngoscope, 87:1904, 1977.

Holinger, P.H., and Schild, J.A.: The Zenker's (hypopharyngeal) diverticulum. Ann. Otolaryngol., 78:679, 1969.

Kornblut, A., and Kornblut, A.D.: Tonsillectomy and adenoidectomy. In Otolaryngology. 2nd Ed. Edited by M.M. Paparella and D. Shumrick. Philadelphia, W.B. Saunders Co., 1980. pp. 2283–2301.

Lederman, M.: Cancer of the Nasopharynx: Its Natural History and Treatment. Springfield, Illinois, Charles C Thomas, 1961.

McGavram, M.H., et al.: Nasopharyngeal angiofibroma. Arch. Otolaryngol., 90:68, 1969.

Ogra, P.L.: Effect of tonsillectomy and adenoidectomy on nasopharyngeal antibody response to polio virus. N. Engl. J. Med., 284:59–64, 1971.

Parkinson, R.H.: Tonsil and Allied Problems. New York, The Macmillan Company, 1951.

Shah, J.P., Shaha, A.P., Spiro, R.H., and Strong, E.W.: Carcinoma of the hypopharynx. Am. J. Surg., 132:439, 1976.

Whicker, J.H., DeSanto, L.W., and Devine, K.D.: Surgical treatment of squamous cell carcinoma of the tonsil. Laryngoscope, 84:90, 1974.

Chapter 17

LARYNX AND TRACHEA

ANATOMY

The Larynx (Voice Box, Adam's Apple)

The larynx is a protective valve in the form of a box which is open above and below and positioned immediately anterior to the esophageal inlet and the cervical spine. It is composed of many cartilages, delicate muscles, ligaments, and tendons, and its internal surface is lined by a smooth mucous membrane. There are two large cartilages: the thyroid and cricoid. The keel-like thyroid cartilage consists of two flat lamina (ala) that are fused in the midline anteriorly and open posteriorly. The cricoid cartilage looks like a signet ring, with a broad, flat, posterior lamina. The cricoid cartilage is the only complete cartilaginous ring and, therefore, the only rigid area in the respiratory tree (Figure 17.1). The arytenoid cartilages are small and pyramid-shaped and perch on top of and articulate with the lamina of the cricoid cartilage by the synovial cricoarytenoid joints. Each arytenoid cartilage has two projections or processes: a vocal process, to which the posterior end of the vocal ligament is attached, and a muscular process, to which the posterior cricoarytenoid muscle is attached. When the posterior cricoarytenoid muscle contracts, the arytenoid cartilages slide and rotate, pulling the vocal cords laterally

(abduction), which opens the glottis (Figure 17.2). Closure of the glottis is accomplished by contraction of the other intrinsic laryngeal muscles. The tiny corniculate cartilages sit on top of the arytenoid cartilages, and the tiny cuneiform cartilages are in the aryepiglottic folds. The epiglottis is a pear-shaped, curved plate of cartilage covered by mucosa on both surfaces and attached to the inner aspect of the anterior thyroid cartilage. The superior half of the epiglottis, above the level of the hyoid bone, projects freely into the oropharynx. The inferior half is posterior to the hyoid bone, thyrohyoid membrane, and the thyroid cartilage and is separated

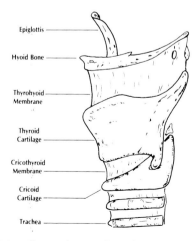

Epiglottis

Hyoid Bone

Thyrohyoid
Membrane

Thyroid
Cartilage

Cricothyroid
Membrane

Cricoid
Cartilage

Trachea

Fig. 17.1. The cartilages and membranes of the larynx.

187

from these structures by the fat-filled pre-epiglottic space. The hyoid bone, which is usually considered with the larynx, forms the junction between the larynx and tongue. This bone provides a solid structure for attachment of the musculature of the tongue and for suspension of the larynx. The hyoid bone also maintains the shape of the pharyngeal lumen.

MUSCLES, LIGAMENTS, AND MEMBRANES OF THE LARYNX. The laryngeal membranes are thin but tough. They close the spaces between the cartilages (Figure 17.3). The three most important membranes are the thyrohyoid membrane between the hyoid bone and thyroid cartilage, the cricothyroid membrane between the cricoid and thyroid cartilages, and the thin conus elasticus whose free edge thickens to form the vocal ligament. Two horizontal ligaments occur on each side: the vocal ligament between the arytenoid and thyroid cartilages and the false vocal cords

or ventricular bands, which are primarily muscular.

The cricothyroid membrane is particularly important because at this point the lumen of the airway is closest to the skin of the neck and, therefore, most accessible in an emergency.

There is an intricate pattern of small muscles in the larynx and most of them are on the luminal side of the cartilages, which control opening and closing of the glottis. The most important of these muscles are the thyroarytenoid or vocalis muscle, the external cricothyroid muscle, and the posterior and lateral cricoarytenoid muscles.

The mucosa of the larynx is lined by a ciliated, columnar, respiratory-type epithelium that changes to squamous epithelium over the vocal cords. The mucosa is thrown into prominent folds over the muscles and ligaments described above. The most important of these are the vocal cords (vocal folds) and the ventricular bands

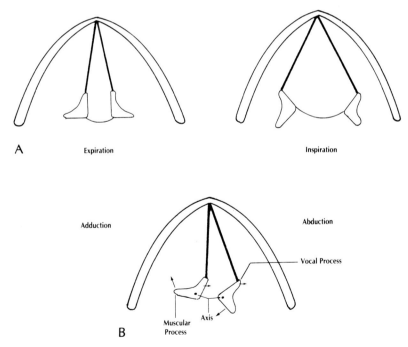

Fig. 17.2. A. Diagram demonstrating the motion of the vocal cords. The arytenoids rotate and slide. B. The motion of the cricoarytenoid joints. The adductor group of muscles pull the muscular process of the arytenoid cartilage anteriorly, while the abductors pull the muscular process posteriorly. The movements of the vocal process swing the cord medially and laterally, respectively.

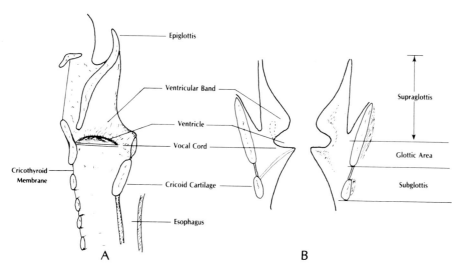

Fig. 17.3. A. Sagittal section of the larynx. The epiglottis is attached to the deep surface of the thyroid cartilage. Note that the cricoid cartilage forms the only completely rigid area in the larynx and trachea. Note also that the airway is most easily accessible through the cricothyroid membrane. B. Coronal section of the larynx. The vocal ligament represents a thickened edge of the fibrous conus elasticus.

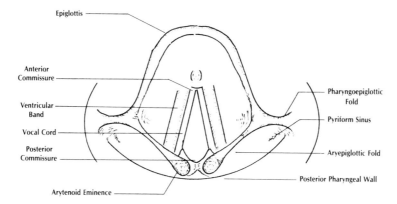

Fig. 17.4. View of the larynx from above. The vocal cords are taut, white bands, while the ventricular bands are pink, thick, muscular structures.

(false cords) (Figure 17.3). The two vocal cords consist of muscles and ligaments that are covered by mucosa and extend from the vocal processes of the arytenoid cartilages to meet at the anterior commissure, where they are anchored to the thyroid cartilages. The ventricular bands, or false vocal cords, are thicker, rounded, and more muscular bands that are above the level of the true cords (Figure 17.4). The ventricles are mucosa-lined spaces between the true and false cords. The aryepiglottic folds are thin mucosal folds containing slender muscles that extend from the lateral edges of the epiglottis to the arytenoid cartilages. The mucous glands of the ventricles secrete mucus to keep the surface of the larynx moist. The larynx is comparatively smaller in infants and children and is generally smaller in females.

NERVE AND BLOOD SUPPLY AND THE LYMPHATIC DRAINAGE OF THE LARYNX. The recurrent laryngeal nerves provide the motor supply to the intrinsic muscles of the larynx and sensory innervation to the subglottis. The superior laryngeal nerves are the motor nerves of the cricothyroid muscles and provide the sensory supply to the supraglottis.

The vocal cords have few lymphatic spaces and poor lymphatic drainage. In contrast, both the supraglottic and subglottic areas are richly supplied with lymphatic vessels. The lymphatic vessels of the supraglottis drain into the ipsilateral midjugular lymph nodes, and those from the subglottis empty into the paratracheal nodes. The lymphatic vessels of the anterior subglottis may drain into the Delphian node, which lies on the anterior surface of the cricothyroid membrane. Malignancies of the vocal cord, therefore, metastasize late, while tumors of the supraglottis and subglottis metastasize early.

The following is a list of pertinent laryngeal anatomic terminology:

Glottis
—the space between the vocal cords.

Supraglottis
—that part of the larynx above the level of the vocal cords. The supraglottis consists of the epiglottis, the aryepiglottic folds, the arytenoid eminences, and the ventricular bands.

Subglottis
—that part of the larynx below the level of the vocal cord, which is bounded by the cricoid cartilage and cricothyroid membrane and delineated inferiorly by the lower border of the cricoid cartilage.

The Trachea (Windpipe)

The trachea is a tubular conduit for air that extends from the lower border of the cricoid cartilage to the carina, where it bi-furcates into right and left mainstem bronchi. The walls of the trachea consist of incomplete rings of cartilage that are open posteriorly, where the ring is completed by muscle. The spaces between the cartilages are sealed by elastic membranes. The lumen of the trachea is lined by a ciliated, columnar, respiratory-type mucosa. The structure of the trachea, therefore, allows it to be a flexible, elastic, distensible organ, while the ringlike cartilages ensure the integrity of its lumen. The infant's trachea is particularly soft and pliable.

The trachea traverses both the neck and superior mediastinum and is immediately anterior to the esophagus and vertebral column. The carotid sheaths and the arch of the aorta are lateral to the trachea. The recurrent laryngeal nerves run in the tracheoesophageal grooves. The lobes of the thyroid gland are anterolateral to the upper trachea, while the isthmus of the thyroid crosses anterior to the third, fourth, and fifth tracheal cartilages. The strap muscles are anterior to the thyroid gland.

The upper end of the trachea is easily palpable in the midline of the neck. As it progresses inferiorly, however, the trachea is more posteriorly placed so that in the young adult male the trachea is about 3 to 5 cm deep to the skin of the suprasternal notch.

PHYSIOLOGY

The Larynx

The larynx has the following functions:

1. To protect the lower respiratory passages.
2. To conduct air to and from the lungs.
3. To function as a vocal organ.
4. To fix the chest in heavy physical effort.
5. To humidify and cleanse inspired air (this is a minimal function).

The primary function of the larynx is its protective, sphincteric action. Vocalization is a secondary function. There are three levels at which closure of the larynx is possible: at the aryepiglottic folds and epiglottis, at the ventricular bands, and at the glottis. During heavy physical effort, the chest wall and diaphragm must be fixed to provide a rigid structure for efficient functioning of the muscles of the trunk. Fixation is achieved by closure of the glottis, which momentarily stiffens the thoracic cage in one position.

The larynx is really a muscular organ and should be considered in the same dimension as the heart, diaphragm, and intercostal muscles, all of which are in constant activity during life. The recurrent laryngeal nerves control the function of the vocal cords, posterior and lateral cricoarytenoid, and the interarytenoid muscles. The superior laryngeal nerve controls the aryepiglottic folds and cricothyroid muscles. Although laryngeal functions would seem to be involuntary (based solely on reflex mechanisms), all laryngeal muscles are striated voluntary muscles. Therefore, nonfunction of the nerve supply causes complete loss of function of the ipsilateral larynx. Movement of the vocal cords toward the midline is known as adduction and movement away from the midline as abduction (Figure 17.2). Adduction, therefore, closes the glottis and abduction opens it. There is only one abductor muscle on each side—the posterior cricoarytenoid.

Voice is produced during expiration by the vibration of the vocal cords, which modulate the periodicity of the column of air. The vocal cords, like any other solid structure, have a natural frequency (i.e., a frequency at which they vibrate most efficiently). This frequency varies with sex and age. In the young adult male the frequency is around 125 Hz, and in the female the frequency is 250 Hz. The proximity and tensions of the vocal cords modify the fundamental, tone-producing, harmonic overtones, which are further modified by the pharynx, palate, tongue, teeth, and skull. The result is a voice that is highly characteristic for each individual. The whole mechanism is finely tuned so that the slightest, most subtle, dysfunction becomes apparent to the speaker.

The Trachea

The trachea is primarily a conduit for air to and from the lungs.

DISORDERS OF THE LARYNX AND TRACHEA

Symptoms of Laryngeal Disorders

Hoarseness, cough, odynophagia, local pain, local swelling, referred otalgia, and aspiration pneumonitis are all possible symptoms that occur either singly or collectively in disorders of the larynx.

Almost all disorders of the larynx cause hoarseness, and the most minimal organic or functional changes will cause subjective changes in the quality of the voice.

In addition to hoarseness, any compromise in the lumen of the larynx will result in stridor. Stridor is a symptom. It is the term that is applied to harsh, noisy inspiration. Expiration is usually less noisy. Stridor is an ominous phenomenon.

Dyspnea can be a symptom of laryngeal compromise and is usually worsened by exertion. Odynophagia is the phenomenon of painful swallowing and is caused by acute inflammatory conditions and some neoplastic lesions of the larynx and pharynx. Aspiration occurs when the sphincteric mechanism of the larynx malfunctions. Attempts at swallowing cause food to pass into the upper trachea, which excites violent coughing. Chronic aspiration causes loss of weight and eventually a pneumonitis. Pain is an uncommon complaint. The patient, however, might complain of a deep-seated soreness of the throat, which is aggravated by swallowing and, sometimes, by speaking. Laryngeal pain is frequently referred to the ear because of common sensory innervation by the vagus nerve. Nonproductive cough is a common symptom of inflammatory laryngeal disease. This is not to be confused with the food-related cough of aspiration.

Physical Findings in Laryngeal Disease

A thorough physical examination of the larynx must include assessment for a shift in position from the midline and external palpation of the larynx, trachea, and the rest of the neck, especially the thyroid gland. Indirect laryngoscopy must be performed, and the chest should be examined in pertinent cases. Obstruction of the upper airway, particularly at the laryngeal level, causes difficulty with inspiration, while obstruction to the lower airway at the level of the mainstem bronchi and more peripherally tends to cause expiratory difficulty and wheezing. With respiratory obstruction, the patient complains of difficulty with breathing, tends to sit or lie quietly, and, if the problem is acute in onset, becomes most apprehensive and anxious. With inspiratory difficulty, retraction of the suprasternal, supraclavicular, and intercostal spaces develops. The patient tends to breathe through his mouth to lessen resistance and fixes his arms by holding the sides of the bed because fixation of the arms assists in expansion of the chest. Examine the patient for cyanosis of the lips and nailbeds, and assess the status of the veins in his neck. The veins in the neck and upper arms dilate and become prominent with an increase in venous pressure. Carefully record the blood pressure and pulse rate because increasing respiratory difficulty speeds up the pulse rate.

The radiology of the larynx has already been discussed in Chapter 2; however, it should be remembered that the subglottic area and the cervical esophagus are not accessible to the examiner by indirect laryngoscopy. Therefore, these areas should be examined radiologically before invasive methods are contemplated.

DIRECT LARYNGOSCOPY (see Chapter 22). As its name implies, indirect laryngoscopy is examination of the larynx by way of reflected light. Direct laryngoscopy is a direct examination through instruments that are passed to the level of the larynx and is performed when the larynx cannot be adequately evaluated by indirect laryngoscopy, or when a biopsy is necessary. Direct laryngoscopy is accomplished through a lighted, tubular laryngoscope that is passed through the mouth or by the use of a fiberoptic instrument that is usually passed transnasally.

Congenital Disorders of the Larynx

Congenital disorders of the larynx are not common but do occur. Only brief descriptions of these disorders are possible in this chapter.*

Infants with congenital stridor might require immediate evaluation; those with cyanosis may need urgent intubation or tracheostomy for survival. If, however, the infant is stridulous but is well oxygenated, a more conservative, less hurried approach is advised. Radiologic examination of the neck and chest might be helpful in identifying an obstructing lesion, or a barium study of the pharynx and esophagus can be diagnostic (e.g., a tracheoesophageal fistula). Occasionally, angiography is indicated to delineate vascular anomalies such as aberrant, large vessels or vascular rings. The symptoms of many congenital anomalies might improve with time, but, alternatively, too-early instrumentation could precipitate the necessity for intubation or tracheostomy, and both of these are best avoided in the infant.

LARYNGOMALACIA. Laryngomalacia is a condition in which the supraglottic tissues lack resiliency. This causes the epiglottis to be sucked into the airway on inspiration. The infant is, therefore, stridulous but is usually not cyanotic, and the stridor can be relieved by lying the infant on its abdomen. These children do not have difficulty with feeding and do not

---

*For a discussion of tracheoesophageal fistulae, see Chapter 18.

aspirate their food. Laryngomalacia is easily diagnosed on direct laryngoscopy because the stridor is immediately relieved by holding the epiglottis forward. Laryngomalacia improves spontaneously and is usually substantially resolved by the time the infant is 1 year old.

CONGENITAL GLOTTIC WEBS. Fine webs between the vocal cords are not uncommon. They may be short and confined to the anterior cords or much larger, reducing the glottis to a small, posteriorly placed aperture (Figure 17.5). Glottic webs cause hoarseness or a voice of a higher pitch. They are treated surgically by lysis, and the cut edges are kept apart by a thin splint of alloplastic material. Unless the patency of the glottis demands early attention, surgical correction of glottic webs is best performed on an older child or even a young adult.

CONGENITAL STENOSIS OF THE LARYNX. Fortunately, congenital stenosis of the larynx is rare. Stenosis occurs at the glottic and subglottic levels and in varying degrees from mild to complete obstruction of the laryngeal lumen. Severe forms require immediate tracheostomy (see Chapter 22).

CONGENITAL HEMANGIOMA. Hemangiomas may occur in the larynx of the newborn. They are usually, but not always, associated with hemangiomas elsewhere. The infant might not have any difficulty initially but develops progressive stridor over the course of a few weeks, or stridor is precipitated by the first respiratory tract infection. Congenital hemangiomas might regress spontaneously but must be treated if the airway is excessively compromised. Treatment might be by corticosteroids, radiation therapy, or excision with a CO_2 laser.

VASCULAR ANOMALIES. Anomalies of the major arteries of the neck and thorax might compromise the lumen of the trachea and cause dyspnea in the neonate and young child. A number of anomalies of the major branches of the aortic arch are possible. Most of these anomalies are rare and the most important involve the subclavian artery. The right subclavian artery sometimes arises from the left side of the aortic arch and then courses between the trachea and esophagus. In this position the

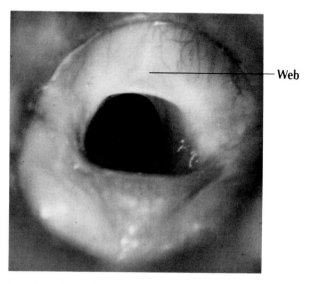 — **Web**

Fig. 17.5. Anterior glottic web. A thin web is present between the anterior two-third of the vocal cords (photo courtesy of G. Healy, M.D.).

vessel produces a pulsating prominence in the anterior wall of the esophagus and a similar prominence on the posterior wall of the trachea. Patients with this disorder may have difficulty with swallowing or breathing, depending on which channel is more compromised. Dysphagia might present in middle or old age.

Diagnosis is usualy first made on endoscopy and confirmed with angiography. Treatment is by ligature of the subclavian artery. Occasionally, a prosthetic bypass is necessary.

In rare cases the subclavian artery or the aorta bifurcates to form an arterial ring around the trachea, which is severely constricted just above the carina.

CONGENITAL CYSTS. In rare cases embryonal cysts may cause laryngeal obstruction in the neonate. They are treated by marsupialization.

Trauma to the Larynx

Laryngeal trauma can be either external or internal. The incidence of trauma to the larynx is increasing because of the greater use of endotracheal tubes and the rising numbers of vehicular accidents. External trauma usually occurs from blunt instruments and might consist of a variety of injuries. The commonest and least dangerous is slight bruising of the soft tissues. Alternatively, excessive bleeding into the laryngeal tissues might occur, with acute luminal obstruction. The laryngeal cartilages fracture if sufficient force is applied. Compromise of the airway results from the displacement of fragments, swelling of soft tissues, or from dysfunction of the vocal cords. Subcutaneous emphysema develops if the laryngeal or pharyngeal mucosa is torn. Laryngeal trauma is one of the causes of rapid roadside death after automobile accidents. Any patient with a history of trauma to the neck should be evaluated for laryngeal injury and should be examined for hoarseness, swelling of the neck, particularly around the larynx, and subcutaneous emphysema. The laryngeal prominence might be flattened (Figure 17.6). All injuries cause hoarseness or even aphonia. If a laryngeal injury is suspected, indirect laryngoscopy should be attempted gently. The patient should not be left unattended, and the facilities for an immediate intubation and/or tracheostomy must be available. Mild injuries can be treated expectantly, but more severe injuries, and especially fractures, will require tracheostomy followed by open reduction of fragments, repair of mucosal tears, and intraluminal splints, as indicated.

LARYNGEAL TRAUMA FROM INTUBATION. Probably the most common

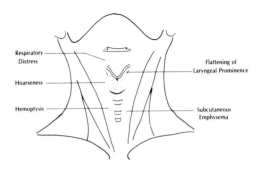

Fig. 17.6. Important points in the diagnosis of fractures of the larynx. Subcutaneous emphysema can be massive.

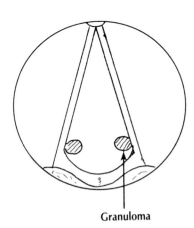

Fig. 17.7. Intubation granuloma. These characteristically develop at the tips of the vocal processes and are usually caused by pressure necrosis.

cause of laryngeal trauma today is the use of the endotracheal tube. Trauma is more likely when relatively larger tubes and vigorous manipulation are used. Two sites of injury are possible: the tips of the vocal processes, at the junction of the posterior and middle thirds of the vocal cords, and the subglottic area. Granular polyps develop on the vocal processes (intubation granulomas), cause hoarseness, and may persist unless removed surgically (Figure 17.7).

An excessively large tube will erode the mucosa of the subglottic area at the level of the rigid cricoid cartilage. An annular stricture forms within a few weeks of extubation. Some of these strictures respond to periodic dilatation and local infiltration with corticosteroids, while others require extensive surgery. Excision of the stricture with a CO_2 laser via an endoscope seems to hold great promise.

VOCAL CORD NODULES (SINGER'S NODES). These are small masses of fibrous tissue that represent organized hematomas and characteristically develop at the junction of the anterior and middle thirds of the free edge of the vocal cords (Figure 17.8) (i.e., at the maximum point of vibration on the cords). Nodules are caused by trauma from vocal abuse and frequently occur in professional singers. Nodules are removed surgically, one side at a time,

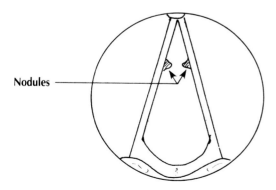

Fig. 17.8. Nodules on the vocal cords. The characteristic position is on the free edge of the cord at the junction of anterior and middle thirds.

preferably with the aid of the operating microscope for accuracy and to prevent "notching" of the free edge of the cord.

Inflammatory Diseases of the Larynx

Inflammatory diseases of the larynx might be either infective or allergic. The infection might be viral, bacterial, or fungal.

Symptoms

Hoarseness, soreness of the throat, pain on swallowing, respiratory difficulty, including stridor, nonproductive cough, and fever are all symptoms that are possible with laryngitis. Stridor and severe pain are ominous signs, which are usually associated with epiglottitis.

Viral Infections

Viral infection is by far the commonest cause of laryngitis and is more frequently associated with upper and lower respiratory tract infections (laryngotracheobronchitis). The patient complains of a sore throat, hoarseness, mild fever, and a dry, nonproductive cough. The pharyngeal and laryngeal mucosa are minimally hyperemic and lose their luster. Treatment is primarily symptomatic because the condition resolves spontaneously in 5 to 10 days. Gargling with warm, diluted, saline solution and various lozenges are soothing. Use of a humidifier (vaporizer) is advised, and steam inhalations are soothing.

Bacterial Infections

Bacterial infections of the larynx are, fortunately, not as common as viral infections. β-hemolytic streptococci and Hemophilus influenzae are usually the offending organisms. There is fever, severe odynophagia, hoarseness, and coughing. The patient is much more ill than he would be with viral laryngitis. The arytenoid eminences are red and swollen and the vocal cords are edematous but mobile. Treatment is with antibiotics given in large doses, preferably intravenously. All patients with acute bacterial laryngitis should be kept under close observation because of the danger of acute obstruction of the airway. Abscesses sometimes develop.

ACUTE EPIGLOTTITIS (ACUTE SUPRAGLOTTITIS). This is a most dangerous condition, which primarily afflicts children but may also affect adults. The usual infecting organism is Hemophilus influenzae. There is cherry red swelling of the epiglottis, aryepiglottic folds, arytenoid eminences, and ventricular bands (Figure 17.9). Edema might increase rapidly. The child complains of a sore throat and pain on swallowing, is febrile and lethargic, and has increased salivation and drools. He becomes stridulous and apprehensive and sits upright with his neck extended for easier breathing. The diagnosis of epiglottitis must be made on the history and clinical picture because even gentle depression of the tongue might precipitate acute obstruction of the airway. Once the diagnosis is made, the patient should be admitted to a hospital. If the symptoms are still mild, obtain a lateral roentgenogram

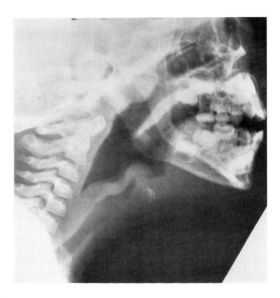

Fig. 17.10. Acute epiglottitis. Lateral roentgenogram of the neck in a 4-year-old child with acute epiglottitis. The epiglottis and aryepiglottic folds are swollen. The hypopharynx is widely dilated, which is a sign of obstruction at the laryngeal level. Note the extended position of the head and neck.

of the neck (Figure 17.10) and begin treatment immediately with intravenous ampicillin or chloramphenicol. If, however, there is severe compromise of the airway the child should be intubated with a nasotracheal tube or a tracheostomy should be performed. These procedures are best undertaken in an operating room under general anesthesia administered by an experienced anesthetist. Intubation is usually required for 3 to 5 days. Extubation should be done under ideal conditions in an operating room because reintubation or a tracheostomy might be necessary.

Acute epiglottitis must always be considered to be a dire emergency because of the danger of sudden respiratory obstruction and death.

CROUP. Like stridor, croup is a symptom that is characterized by hoarseness, a resounding dry cough, and difficulty with breathing. Croup is caused by subglottic

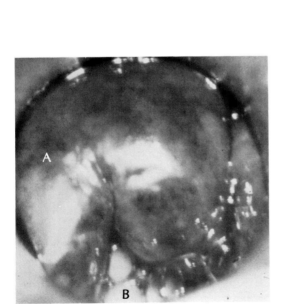

Fig. 17.9. Acute epiglottitis. The epiglottis is grossly swollen, red, and fluctuant. A. Swollen epiglottis. B. Endotracheal tube. The child has been intubated (photo courtesy of G. Healy, M.D.).

swelling, is common in children, and is usually caused by viral laryngotracheo-bronchitis. Although most cases of inflammatory croup run a benign course, a few progress to respiratory obstruction. The child with croup should, therefore, be assessed carefully and should be hospitalized for close observation if indicated. Treatment is with high humidity in a mist tent, antibiotics, and corticosteroids. If respiration becomes increasingly difficult, as indicated by a rise in respiratory and pulse rates, the child should be intubated with a small nasotracheal tube or a tracheostomy performed.

SPASMODIC CROUP (LARYNGISMUS STRIDULUS). This is not truly a croup. It afflicts infants, young children, and even adults. Characteristically, nocturnal episodes of abrupt onset of stridor occur that persist until the patient beomes exhausted and then suddenly regress spontaneously. Laryngismus stridulus can be secondary to hypocalcemia, such as occurs in hypoparathyroidism, or might be idiopathic. A thorough, direct examination of the larynx must be performed to rule out organic lesions.

DIPHTHERIA. Diphtheria is not a disease of the past. Its clinical presence is entirely dependent on effective immunization programs. If immunization lapses within a community, diphtheria quickly recurs.

Diphtheria is an infection caused by a virulent form of Corynebacterium diphtheriae. The common sites of involvement are the oropharynx, larynx, tracheobronchial tree, and nose. Shallow ulcers covered by an adherent, dirty-gray membrane develop, which bleed easily if the membrane is removed. Fetor oris and marked toxicity are also present. If the larynx is involved, there is great danger that respiratory obstruction will occur, which would demand intubation or a tracheostomy. Treatment is with antitoxin serum and high doses of penicillin given intravenously.

SYPHILITIC LARYNGITIS. Syphilis might affect the larynx in either its secondary or tertiary phases. Secondary syphilis causes an acute inflammatory reaction that might even mimic acute epiglottitis. In tertiary syphilis gummas are present, which are extremely destructive and may cause necrosis of the laryngeal cartilages. The larynx becomes grossly distorted with scars and adhesions. Serologic tests for syphilis are positive. Treatment is with large doses of penicillin given parenterally (2.5 million units weekly for three doses).

TUBERCULOUS LARYNGITIS. Tuberculosis of the larynx is usually secondary to advanced pulmonary tuberculosis. The patient complains of horseness and sometimes of pain. The laryngeal mucosa at first becomes reddened and swollen, particularly over the vocal cords and ventricular bands. Ulcers typically develop at the posterior commissure.

Treatment is with antituberculous medications such as streptomycin, isoniazid, and ethambutol.

Fungal Infections (Candidiasis, Blastomycosis)

Fungal infections of the larynx are uncommon; however, an increasing incidence is probably occurring secondary to immunosuppression by chemotherapy and radiation therapy for malignancies. The commonest organisms in these cases are the Candida species, which causes superficial ulcers on the epiglottis, ventricular bands, and even the subglottic area. The patient complains of a sore throat, hoarseness, and odynophagia. Frequently, concomitant lesions are present in the mouth. Diagnosis is made by indirect laryngoscopy, by sampling of sputum, and swabs from the larynx for microscopic examination and culture. Treatment is with amphotericin B.

Chronic Laryngitis

Chronic laryngitis is a somewhat ill-defined term that covers many different entities. Patients have long-standing hoarseness, with a rough gravelly voice but without local or referred pain. Chronic laryngitis may be caused by abuse of the voice or by irritative factors such as tobacco, alcohol, or gastroesophageal reflux, which might occur even in the young child. Children with cleft palates are prone to chronic laryngitis and develop vocal cord nodules because of their inherent difficulty with speech.

In chronic laryngitis the laryngeal mucosa is generally thickened, and the vocal cords are pink and slightly swollen but are mobile.

CONTACT ULCERS. Severe, persistent, vocal cord abuse may cause ulceration at the tips of the vocal processes. These are known as contact ulcers. Contact ulcers are shallow, covered by a white or yellow membrane, and may cause pain on speaking and swallowing. They are sometimes also secondary to gastroesophageal reflux.

All cases of chronic laryngitis should be thoroughly investigated for causative factors. A detailed history, including personal habits, use of the voice, and symptoms of stomach disorders, is essential. Contrast radiography of the upper gastrointestinal tract with the appropriate positional maneuvers are sometimes diagnostic. Direct laryngoscopy and biopsy should be performed in the high-risk, heavy consumer of alcohol and tobacco. Persistent contact ulcers should also be biopsied.

The treatment of chronic laryngitis depends on its cause. All irritative factors should be eliminated. The voice should be rested for 6 to 8 weeks, and intensive speech therapy is helpful in most cases, particularly for contact ulcers.

Vocal Cord Polyps

Polypoid degeneration of the vocal cords is a disorder of middle age and is more prevalent in females. Polyps might involve the entire length of the anterior two-thirds of the true vocal cords but can be localized to a smaller area. Polyps are caused by edema of the subepidermal space, "Reinke's space," but the cause of these changes is unknown. Many, but not all, patients with polypoid laryngitis are heavy smokers and some are long-term vocal cord abusers. Vocal cord polyps are benign and almost never become malignant. They may stay at the same size for a long time. Some grow slowly but seldom cause respiratory obstruction.

Vocal cord polyps are treated by stripping the edematous epithelium from the vocal cords, one cord at a time, with a 6-week interval.

Neoplasms of the Larynx

The majority of neoplasms of the larynx are squamous cell carcinomas. Benign neoplasms are comparatively uncommon if polyps are considered to be non-neoplastic.

Smoking predisposes to carcinoma of the larynx. A twofold increase in risk occurs with consumption of 30 cigarettes per day. Therefore, persistent hoarseness in a heavy smoker must be viewed with suspicion. Moderate to heavy, regular consumption of alcohol acts synergistically with smoking to increase the incidence of carcinoma of the larynx.

Symptoms

Neoplasms of the larynx cause hoarseness early if they involve the vocal cords or cricoarytenoid joints. If, however, they do not originate in these areas, hoarseness might be a comparatively late symptom. Other symptoms that occur late are pain in the throat, referred otalgia, dysphagia, and respiratory obstruction.

Physical examination must include indirect laryngoscopy, palpation of the laryngeal cartilages and neck, and examination of the nose, oral cavity, and pharynx. Ancillary techniques are necessary to determine the extent of the tumor. These techniques include direct laryngoscopy under anesthesia, laryngography, and multidirectional and/or computed tomography. Ten percent of patients with carcinoma of the larynx develop a synchronous or metachronous secondary primary bronchial malignancy. Therefore, the lungs of these patients must always be thoroughly examined. Radiography of the chest and bronchosocopy are minimal investigative requirements.

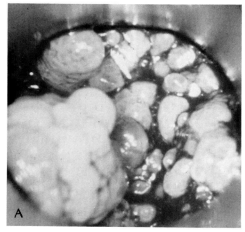

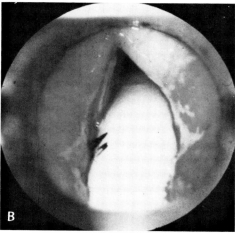

Fig. 17.11.   A. Juvenile laryngeal papilloma. Masses of papillomatous growths are present on the vocal cord. These caused hoarseness and obstruction of the airway (photo courtesy of G. Healy, M.D.). B. Same case as in Figure 17.11A. The vocal cords after removal of papillomas with the CO_2 laser. An endotracheal tube is positioned in the posterior glottis.

Benign Neoplasms

The most frequent benign neoplasms of the larynx are squamous papillomas. Papillomas occur in the larynx in two age goups: the young child and in the middle-aged to elderly. The pattern suggests two different diseases, although the lesions are identical histologically.

JUVENILE PAPILLOMAS. Juvenile papillomas occur on the larynx, palate, and pharynx in young children, even in the newborn. There is a definite relationship between maternal condyloma acuminata and the incidence of juvenile papillomas. Both are probably caused by a papova-type virus. Juvenile papillomas usually present with progressive hoarseness and later with increasing respiratory difficulty. Therefore, every young child who presents with progressive hoarseness is suspected of having laryngeal papillomas. These lesions are pink, sessile, cauliflower-like masses that grow profusely on the vocal cords and supraglottic areas (Figure 17.11). They then spread inferiorly into the subglottis and trachea and even to the bronchi. Treatment is by surgical removal, and the CO_2 laser is now the instrument of choice because of its accuracy. Treatment with vaccines has had varying results and is still being evaluated. Papillomas quickly implant on traumatized mucosa, and, as far as is possible, trauma to the respiratory mucosa should be avoided. Tracheostomy is performed only if absolutely necessary. In a number of patients spontaneous regression occurs in puberty, while in other patients the papillomas persist into adulthood. A small number of juvenile papillomas become malignant.

Papillomas occurring in middle-aged to elderly adults tend to be more localized, confined to the vocal cords, and have little tendency to spread to the lower respiratory tract.

Many other benign tumors of the larynx have been described: neuromas, chondromas, fibromas, and granular cell myoblastoma. Most of these tumors cause hoarseness or respiratory obstruction and are treated by surgical excision.

Malignant Neoplasms

For a more general discussion of head and neck cancer, including malignant neoplasms of the larynx, see Chapter 20. Laryngeal carcinoma accounts for about 4% of all malignancies. Males predominate, with a 7:1 ratio, and 80% of laryngeal cancers occur in the 50- to 70-year-old age group. Carcinoma of the larynx is clinically subdivided into glottic, supraglottic, and subglottic in descending order of incidence. "Glottic" refers to lesions on the vocal cords. Supraglottic refers to lesions above the level of the vocal cords, and subglottic refers to lesions in the subglottic space, whose lower limit is the inferior border of the cricoid cartilage.

CARCINOMA OF THE VOCAL CORDS. Carcinoma of the vocal cords is frequently unilateral and usually begins on the free edge of the anterior two-thirds of the cord. Leukoplakia or dyskeratosis might precede frank malignancy.

Initially, part of the anterior two-thirds of the cords becomes pink, with a rough-ened, pebbly surface. Even at this early stage, the patient recognizes a change in the quality of his voice. Tumefaction occurs at one area, usually along the free edge of the cord (Figure 17.12). Exophytic tumors grow toward the glottis and prevent complete apposition of the cords, which increases hoarseness. Ulcerative lesions infiltrate into the thyroarytenoid (vocalis) muscle and thereby cause a loss of mobility (fixation) of the cord.

Glottic lesions are classified in the TNM system according to the size of the lesions, and the mobility of the vocal cord, as discussed in Chapter 20.

There are few lymphatic channels in the vocal cords, while the paraglottic laryngeal muscles are richly supplied with lymphatic vessels. Therefore, lesions confined to the vocal cord have a low incidence of metastases, while tumors that have spread beyond the cords metastasize more readily. Accordingly, the five-year survival rates fall off precipitously from 85% for cordal lesions to 20% if there are nodal metastases at the time of diagnosis. Thus, early diagnosis is obviously the key to successful treatment of glottic carcinoma.

The patient complains of hoarseness early in the disease. Hoarseness persists and progresses gradually. Pain is a late symptom. Larger tumors eventually cause respiratory obstruction. Later, the tumor metastasizes, first to the midjugular lymph nodes of the neck and then to more distant sites (e.g., the lung).

The treatment of glottic lesions depends on the stage of disease at presentation. T1 lesions (i.e., lesions that are confined to a mobile vocal cord) are treated with equal success by surgery or radiation therapy and have an 85% cure rate. Radiation therapy has become the modality of choice because it preserves the vocal mechanism. Surgery consists of a cordectomy, usually via a "laryngofissure" in which the thyroid cartilage is split anteriorly for access. Alternatively, a cordectomy can be performed via a laryngoscope with a CO_2 laser.

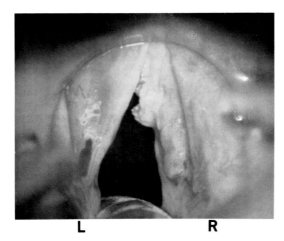

L   R

Fig. 17.12. Carcinoma of the right vocal cord. A granular exophytic lesion involves the anterior two-thirds of the cord (photo courtesy of C. Vaughan, M.D.).

T2 lesions are usually treated by radiation therapy, with surgery reserved for recurrence of disease. In some centers, however, T2 lesions are treated primarily by more extensive surgery that consists of a vertical hemilaryngectomy (see Chapter 22).

T3 lesions are treated with a combination of surgery and radiation therapy. Surgery consists of a total laryngectomy with or without a radical neck dissection (see Chapter 22).

CARCINOMA OF THE SUPRAGLOTTIC LARYNX. Supraglottic lesions are usually more aggressive than glottic lesions and tend to metastasize earlier. They may cause symptoms, as described above, but might be asymptomatic, presenting only when a metastasis to a cervical node becomes obvious. Small T1 lesions are treated with radiation therapy. Larger lesions that are confined above the level of the mobile vocal cords are treated by surgery. The preferred surgical procedure is a supraglottic laryngectomy (see Chapter 22). This is really a horizontal hemilaryngectomy with removal of the epiglottis and all other tissue above the level of the vocal cords. The vocal cords and arytenoid cartilages are left in place. A supraglottic laryngectomy is usually, but not always, performed in continuity with a radical neck dissection.

CARCINOMA OF THE SUBGLOTTIS. Subglottic lesions are, fortunately, rare. They are aggressive and tend to metastasize early to the paratracheal lymph nodes. They carry a poor prognosis and are best treated by a wide-field laryngectomy, followed by radiation therapy.

Cysts of the Larynx

A variety of cysts and cystlike structures may be found in the larynx. Mucous retention cysts occur on the vocal cords, ventricular bands, and epiglottis. Laryngeal cysts are treated by excision or marsupialization.

LARYNGOCELE. A laryngocele is an idiopathic, probably developmental, dilatation of the laryngeal ventricle that usually presents in middle-aged adults. The dilated sac, which communicates with the saccule of the ventricle, expands laterally and may herniate through the thyrohyoid membrane. This sac then becomes visible as an elastic swelling, adjacent to the larynx, which bulges on coughing. On laryngoscopy there is smooth, rounded expansion of the ipsilateral ventricular band. Patients may present because of swelling in the neck or dyspnea. The laryngocele may become acutely infected, with rapidly progressive respiratory obstruction and should, therefore, be excised electively.

Neoplasms of the Trachea

Fortunately, neoplasms of the trachea are rare. They present with asthma-like symptoms and, therefore, remain unrecognized until the tracheal lumen is severely compromised. Most tracheal neoplasms are malignant and few are surgically resectable at diagnosis. Radiation is, therefore, the usual form of therapy.

Paralysis of the Vocal Cords

Paralysis of the vocal cords is caused by dysfunction of the motor nerves, disorders of the cricoarytenoid joints, and disorders of the intrinsic musculature of the larynx. Paralysis might be unilateral or bilateral. Unilateral paralysis is more frequent, and the left cord is more usually involved.

There are five positions in which the vocal cord might come to rest: median, paramedian, intermediate, slight abduction, and full abduction. Clinically, only three are relevant: median, paramedian, and abduction (Figure 17.13). The paralyzed vocal cord generally adopts a position off the median. There are, however, no rules that determine the ultimate position of the paralyzed cord. In unilateral paralysis the voice is hoarse and breathy because of "air waste" during phonation with one cord in abduction. If the cord is in the median position, the voice might be

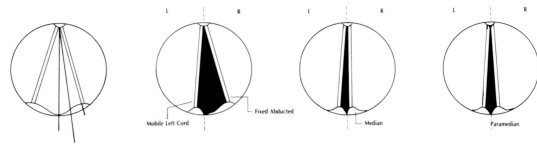

Fig. 17.13. The more frequent positions adopted by a paralyzed vocal cord (here, the right cord). Note the relative sizes of the glottis with the mobile left cord in the medial "phonatric" positions.

quite normal. Breathing is usually unaffected with unilateral paralysis.

If both cords are paralyzed, they usually adopt a median or paramedian position. Voice remains adequate but somewhat flat. Breathing is a problem, and dyspnea might occur, even at rest, in which case a tracheostmy is necessary.

Both unilateral and bilateral paralysis of the vocal cords may be associated with aspiration of saliva and food.

NEUROGENIC PARALYSIS. The motor nerves of the vocal cords are the recurrent laryngeal nerves, which are branches of the vagus nerves. The superior laryngeal nerves are mixed nerves that are primarily sensory to the supraglottis and motor to the cricothyroid muscles, which tense the vocal cords but are not involved in cord motion. Therefore, any lesion along the pathway of the upper vagus and recurrent laryngeal nerves will cause paralysis of the ipsilateral vocal cord. At the level of the brainstem and jugular foramen other associated neurologic deficits are easily identified. In the posterior cranial fossa and in the jugular foramen, dysfunction of the vagus nerve is most frequently caused by neoplasms. In the neck the vagus nerve might be involved by primary neurogenic tumors or primary and metastatic carcinoma. Penetrating injuries may injure the vagus nerve. In the superior mediastinum both the vagus and recurrent laryngeal nerves might be involved by primary tu-

mors or an expanding aneurysm of the aortic arch.

The recurrent laryngeal nerves travel for long distances when they leave the main trunk of the vagus to their destination in the endolarynx. The left recurrent nerve hooks around the aortic arch, and the right nerve hooks around the right subclavian artery. In the chest the left recurrent laryngeal nerve is sometimes compressed by a dilated left cardiac atrium (e.g., in mitral valve stenosis) or by expanding hilar lymphadenopathy (e.g., from bronchial carcinoma). Both recurrent nerves might be involved in peripheral-type carcinoma of the apices of the lung or malignancies of the esophagus and thyroid glands. Both nerves are also vulnerable during surgery on the thyroid gland. A significant number of unilateral, particularly left-sided, paralyses of the vocal cords are idiopathic, possibly viral. Other causes of recurrent nerve dysfunction are diabetic neuropathy, pressure from the cuff of endotracheal tubes, and during cardiovascular surgery.

DISORDERS OF THE CRICOARYTENOID JOINTS. The arytenoid cartilage might be dislocated during endotracheal intubation. This is more likely to occur in difficult or emergency intubations. The arytenoid cartilage is displaced to one side, usually laterally. The usual eminence of the arytenoid becomes more rounded, and the vocal cord is fixed in an intermediate position. The cricoarytenoid joint might be acutely involved in rheumatoid arthritis that has usually been previously documented in other joints. Patients complain of acute onset of hoarseness and pain on swallowing. The arytenoid eminences are red and edematous. Later, the joint becomes fixed.

The intrinsic musculature of the larynx becomes nonfunctional from invasion by neoplasm. In rare cases laryngeal muscle dysfunction is an expression of myasthenia gravis, in which case the voice gradually weakens during conversation.

As can be seen, paralysis of the vocal cord may be caused by many factors occurring over a wide anatomic area. Investigation, therefore, requires a thorough physical examination of the larynx, cranial nerves, neck, thyroid gland, heart, and lungs. Roentgenographic study of the skull, including the skull base and jugular foramina, esophagus, and chest, are essential. Radioactive studies of the thyroid gland should be performed. Routine blood studies, including a glucose tolerance test, are indicated.

The treatment of paralysis of the vocal cord depends on its cause. A number of idiopathic paralyses recover spontaneously. Compression lesions of recent onset might recover with relief of the pressure. Paralysis from neoplastic infiltration and surgical or traumatic incision do not recover. End-to-end anastomosis of the freshly sectioned recurrent laryngeal nerve might work but is seldom possible.

In unilateral paralysis the quality of the voice can be improved by the injection of Teflon paste into the paralyzed cord so that the edge of the cord lies closer to the median position. In bilateral abductor paralysis dyspnea usually necessitates a tracheostomy. The voice, however, is acceptable. Breathing can be significantly improved by the King procedure, in which one arytenoid cartilage is anchored laterally to provide a 4 mm wide glottis. The quality of the voice diminishes, but the tracheostomy can be removed.

Disorders of Speech

Speech is an acquired function. It is not instinctive. The development of speech depends on the ability to hear. The infant first hears sounds that are repeated many times. He associates these sounds with pleasant or unpleasant circumstances, and eventually he becomes aware of his own ability to produce a noise. Infants begin to babble and "coo" around the age of 6 months. The child soon begins his own attempt at speech by mimicking what he hears. "Mama" or "dada" are the easiest and usually the first words, spoken around the age of 1 year. At around 20 months the child has developed a vocabulary of about 20 words, but his understanding of the spoken word improves much faster so that he can follow simple requests and commands. By the age of 30 months the child uses a few sentences, and by the age of 40 to 50 months he can hold a simple conversation.

A child who does not hear has great difficulty in learning speech. Therefore, if a young child shows no development of speech, the first step is to evaluate his hearing. By the same token, the development of speech, even in an otherwise normal child, depends on constant stimulation. Lack of stimulation results in poor, and sometimes grossly retarded, speech patterns. Poor articulation is also caused by defective hearing, particularly if the child has great discrepancies in auditory thresholds for low and higher frequencies so that only part of a spoken word is heard. If hearing loss is documented, a hearing aid or other form of management must be provided immediately and speech therapy begun. Speech might not develop in the severely mentally retarded or autistic child.

APHASIA AND DYSPHASIA. Aphasia is the loss of language, and dysphasia is a difficulty with language. Both conditions are disorders of the central nervous system and are usually brought on by sudden dysfunction of the speech centers (Broca's area) (e.g., as occurs in stroke). Dysphasia can be simply classified into two types: motor and sensory. In motor dysphasia the patient may understand the spoken or written word but has difficulty in expressing his thoughts. For instance, he may wish to say "come here" but says "Tuesday" instead. In sensory dysphasia, on the other hand, the patient has difficulty in understanding spoken or written language but can speak and express his own thoughts. Fortunately, acute dysphasia from a stroke frequently resolves spontaneously.

Disorders of Voice

Hoarseness is the most frequent voice disorder. Hoarseness might be caused by a variety of factors: congenital webs, inflammatory disorders, trauma to the larynx, neoplasms, paralysis of the vocal cords, and can even be psychosomatic.

APHONIA AND DYSPHONIA. The sudden loss of voice or difficulty in producing a voice is usually a psychosomatic (functional) problem. Functional dysphonia is much more prevalent among young women and presents as a sudden loss of voice, usually after emotional trauma. On indirect laryngoscopy the vocal cords look normal and have normal motion. They approximate normally with coughing. Treatment is directed at the underlying problem.

SPASTIC DYSPHONIA. Spastic dysphonia is characterized by a spasmodic, tight, quivering, jerky voice that seems to require great effort. It is a disorder of middle-aged men and women. The vocal cords do appear to be in a constant, jerky, fluttering, asynchronous motion. The cause of spastic dysphonia is not clear, but evidence suggests neuronal degeneration. Severe spastic dysphonia can be helped by section of one recurrent laryngeal nerve.

DYSPHONIA PLICAE VENTRICULARIS. This is a somewhat ill-defined entity in which excessive approximation of the ventricular bands (false cords) occurs. The voice is rough and flat and has many overtones. Dysphonia plicae ventricularis is helped by intensive speech therapy.

The Management of Acute Obstruction of the Upper Airway

Obstruction of the upper airway can be diagnosed by observation and listening to the patient's pattern of breathing. The following is a list of the signs of respiratory insufficiency:*

1. Visual signs
   —abnormal rate of respiration
   —gasping and breathing with great effort
   —retraction of intercostal, suprasternal, and substernal tissues
   —cyanosis
   —sweating
   —obvious fright and apprehension
   —prominent contraction of the sternocleidomastoid muscles and other muscles of the neck
2. Tactile signs
   —pulse very fast, very slow, or irregular
   —cold, clammy skin
3. Auditory signs
   —silence
   —stridor
   —wheezing
   —gurgling

The following is a list of the equipment that is required to manage upper airway obstruction:

Ambu bag
Face masks
Oral airway
Nasopharyngeal airway
Endotracheal tubes
Laryngoscope
Suction apparatus
Tracheostomy set

---

*(Adapted from Applebaum, E.L. and Bruce, D.L.: Tracheal Intubation. Philadelphia, W.B. Saunders, 1975.)

Tracheostomy tubes
Instruments for cricothyrotomy

In all hospitals and clinics this collection of equipment should be kept on a mobile emergency cart.

In the management of acute obstruction of the airway the primary objective is to ensure that sufficient air/oxygen gets to the lungs. Diagnosis is essential and must be made promptly because related treatment must be equally swift and efficient. For instance, a foreign body in the pharynx is best treated by immediate manual removal and not by attempts at endotracheal intubation.

If adequate inflation of the lungs can be achieved by use of an ambu bag and face mask, this should be used until further help is obtained because attempts at manipulation of the airway under adverse conditions might be disastrous.

The first and preferable line of defense in the management of acute respiratory insufficiency is the use of the pressure bag and face mask. Every physician should be familiar with the use of the pressure bag. Two points are important in the use of the pressure bag: the mask must be of adequate size and fit with an airtight seal on the face and the mandible must be pulled forward to prevent the tongue from falling backward. The pharynx should be suctioned clean and an oral airway inserted as soon as possible.

Obstructions can be either bypassed or traversed. Nasal obstructions (e.g., in the neonate) are bypassed with an oropharyngeal airway. Oral cavity obstructions are circumvented with a nasopharyngeal or nasotracheal airway. Laryngeal obstructions are traversed by an endotracheal tube if this is possible (e.g., in supraglottitis) or may be bypassed with a tracheostomy or cricothyrotomy.

LARYNGOSCOPY AND ENDOTRACHEAL INTUBATION. All aspiring physicians must be adept at the technique of laryngoscopy and endotracheal intuba-

tion. The laryngoscopes that are provided usually have flat, straight, or curved blades and distal lighting. For endotracheal intubation the patient is placed in a flat, supine position with his head slightly elevated and extended and the neck slightly flexed. The operator stands behind the patient's head. The mouth is opened with one hand, and the laryngoscope is held in the other hand. The tip of the blade is passed over the dorsum of the tongue into the vallecula. The vector of pull on the base of the tongue is in an anterior and inferior direction relative to the patient. The laryngoscope is *not* rotated with the upper teeth as a fulcrum. The idea is almost one of lifting the patient with the laryngoscope. Secretions and vomitus should be sucked away quickly. The epiglottis and arytenoid eminences are identified, as well as the vocal cords and glottis (possibly). The appropriate size, bevel-ended endotracheal tube is then inserted between the cords into the trachea. If the tube is cuffed, the cuff is inflated and a source of oxygen and air connected to the tube, which is then anchored to the cheek with tape. Intravenous lines are established and blood is drawn for analysis, as indicated.

CRICOTHYROTOMY. Cricothyrotomy is the surgical technique of creating an opening into the airway through the cricothyroid membrane. The cricothyroid membrane is sandwiched between the skin and subcutaneous tissues and the mucosa of the larynx. The lumen of the airway is, therefore, most accessible at this point. Cricothyrotomy should be used only in a dire emergency when no other techniques are available or advisable. Special trocar and cannula-like instruments are available for cricothyrotomy. Alternatively, any sharp blade can be used.

TECHNIQUE. Palpate the prominence of the thyroid cartilage with the left hand and identify the cricothyroid notch. At this point, hold the larynx between the thumb and index finger of the left hand and elevate to stretch the overlying skin. Sharply incise the skin and with the same motion open the cricothyroid membrane with a stabbing action. If the blade is thick, it can then be rotated to open the space. Otherwise, a hemostat or the handle of a spoon can be used to keep the space open.

Cricothyrotomy should be followed immediately by a tracheostomy because there is a substantial risk of subglottic stenosis after cricothyrotomy.

BIBLIOGRAPHY

Baugh, R., and Baker, S.: Epiglottitis in children. Otolaryngol. Head Neck Surg., 90:157–162, 1982.

Bryce, D.P.: The management of laryngeal cancer. J. Otolaryngol., 8:105–126, 1979.

Burns, H.P., et al.: Laryngotracheal trauma: Observations on its pathogenesis and its prevention following prolonged orotracheal intubation in the adult. Laryngoscope, 89:1316–1325, 1979.

Fink, R.B.: The Human Larynx—A Functional Study. New York, Raven Press, 1975.

Holinger, L.D.: Congenital anomalies of the larynx. In Otolaryngology. Edited by G.M. English. Hagerstown, Maryland, Harper and Row, Inc., 1976. pp. 1–6.

Jackson, C.: Acute infectious laryngitis. In Diseases of the Nose, Throat, and Ear. 2nd Ed. Edited by C. Jackson and C.L. Jackson. Philadelphia, W.B. Saunders Co., 1959. pp. 577–595.

Jackson, C., and Jackson, C.L.: Paralysis of the larynx. In Diseases of the Nose, Throat, and Ear. 2nd Ed. Edited by C. Jackson and C.L. Jackson. Philadelphia, W.B. Saunders Co., 1959.

Negus, V.E.: The Comparative Anatomy and Physiology of the Larynx. New York, Grune and Stratton, 1949.

Olson, N.R.: Surgical treatment of acute blunt laryngeal injuries. Ann. Otol. Rhinol. Laryngol., 87:716–721, 1978.

Ward, P.H., Zwitman, D., Hanson, D., and Berci, G.: Contact ulcers and granulomas of the larynx: New insights into their etiology as a basis for more rational treatment. Otolaryngol. Head Neck Surg., 88:262–269, 1980.

Wynder, E.L., et al: Epidemiologic investigation of multiple primary cancer of the upper alimentary and respiratory tracts. Cancer, 24:730–739, 1969.

Chapter 18

THE ESOPHAGUS

ANATOMY AND PHYSIOLOGY

The esophagus is a muscular tube lined by a thick mucosa that extends from the hypopharynx to the stomach. For descriptive purposes, the esophagus is divided into three parts: cervical, thoracic, and abdominal, or upper, middle, and lower thirds. There are four areas of comparative narrowing: at the upper end, where the aorta crosses, where the left mainstem bronchus crosses, and at the gastroesophageal junction. The primary functions of the esophagus are as a conduit and propellor of food into the stomach. The lumen of the esophagus is normally closed and does not contain air, and the musculature is relaxed. The cricopharyngeus muscle at its upper end acts as a sphincter and is closed at rest, opening only in concert with the act of swallowing. At the gastroesophageal junction a functional, although not anatomically discrete, sphincter and a number of valvelike mucosal folds are present that protect the esophagus from the acidic gastric contents.

During swallowing, the pharyngeal constrictors contract around the bolus of food, the cricopharyngeus muscle relaxes, and the bolus is pushed into the upper esophagus. Immediately, a peristaltic wave is initiated in the esophagus. This primary wave, which is centrally mediated, pro-pels the bolus progressively along the length of the esophagus. The gastroesophageal sphincter relaxes to allow the bolus to pass. Therefore, the pharynx and esophagus and their sphincters function in unison.

In most of its course the esophagus is not amenable to direct examination. The esophagus, therefore, is studied radiologically using barium as a contrast medium, directly by esophagoscopy, or by manometry, which is the measurement of intraluminal pressures. The esophagus is a soft structure and is easily damaged by manipulation.

DISORDERS OF THE ESOPHAGUS

Only the more common pertinent disorders of the esophagus will be discussed briefly in this chapter.

Congenital Atresia

Esophageal atresia is a congenital anomaly in which the esophagus is narrowed or there is segmental absence of the lumen. Atresia of the esophagus occurs in 1/3000 births and is frequently, but not always, associated with a tracheoesophagel fistula. Esophageal atresia is life-threatening unless promptly recognized and treated. There are five types of atresia of the esophagus and four are associated with tracheoesophageal fistulae. The types, in

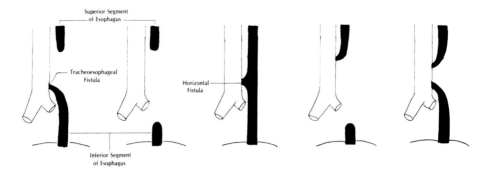

Fig. 18.1. The five types of esophageal "atresia" in order of frequency of occurrence. Four types are associated with tracheoesophageal fistulae (see Chapter 17).

order of frequency, are as follows (Figure 18.1):

1. The upper third of the esophagus ends in a blind pouch, while the middle segment opens into the trachea.
2. Both upper and lower segments end blindly.
3. A short horizontal communication exists between the esophagus and trachea.
4. The upper esophagus forms a fistula with the trachea and the lower segment is blind.
5. Both segments of the esophagus open into the trachea.

By far the commonest atresia is Type 1. At birth the infant drools excessively and the stomach quickly distends with air passing from the trachea. Diagnosis, which must be prompt, is confirmed by the obstruction of the passage of a soft catheter. Diagnosis, however, is best made with contrast radiography, using barium sulphate introduced through a catheter, and fluoroscopic techniques.

The treatment of esophageal atresia depends on the type of anomaly. Generally, the first steps are to keep the upper pouch suctioned and perform a gastrostomy for decompression of the stomach and feeding. More definitive surgery is undertaken later when the infant has stabilized.

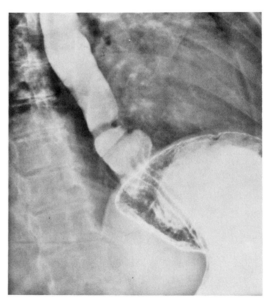

Fig. 18.2. Gastroesophageal reflux and a hiatus hernia in a 70-year-old woman who complained of epigastric discomfort. A small segment of stomach is positioned above the diaphragm.

Gastroesophageal Reflux

Reflux of gastric contents into the esophagus is a common problem in adults but also occurs in infants and young children.

Incompetence of the gastroesophageal sphincter allows the acidic gastric contents to pass upward into the esophagus. The acidity is intensely irritating to the esophagus and causes heartburn and even retrosternal pain. Symptoms, however, might be referred to the throat and neck, and gastric contents might even reflux as far as the larynx, causing chronic laryngitis and contact ulcers of the vocal cords. Gastroesophageal reflux is a common cause of recurrent or refractory pneumonia in the first year of life. In adults the reflux is frequently associated with a hiatus hernia and is more common in overweight middle-aged and elderly patients (Figure 18.2). Reflux is treated with antacids and by elevating the head of the bed.

Achalasia (Megaesophagus)

The characteristic feature of achalasia is a massively dilated esophagus. In achalasia the lower esophageal sphincter fails to relax, while the esophagus itself contracts purposelessly. The dilated esophagus fills with fluid and undigested food, which might spill into the larynx. Achalasia occurs in all age groups but only rarely in children. Histologically, there is a lack of ganglion cells in Auerbach's plexus, the cause of which is unknown.

Patients complain of dysphagia, may have substernal discomfort and spells of coughing, and are chronically underweight. Diagnosis is made by roentgenography but must be differentiated from neoplasm and stricture. The dilated esophagus with fluid levels is seen on routine chest roentgenograms and is confirmed by barium study. Achalasia is treated by dilation of the lower end of the esophagus. This is not as easy as it sounds and should not be attempted by the inexperienced physician. Alternatively, Heller's gastroesophageal myotomy can be performed.

Foreign Bodies

Swallowed foreign bodies frequently lodge in the esophagus, usually at one of three levels: at the cricopharyngeus muscle, where the left mainstem bronchus crosses, and where the esophagus penetrates the diaphragm. Foreign bodies are more common among children and the edentulous elderly.

Impaction of a foreign body occurs during the act of swallowing and can be accurately timed by the patient. The individual complains immediately of "something sticking," begins to salivate profusely, and can usually identify the level of obstruction. An impacted foreign body that causes intense pain probably has sharp edges and is potentially dangerous.

INVESTIGATION. Roentgenograms of the neck and chest should be obtained immediately (Figure 18.3). Radiopaque bodies are easily identified and, in addition, a column of air is frequently present above the foreign body, which is a diagnostic sign. Barium studies are somewhat controversial. They do outline the foreign body but also leave a white deposit on the esophagus, which is troublesome during the removal of the object. A cotton pledget soaked in barium might be caught on a foreign body, and, therefore, will identify a radiolucent foreign body.

TREATMENT. Most foreign bodies that lodge in the esophagus must be removed by esophagoscopy. Those that penetrate the esophagus may cause periesophagitis, abscess formation, and mediastinitis, all of which are potentially fatal. Sharp-pointed foreign bodies, therefore, should be removed as soon as possible. A bolus of meat or other soft material might pass spontaneously after the patient has been relaxed with intramuscular morphine. Digestive enzymes are no longer in use.

Neoplasms

Most neoplasms of the esophagus are malignant, and the majority, by far, are squamous cell carcinomma.* The commonest site is the lower third of the esophagus, followed by the middle and upper

---

*For a more general discussion of head and neck cancer, including neoplasms of the esophagus, see Chapter 20.

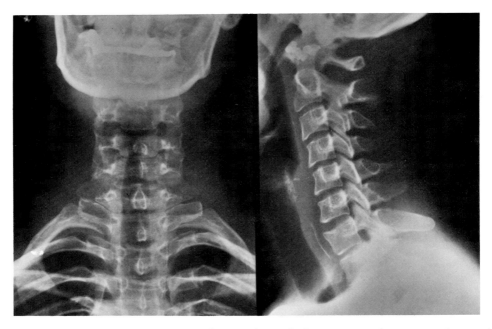

Fig. 18.3. Foreign body in the esophagus. A radiopaque foreign body is present in the upper esophagus, which is visible on the lateral but not on the anteroposterior roentgenogram. The small calcified mass immediately anterior to C5 is the calcified arytenoid cartilage and not a foreign body.

thirds. Tumors of the esophagus are common in certain parts of the world, for example, northeast Iran, Scandinavia (upper third of the esophagus), and parts of East Africa and China. A relationship with diet seems to exist, particularly with a high intake of nitrosamines, and in one area of China a relationship has been found between esophageal tumors and endemic fungus. Neoplasms of the esophagus are asymptomatic until they cause significant compromise of the lumen. The patient complains of dysphagia, which rapidly proceeds to complete obstruction. Occasionally, a neoplasm is heralded by hoarseness, which is caused by involvement of a recurrent laryngeal nerve. Esophageal tumors are delineated by barium studies (Figure 18.4) and further assessed by esophagoscopy and biopsy. Treatment is by a combination of surgery and/or radiation therapy. Prognosis is uniformly poor.

Caustic Burns

The esophagus is vulnerable to concentrated acids and alkalies. Burns occur at the upper end and where the left bronchus crosses and indents the esophagus. The lower third of the esophagus is seldom involved. Diagnosis is made by history, and the absence of burns in the oral cavity or pharynx is not an indication that the esophagus has been spared. The patient usually salivates profusely and complains of pain in the neck or chest and might rapidly go into shock from severe burns. Perform an esophagoscopy but only to the upper margin of the burn. Do not pass instrument through the burned segment.

This is a serious problem that demands prompt treatment. The immediate danger of a caustic burn is perforation of the esophagus and mediastinitis. Later, a stricture might form at the site of the burn. Immediate therapy of the ingestion of

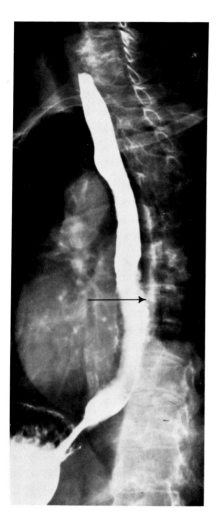

Fig. 18.4. Carcinoma of the esophagus. A barium-contrast roentgenogram outlines a large exophytic lesion at the middle third of the esophagus.

caustics must be concerned with patient survival. Shock is treated vigorously with intravenous fluids and other measures, and the airway is secured. No manipulations of the esophagus are performed until the patient's general condition stabilizes. Nasogastric tubes must not be passed

blindly. A roentgenogram of the chest is obtained as soon as is possible. When the patient's status permits, esophagosopy is performed to assess the level and depth of injury. The esophagoscope, however, is passed only to the upper limit of the burn but is not advanced through the burnt areas for fear of perforating the esophagus.

Limited superficial mild burns are treated with intravenous antibiotics and fluids only by mouth for 10 days. Extensive deep lesions are more likely to cause leakage into the mediastinum and, therefore, should not be treated with corticosteroids, nor should a nasogastric tube be passed. The patient is supported with intravenous fluids and massive doses of antibiotics and is closely monitored by serial roentgenograms of the chest. Burns of moderate extent and depth are best treated with antibiotics given intravenously and parenteral corticosteroids in a sliding dose schedule. If swallowing is too painful, a soft-weighted silicone nasogastric tube is gently passed. The tube is left in place as a guide for subsequent esophagoscopy which is repeated in 2 weeks. Strictures are then dilated with great caution.

BIBLIOGRAPHY

Cassella, R.R., Brown, A.L., Sayre, G.P., and Ellis, F.H.: Achalasia of the esophagus. Ann. Surg., 160:474, 1964.

Code, C.F., et al.: An Atlas of Esophageal Motility in Health and Disease. Springfield, Illinois, Charles C Thomas, 1958.

Darling, D.B.: Hiatal hernia and gastroesophageal reflux in infancy and childhood. Analysis of radiologic findings. Pediatrics, 54:450, 1974.

Holder, T.M., Leape, L.L., and Mann, C.M.: Esophageal atresia, tracheoesophageal fistula, and associated anomalies. Thorac. Cardiovasc. Surg., 63:838, 1972.

Holinger, P.H.: Foreign bodies in the air and food passages. Trans. Am. Acad. Ophthalmol. Otolaryngol., 66:193–210, 1962.

Ingelfinger, F.J.: Esophageal motility. Physiol. Rev., 38:533, 1958.

Chapter *19*

THE NECK

ANATOMY

The neck is enveloped by skin, subcutaneous tissue, and fascia. The deep fascia of the neck splits into many layers, which enclose different compartments. The important contents of the neck are contained in visceral, neurovascular, and muscular compartments (Figure 19.1). The visceral compartment is in the anterior midline and contains the pharynx, larynx, trachea, thyroid, parathyroid glands, recurrent laryngeal nerves, and cervical esophagus. The neurovascular compartment (parapharyngeal space) runs the length of the neck from the base of the skull to the thoracic inlet immediately lateral to the visceral compartment and deep to the sternocleidomastoid muscle. It contains the common, external, and internal carotid arteries, the internal jugular vein, the vagus nerve, and the jugular lymph nodes. There are two muscular compartments on each side. The sternocleidomastoid muscle is in a separate compartment. The other compartments are the posterior blocks of muscles that are lateral to each side of the cervical spine.

The brachial plexus, phrenic nerves, and cervical plexus are contained in the posterior muscular compartment.

For descriptive purposes, the surface anatomy of the neck is divided by the ster-

nocleidomastoid muscle into anterior and posterior triangles. The anterior triangle is further subdivided by the digastric and omohyoid muscles into submental, submandibular, and carotid triangles (Figure 19.2).

DISORDERS OF THE NECK

The neck is subject to many complicated problems, but only the most frequent of these will be discussed.

Congenital Disorders

Most of the head and neck is developed from the branchial arch apparatus. The

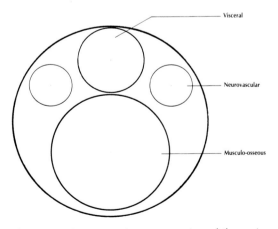

Fig. 19.1. Diagrammatic representation of the major fascial compartments of the neck. There are less-defined spaces (e.g., around the sternocleidomastoid muscle).

212

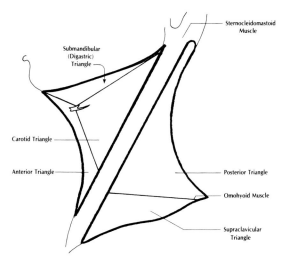

Fig. 19.2. The triangles of the neck. These are arbitrary triangles that are very useful for descriptive purposes.

common anomalies of the branchial apparatus are caused by persistence of the branchial pouches as internal sinuses or cysts, the branchial grooves as external sinuses or cysts, or a combination of internal and external sinuses as fistulae (Figure 19.3). Internal sinuses are exceedingly rare. The third, fourth, and sixth grooves are submerged beneath the operculum, which is a mass of tissue that grows caudally from the lateral aspect of the second branchial arch. The buried ectoderm usually dies but might persist as a branchial cleft cyst.

BRANCHIAL CLEFT FISTULAE. These are long tracts that extend from the anterior border of the lower sternocleidomastoid muscle, pierce the platysma, and run upward and medially between the internal and external carotid arteries to enter the oropharynx in the tonsillar fossa (Figure 19.4). The fistula produces mucus and might be cosmetically unacceptable. Fistulae can be removed surgically. The tract is dissected up to the pharyngeal musculature and ligated at that point. Two short horizontal incisions at different levels of the neck are usually required.

BRANCHIAL CLEFT SINUSES. These are shallow mucus-producing tracts along the anterior border of the sternocleidomastoid muscle at the level of the thyroid or cricoid cartilages. They are about 2 to 3 cm long and are easily removed surgically.

BRANCHIAL CLEFT CYSTS. Cysts may develop from any of the branchial clefts. The term "branchial cleft cyst" is, however, generally used to denote a cyst of the second cleft (which is the most frequent type). This typically presents as a painless, mobile, cystic mass deep to the upper sternocleidomastoid muscle at about the level

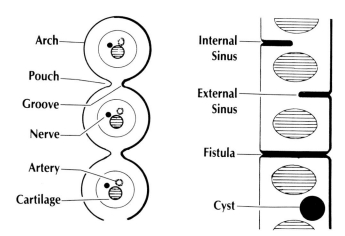

Fig. 19.3. Stylized diagram of the branchial apparatus and associated anomalies of development.

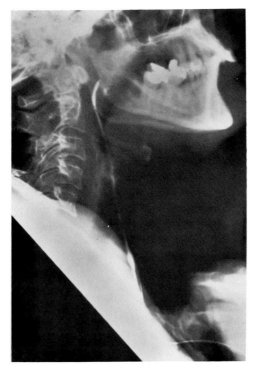

of the hyoid bone (Figure 19.5). Branchial cleft cysts present in children or in adults around the fourth decade of life and are probably excited by mild infection. Occasionally, a branchial cleft cyst presents as an acutely infected, painful, erythematous, tender, fluctuant mass in the same position.

Branchial cleft cysts are treated surgically. Acutely inflamed cysts are treated

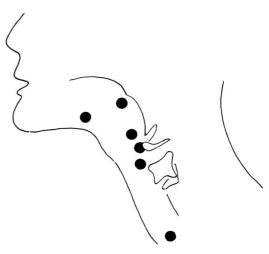

Fig. 19.4. Fistula of the second branchial cleft. Radiopaque contrast has been injected into the lower end and exits through the upper end in the tonsillar fossa.

Fig. 19.6. Sites of presentation of thyroglossal duct cysts. The most frequent site is anterior to the larynx.

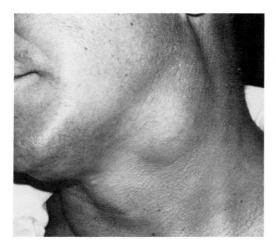

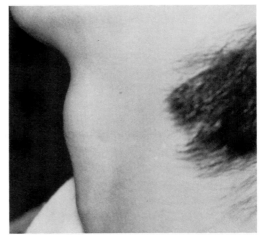

Fig. 19.5. Cyst of the second branchial cleft. This is the most common cystic anomaly of the branchial apparatus

Fig. 19.7. Thyroglossal duct cyst in a 16-year old boy. A painless, fluctuant swelling is anterior to the thyrohyoid membrane.

vigorously with antibiotics before surgery is undertaken. Cysts are removed by an external approach through an oblique incision and usually dissect out easily. A connection with the pharynx might be present, and this must be followed and ligated where it penetrates the constrictor muscle.

THYROGLOSSAL DUCT CYSTS. Thyroglossal duct cysts develop in the remnants of the thyroglossal duct, which is the embryonic tract along which the thyroid and parathyroid glands descend from the foramen cecum of the tongue to the lower anterior neck. Although the duct usually atrophies, ductal remnants and, therefore, cysts may be found anywhere along its course (Figure 19.6). A thyroglossal duct cyst typically develops in childhood as a painless, cystic mass in the midline or just off the midline of the neck at the level of the thyrohyoid membrane (Figure 19.7). The cysts usually expand slowly but might become acutely infected and expand rapidly. Cysts occasionally first present in adults.

Thyrogossal duct cysts are removed surgically by the Sistrunk procedure. This consists of excision of the cyst in continuity with the central segment of the hyoid bone and a core of the substance of the tongue up to the foramen cecum. Incision

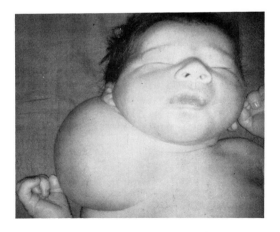

Fig. 19.8. Cystic hygroma in the neck of a neonate.

of these cysts should be avoided because of their tendency to form unsightly draining sinuses through the skin of the neck.

CYSTIC HYGROMA. Cystic hygromas and lymphangiomas are painless, soft, compressible, translucent masses that consist of dilated lymphatic channels. A cystic hygroma is a congenital mass of wide, almost cystic, lymphatic channels that is more commonly found in the neck, face, or chest of neonates (Figure 19.8). They are formed as a result of the failure of the embryonic lymph channels to establish communication with the venous system. Hygromas may be of enormous size and might involve the full thickness of the neck, extending from the skin to pharyngeal mucosa. They require careful surgical excision with preservation of vital structures.

LYMPHANGIOMA. Lymphangiomas are histologically similar to cystic hygromas but consist of smaller lymphatic channels and may contain components of angiomatous malformations. Most lymphangiomas are, therefore, lymphangiohemangiomas. Lymphangiomas may present as a small excrescence on the skin or involve deeper structures, even the mucosa of the aerodigestive tract. They may present for the first time in adults. They are treated by wide local excision if this can be done without jeopardizing important anatomic structures.

HEMANGIOMA. Congenital hemangiomas are not uncommon in the head and neck, particularly in the area of the parotid gland. It is the most common mass lesion in the parotid gland of the newborn infant and young child (Figure 15.2). Hemangiomas present as an obviously vascular mass or as a painless, soft, compressible lump with a few dilated veins in the overlying skin. A bruit might be audible. The facial nerve is usually not affected. Diagnosis is easily confirmed by computed tomography with the simultaneous intravenous infusion of contrast material. Congenital hemangiomas may subside spontaneously. Therefore, it is best to wait about 6 months before beginning treatment. Alternatively, some evidence suggests that the administration of high doses of corticosteroids might hasten resolution. Surgical excision is extremely difficult.

Trauma to the Neck

This section will deal primarily with trauma to the soft tissues of the neck. The danger of trauma to the neck is the possibility of injury to the major vessels or to the viscera. The major vessels are usually injured by incisional or penetrating injuries, while the viscera can be damaged by incisional, penetrating, or blunt trauma. If a major vessel is injured, the neck swells rapidly and substantial bleeding into the soft tissue occurs, which could compromise the airway.

PENETRATING INJURIES. Penetrating injuries of the neck are dangerous and should be viewed with suspicion. Never assume that a penetrating injury of the neck is superficial; if possible, determine the direction of penetration by taking a careful history. Injury to the viscera causes subcutaneous emphysema and, possibly, respiratory obstruction. Injury to a major vessel, particularly a carotid artery, causes leakage of blood into the soft tissues. Swelling might be minimal initially and then expand rapidly. If this injury is left untreated, an arteriovenous fistula might develop later. Therefore, if there are indications of damage to the major vessels, the neck should be explored electively, sooner rather than later. Preoperative angiography might not be valuable and might waste precious time. Routine anteroposterior and lateral roentgenograms will identify air in the tissues, indicating injury to the viscera, or swelling of the soft tissues, which is caused by a hematoma. Large defects in the trachea or pharynx should be explored and repaired. Small defects usually seal spontaneously.

BLUNT INJURIES. Blunt trauma, particularly to the anterior neck, which is common in automobile accidents and altercations, can cause fractures of the laryngeal cartilages (see the section on fracture of the larynx in Chapter 17), separation of the trachea, or laceration of the pharynx. The patient might become hoarse immediately and quickly develop rapidly progressive subcutaneous emphysema. Routine radiologic studies confirm the clinical findings, demonstrating air in the tissue planes. It is important to remember that severe blunt injury to the neck is frequently associated with injury to the cervical spine, which should, therefore, be carefully assessed before the patient is manipulated.

If there is rapidly expanding emphysema and increasing respiratory difficulty, a tracheostomy must be performed. Most mucosal tears will heal spontaneously.

Inflammatory Disorders

The most frequent mass lesion in the neck is lymphadenitis of the upper jugular chain, particularly of the jugulodigastric nodes.

Infections of the Parapharyngeal Space

Infections of the soft tissues of the neck are mainly bacterial. Spontaneous "infections" that are not associated with trauma are usually secondary to hematogenous spread. The major vessels in the neck are contained in the carotid sheath that is alongside the jugular lymph nodes (Figure 19.1). The carotid sheath and jugular nodes are themselves contained in a potential space that is immediately lateral to the pharynx, which is known as the parapharyngeal space. The parapharyngeal space extends from the base of the skull to the superior mediastinum. There are no natural fascial barriers in the space. Therefore, infection in the parapharyngeal space can spread rapidly and cause mediastinitis. Superiorly, the space is deep to the ramus of the mandible and masseter muscles; more inferiorly, it is covered by the sternocleidomastoid muscle. The roof of the space is the external auditory canal.

Infection in the parapharyngeal space is usually secondary to a primary source in the pharynx, external auditory canal, or parotid gland. Fever, pain in the neck and throat, and rapid development of a tender swelling of the upper neck occur, with lateral displacement of the sternocleidomastoid muscle and medial displacement of the pharyngeal wall and tonsil without the edema of the soft palate that is seen with a peritonsillar abscess. Trismus might be present, and usually some spasm of the muscles of the neck develop.

Differential diagnosis includes peritonsillar abscess, acute discrete lymphadenitis, and rapidly growing neoplasms. Treatment is with intravenous antibiotics (e.g., ampicillin or cephalosporin). Localized abscesses are drained surgically via an external approach.

Infections of other Spaces of the Neck

There are other named, potential spaces in the neck (Figure 19.9). These are important only because they tend to become infected, and the infection might be confined by their fascial boundaries.

SUBLINGUAL SPACE (SUBMENTAL SPACE) (LUDWIG'S ANGINA). The roof of the sublingual space is the mucosa of the anterior floor of the mouth, and the floor of the sublingual space is the mylo-hyoid muscle. Infection of the sublingual space is known as Ludwig's angina. The primary site of infection is usually a carious tooth, and the bacterial flora is mixed.

Patients complain of a painful, tender, rapidly expanding swelling below the chin (Figure 19.10). Fever and polymorphic leukocytosis are present. The floor of the mouth is swollen and tender with a soft, watery edema, and the tongue is displaced superiorly and posteriorly. The patient quickly becomes toxic. Respiratory obstruction might develop precipitously from displacement of the tongue.

Initially, a soft, doughy edema of the submental area develops, with redness of the overlying skin. The floor of the mouth is exquisitely tender. The source of infection can usually be identified either clinically or by radiologic examination. Later, as an abscess localizes, the swollen area becomes fluctuant. The airway must be carefully and constantly monitored, and facilities for endotracheal intubation and tracheostomy should be readily available.

In the early stages vigorous treatment with a broad-spectrum antibiotic, such as an intravenous cephalosporin, might abort the infection. If an abscess develops, it must be drained by a curvilinear incision

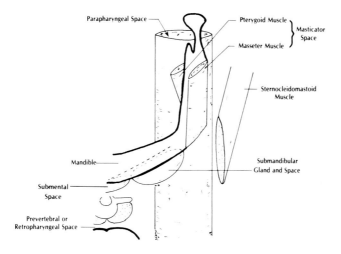

Fig. 19.9. Diagrammatic representation of the potential fascial spaces of the upper neck. The parapharyngeal space communicates directly with the superior mediastinum.

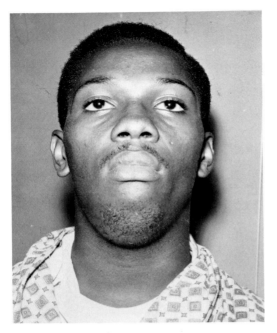

Fig. 19.10. Ludwig's angina in a 24-year-old man. A tender swelling under the jaw and gross edema of the floor of the mouth are present.

that follows the line of the mandible. Treat the infecting tooth as soon as possible either by extraction or pulpectomy.

SUBMANDIBULAR SPACE. The main content of the submandibular space is the submandibular salivary gland, which is bounded laterally by a layer of fascia and sits medially on the hyoglossus muscle and the lingual and hypoglossal nerves. Infection in this space occurs primarily in the salivary gland or submandibular lymph nodes. Alternatively, a dental infection might spread into the submandibular space. Infection in the submandibular gland is by far the most frequent problem, and Staphylococcus aureus is the dominant infecting organism.

Initially, acute pain and tender swelling develop in the area of the submandibular salivary gland. The overlying skin is reddened, and the posterior floor of the mouth is edematous and extremely tender. There is fever and polymorphonuclear leukocytosis. Gentle massage might milk a bead of

pus from Wharton's duct. If an abscess forms, the area becomes fluctuant.

Treatment is first by intravenous antibiotics such as dicloxacillin. Abscesses are drained by external incision.

MASSETER SPACE. The masseter space is the potential space around the masseter muscle, which is bounded medially by the external surface of the ramus of the mandible and laterally by the masseter fascia, which blends inferiorly with the mandibular periosteum. The space contains only the masseter muscle. Infection in the masseter space causes trismus and a tender swelling in the configuration of the masseter muscle. The swelling is sharply delineated inferiorly by the attachment of the fascia to the body of the mandible.

INFRATEMPORAL FOSSA. Although not strictly one of the spaces in the neck, the infratemporal fossa deserves special mention here because of the important anatomic structures that it contains and because of its close relationship to the paranasal sinuses, ear, and jaws. Fortunately, this space rarely becomes infected. The liberal connections between the pterygoid plexus of veins and the veins of the eye and meninges make infections of the intratemporal fossa extremely dangerous. Trismus, caused by spasm of the pterygoid muscles, swelling of the eyelids, chemosis, blindness, and even secondary meningitis develop.

Specific Infections

TUBERCULOUS LYMPHADENITIS. Tuberculous lymphadenitis is characterized by the presence of a firm, sometimes tender, and otherwise asymptomatic mass that usually occurs in the upper and midjugular chain but could develop anywhere in the neck. The mass consists of a single node or a number of nodes matted together. If tuberculous lymphadenitis is suspected, a skin test with purified protein derivatives (PPD) should be performed and a chest roentgenogram obtained. If the PPD is positive, a thin needle aspirate will yield enough material for culture and histologic study. Alternatively, diagnosis may require excision and histologic examination. Tuberculous lymphadenitis demands long-term treatment with antituberculous medications such as isoniazid and ethambutol. Lymphadenitis from atypical, acid-fast bacilli characteristically involves the jugulodigastric or submandibular nodes in the young child. The incidence of lymphadenitis from atypical, acid-fast bacilli is increasing. If localized, atypical, acid-fast lymphadenitis is best treated by excision.

ACTINOMYCOSIS. Actinomycosis is an infection caused by the gram-positive "rayfungus," Actinomyces israelii, which is really an anaerobic bacterium. Infection usually begins in the mouth, sometimes after minor trauma or dental extraction, and spreads into the submandibular area and beyond. Characteristically, a firm, lumpy swelling develops around the mandible. Abscesses then rupture through the skin, forming many sinus tracts. Actinomycosis is an indolent infection and if left untreated, will persist for many years. Diagnosis is easily made by identifying "sulfur granules" on gross or microscopic examination of the purulent material. Confirmation requires histologic examination of biopsies of the walls of the abscesses and culture. The PPD test and the chest roentgenogram are negative. Cultures take a long time and might not be helpful. Actinomycosis usually responds to long-term treatment with high doses of penicillin.

Neoplasms

The following is a list of pertinent points in physical examination:

1. Position—note in which triangle of the neck the neoplasm occurs and its relationship to other structures.
2. Tenderness—usually denotes inflammatory lesions; however, some tumors incite an inflammatory reaction and might be tender.
3. Consistency—a soft mass is usually inflammatory. A firm or hard mass is more likely to be neoplastic.
4. Mobility—fixation usually denotes a neoplasm that is adherent to surrounding structures but can also occur in indolent infections. Masses fixed to the carotid sheath are mobile anteroposteriorly but not vertically, while a mass fixed to the larynx or trachea moves on swallowing.
5. Pulsation—intrinsic or transmitted. Intrinsic pulsation suggests a vascular lesion or an aneurysm. Transmitted pulsation comes from close proximity of the lesion to the carotid arteries.
6. Fluctuation—usually only in a fluid-filled lesion, which could be a cyst, abscess, or necrotic tumor.
7. Bruit—use a stethoscope; a bruit can be heard over a vascular tumor, aneurysm, or arteriovenous fistula.

Neoplasms of the neck may be either benign or malignant. Malignant tumors are far more frequent, and metastatic lesions are the most frequent lesions of all.

Benign Neoplasms

Benign neoplasms of the neck are uncommon. They may be lipomas, lymphangiomas, or hemangiomas (described earlier in this chapter). Neurogenic tumors, although rare, require special attention. Most are schwannomas originating on the vagus nerve. They are asymptomatic and present as painless, firm, mobile masses that are usually deep to the sternocleidomastoid muscle. The vagus nerve continues to function even though the tumor might be of substantial size. Schwannomas are removed surgically with resection of the involved nerve.

TUMORS OF THE CAROTID BODY. The carotid body is a tiny mass of large, polyhedral cells and capillaries that is situtated in the crotch of the carotid bifurcation. This structure is one of a chain of chemoreceptors, which includes the glomus bodies of the jugular bulb, middle ear, aortic arch, and nailbeds. Tumors of these bodies, which are collectively known as chemodectomas or nonchromaffin paragangliomas, are highly vascular and have a similar histologic picture that consists of groups of large cells with clear cytoplasm (zellen bollen) embedded in highly vascular connective tissue. They may secrete catecholamines, particularly norepinephrine, and cause hypertension.

A tumor of the carotid body presents as a firm, but somewhat compressible, pulsatile, slowly expanding, but otherwise asymptomatic, mass that is deep to the sternocleidomastoid muscle at the level of the thyroid cartilage. The tumor is inseparable from the carotid arteries, and a bruit or thrill might be present. Occasionally, firm pressure on a carotid body tumor causes syncope.

Diagnosis is easily confirmed by arteriography, which demonstrates a lacelike vascular mass in the carotid bifurcation, with characteristic spreading apart of the internal and external carotid arteries. These tumors are also easily identified by computed tomography with intravenous contrast.

Carotid body tumors can be removed surgically by careful dissection off the carotid vessels.

Malignant Neoplasms

PRIMARY MALIGNANCIES. Primary malignancies of the neck might arise from any of the basic tissue types of which the neck is composed. Primary malignant tumors of the skin of the neck are uncommon, as are primary malignancies of the cervical muscles and nerves. Probably the most frequent primary malignant neoplasms in the neck are those of the lymph nodes (e.g., malignant lymphomas).

Forty percent of primary Hodgkin's disease presents in the cervical lymph nodes.

HODGKIN'S DISEASE. Hodgkin's disease in the neck presents as enlarged, painless, rubbery, nodular masses that are usually in the jugular chain. The characteristic intermittent (Pel-Ebstein) fever might occur in advanced cases, but most patients are afebrile. A thorough physical examination should be performed to rule out the possibility of the mass being metastatic carcinoma and to check for lymphadenopathy elsewhere and for hepatosplenomegaly. Diagnosis is made by open biopsy. The search for other deposits is helped by scanning with a radioactive isotope of gallium, which is selectively taken up by rapidly dividing leukocytes. Localized Hodgkin's disease is treated with radiation therapy. More widespread disease requires chemotherapy.

NON-HODGKIN'S LYMPHOMA. Non-Hodgkin's lymphoma might also present in the neck, tonsils, and nasopharynx. A firm, painless mass develops, sometimes rapidly, and sometimes even with hyperemia of the overlying skin that mimics infection. Diagnosis is made by biopsy.

Whenever lymphoma is suspected, biopsy material should be handled specifically. A fresh-touch preparation should be made immediately, and sufficient tissue should be taken for B and T lymphocyte marker studies. Non-Hodgkin's lymphomas are treated with radiation therapy and/or chemotherapy.

METASTATIC MALIGNANCIES. Over 90% of the malignancies in the neck are metastases in lymph nodes from a regional or distant source. Metastatic lymphadenopathy presents with enlarged, painless, firm to hard masses in the jugular or spinal accessory chains. They might be the patient's presenting symptom (Figure 19–11). The most frequent sites of the primary neoplasms are in the aerodigestive tracts, particularly the oral cavity, pharynx, and pyriform sinuses. Few of the metastatic foci are free in the soft tissues of the neck, and metastases to the cervical viscera and spine are rare.

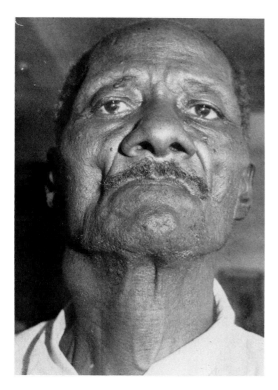

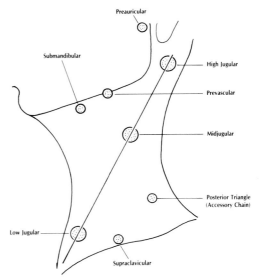

Fig. 19.12. The major groups of lymph nodes in the neck to which metastases spread. The sites of associated primary lesions are not shown.

Fig. 19.11. A 55-year-old man who presented with a painless, slowly expanding "lump in the neck." This was a metastatic lymphadenopathy. The primary tumor was in the ipsilateral pyriform sinus.

The first step after making a clinical diagnosis of a metastatic node in the neck is to search for the primary tumor. A metastatic node should not be explored surgically for biopsy or excision without a prior, thorough search for the primary lesion, 75% of which are in the head and neck. A set plan must be adopted and followed.

Examine in order the skin of the neck, face, and scalp, the salivary glands, lips, oral cavity, nasopharynx, hypopharynx, larynx, and nasal cavity, followed by a thorough general physical examination. If these examinations are all negative, obtain radiologic studies of the paranasal sinuses, esophagus, stomach, and lungs and a thyroid scan and perform a panendoscopy with the patient under general anesthesia. This consists of examining the oral cavity and performing a nasopharyngoscopy, laryngoscopy, bronchoscopy, and esophagoscopy. Biopsies are taken at random from the nasopharynx and base of the tongue. If a primary site is still not identified, only then should the neck mass be sampled by needle aspiration or by open biopsy, being prepared to proceed immediately with a radical neck dissection. The reason for this approach is twofold. First, even if the node is initially found to be metastatic, it will be necessary to search for and treat the primary lesion. Second, an open biopsy contaminates the tissue planes of the neck and makes subsequent radical neck dissection more difficult, with a greater chance of recurrence. In general terms primary tumors and metastatic nodes match as follows (Figure 19.12):

1. Metastases in the higher jugular chain at the level of the mastoid processes are from the nasopharynx and posterior pharyngeal wall.
2. Metastases in the midjugular chain are from the oropharynx, tongue, larynx, and hypopharynx.
3. Metastases to the lower jugular chain

are from the thyroid gland, larynx, hypopharynx, and bronchi.

4. Metastases in the supraclavicular area are from the lung, stomach, genital tract, and breasts.

5. Metastases in the spinal accessory chain are from the nasopharynx and submandibular lymphadenopathy from primary tumors in the floor of the mouth. It is important to remember that primary neoplasms might be as far afield as the uterine cervix.

METASTATIC CERVICAL LYMPHADENOPATHY WITH AN UNKNOWN PRIMARY TUMOR. In 20% of cases of metastatic cervical lymphadenopathy a primary tumor cannot be identified. The philosophy of treatment of these cases varies among medical centers. A radical neck dissection can be performed and should be followed by radiation therapy to the neck and to the regional areas of possible primary sources, including the nasopharynx. Alternatively, radiation therapy can be used as the primary modality of the treatment and again the nasopharynx must be included in the portals. Large, fixed nodes are best palliated with radiation therapy.

Disorders of the Thyroid Gland

THYROIDITIS. Thyroiditis can be acute, subacute, or chronic.

ACUTE THYROIDITIS. Acute thyroiditis is uncommon and is usually caused by a viral or bacterial infection. The patient complains of acute pain in the lower neck or in the throat. One lobe of the thyroid gland is swollen and tender, and the overlying skin becomes reddened. There is fever and leukocytosis. Treatment is with antibiotics (e.g., ampicillin intravenously). Occasionally, an abscess must be drained.

SUBACUTE THYROIDITIS. The patient complains of pain in the neck and usually complains of a constant, ill-defined sore throat. He pinpoints the pain between the throat and the skin and finds the constric-

tion of shirt collars intolerable. Clinically, one or both lobes of the thyroid gland is tender, but tenderness might be elicited only by deep and thorough palpation. T3 and T4 titers might be either low or normal, and ^{131}I scans of the thyroid are usually normal. Subacute thyroiditis is, therefore, primarily a clinical diagnosis.

Treatment is with corticosteroids and thyroid hormone (thyroxine) to suppress the activity of the thyroid gland. The corticosteroids are phased out after the symptoms have abated but the thyroid hormone is continued. Months of treatment might be required to achieve permanent control. Subacute thyroiditis is not accepted as an entity by many endocrinologists; nevertheless, this group of patients will respond to the appropriate treatment.

CHRONIC THYROIDITIS. This condition is also called Hashimoto's disease and Riedel's thyroiditis. These are autoimmune diseases that eventually result in replacement of the thyroid gland by fibrous tissue. The gland becomes hard and almost woody. Treatment is with corticosteroids and a thyroid-replacement hormone (thyroxine).

MALIGNANCIES OF THE THYROID GLAND. Benign goiters are common and will not be discussed here. Malignancies of the thyroid gland may present as a mass in the thyroid, as metastatic cervical lymphadenopathy, or as hoarseness from infiltration of a recurrent laryngeal nerve. Histologically, they are adenocarcinomas and are usually either papillary or follicular. Papillary adenocarcinoma is much more common, occurs in young adults, and tends to be slow growing. It metastasizes to the regional lymph nodes and stays local for a long period of time. Treatment is by surgical resection, radiation therapy, and thyroid hormone therapy.

Follicular adenocarcinoma is much more aggressive and metastasizes to regional and distant sites more readily, especially to bone and the brain. Treatment

Superior wall, which is the inferior surface of the soft palate and uvula

NASOPHARYNX:
Posterosuperior wall
Lateral wall, including fossa of Rosenmüller
Inferior wall, which is the superior surface of the soft palate

HYPOPHARYNX (Laryngopharynx):
Pyriform sinuses
Pharyngoesophageal junction (postcricoid area)
Posterior pharyngeal wall

LARYNX:
Supraglottis
Glottis
Subglottis

Details of the Malignant Process

In the TNM system tumors are recorded as follows:

T =
the extent of the primary tumor

N =
the condition of the regional lymph nodes

M =
the presence of distant metastases

The addition of numbers to these three compartments indicates the extent of malignant disease (T1, T2, etc., N0, N1, etc.). Because of their accessibility, tumors of the upper aerodigestive tracts lend themselves to easy classification. Basically, two methods are used for T classification: absolute size, which is measured in centimeters or the extent of anatomic involvement. Table 20.1 presents staging as it is currently used in head and neck malignancies.

TUMOR MAPS

Neoplasms should always be documented with a tumor map, and stylized preprinted anatomic drawings are usually available in most clinics. The primary tumor is carefully drawn and its determinable measurements recorded. Regional and distant metastases must also be included in the map. Tumor maps are particularly important for future reference, especially where a number of clinicians are collectively involved in patient management (Figure 20.1).

Man obviously is capable of dramatically reducing the incidence of these dreadful lesions by exerting firm controls on his consumption of alcohol and tobacco and by taking the appropriate protective measures in relevant industries. The prevention of malignancies will always be more productive than all our curative attempts.

Table 20.1. Staging Systems for Tumors of the Head and Neck

Size of tumor		Anatomic extent	Stage groups			
T1—up to 2 cm	or	Limited to one anatomic site	Stage I =	T1	N0	M0
T2—2–4 cm	or	Extending into two sites	Stage II =	T2	N0	M0
T3—4⁺ cm	or	Extending beyond the region or fixation of a mobile structure (e.g., vocal cord)	Stage III =	T3	N0	M0
				T1 or 2	N1B	M0
N0 = no palpable regional nodes.			Stage IV =	Any T	N2B	M0
N1 = palpable mobile homolateral nodes.					or	
N1A = nodes not considered to contain tumor.					N3	
N1B = nodes considered to contain tumor.				Any T	Any N	
N2 = bilateral or contralateral mobile nodes.						
N2A = nodes not considered to contain tumor.						
N2B = nodes considered to contain tumor.						
N3 = fixed nodes.						

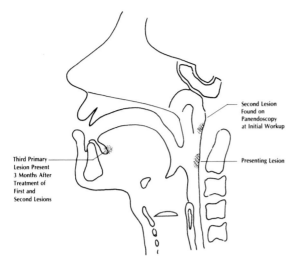

Second Lesion Found on Panendoscopy at Initial Workup

Presenting Lesion

Third Primary Lesion Present 3 Months After Treatment of First and Second Lesions

Fig. 20–1. Tumor map of a 63-year-old patient with multiple primary squamous cell carcinomas of the oral cavity and oropharynx.

BIBLIOGRAPHY

Braumslag, N., Keen, P., and Peterine, H.G.: Carcinoma of the maxillary antrum and its relationship to trace metal content of snuff. Arch. Environ. Health, 23:1–5, 1971.

Chretien, P.B.: Unique immunobiological aspects of head and neck squamous carcinoma. Can. J. Otolaryngol., 4(2):225, 1975.

Epstein, M.A., Achong, B.G., and Barr, Y.M.: Virus particles in cultured lymphoblasts from Burkitt's lymphoma. Lancet, 1:702–703, 1964.

Henle, W., et al.: Antibodies to Epstein-Barr virus in nasopharyngeal carcinoma, other head and neck neoplasms, and control groups. J. Natl. Cancer Inst., 44:225–231, 1970.

Klein, G.: The Epstein-Barr virus and neoplasia. N. Engl. J. Med., 293:1353–1357, 1975.

Lowry, W.S.: Alcoholism in cancer of the head and neck. Laryngoscope, 85:1275–1280, 1975.

Martinez, I.: Factors associated with cancer of the esophagus, mouth, and pharynx in Puerto Rico. J. Natl. Cancer Inst., 42:1069–1094, 1969.

Rothman, K.J.: The effect of alcohol consumption on risk of cancer of the head and neck. Laryngoscope, 88(Suppl. 8):51–55, 1978.

T.N.M. Classification of Malignant Tumors. 2nd Ed. Geneva, International Union Against Cancer, 1974.

Vincent, R.G., and Marchetta, F.: The relationship of the use of tobacco and alcohol to cancer of oral cavity, pharynx, or larynx. Am. J. Surg., 106:501–505, 1963.

Wynder, E.L., et al.: Environmental factors in carcinoma of the larynx. A second look. Cancer, 28:159–160, 1976.

Chapter 21

HEADACHE AND FACIAL PAIN

This chapter will not attempt to describe all aspects of headache and facial pain. Because of space limitations, only the more common problems will be discussed. A few general principles will be presented, as well as a well-defined, orderly plan of action, which should be rigorously followed.

GENERAL POINTS

The following is a list of general points pertaining to headache:

1. Sinusitis and migraine are not common causes of headaches.
2. Tension and other psychosomatic phenomena are the most frequent causes of headache.
3. Headaches may be incapacitating, or they can be easily controlled by minimal medication.
4. Never ignore persistent headaches of recent onset in an otherwise healthy individual.

HISTORY

Obtain a clear, finely detailed history, carefully noting the characteristics of the pain because this might determine the diagnosis. Inquire about the following aspects of the pain:

1. Type and severity.
2. Position—pain in the forehead or face

might be from the paranasal sinuses, while pain in the occiput is likely to be from cervical muscles or the vertebral column.
3. Does the pain radiate?
4. Time of the day—the pain of frontal sinusitis typically begins in the mid-morning.
5. Frequency—is the pain constant, such as with neoplasms, or does it occur at regular intervals?
6. Seasonal variation—suggests allergies.
7. Clustering—clustering of episodes is typical of Horton's syndrome. Are there triggering factors? Pain from temporomandibular joint dysfunction is typically aggravated by chewing.
8. Inquire about associated symptoms such as photophobia, loss of consciousness, vomiting, rhinorrhea or sneezing, lacrimation, scotomata, or other visual disturbances. Has a change in visual acuity occurred?
9. Inquire about medication for relief—will 10 grains (two tablets) of aspirin relieve the symptoms (this suggests mild symptoms)? Do any other maneuvers give relief (e.g., sitting upright, walking, lying down, or physical activity)?
10. Inquire about intercurrent illnesses.

229

Is the patient currently being treated for hypertension, vascular disease, ophthalmic disorders, or sinusitis? Has there been any recent dental problems?

11. Family history—is there a family history of headaches, allergies, vascular disease, or neoplsms?

PHYSICAL EXAMINATION

The following is a list of the steps that should be followed in conducting a physical examination:

1. Look for swelling or signs of inflammation about the scalp and face.
2. Palpate the scalp and over the paranasal sinuses.
3. Carefully palpate the major arteries in the neck, face, and scalp.
4. Examine all cranial nerves.
5. Carefully record the pulse rate and blood pressure readings from both arms.
6. Perform ophthalmoscopy.
7. Examine carefully the nose, oral cavity, nasopharynx, hypopharynx, larynx, and neck.
8. Perform a full physical examination.

Laboratory Tests

Obtain a routine CBC and VDRL. Determine the erythrocyte sedimentation rate, serum electrolytes and fasting blood sugar levels.

CAUSATIVE FACTORS
Psychosomatic

Some determinable basis for headache usually exists, for example, family rifts, problems at work, and so on. Tension-type headaches usually occur in the temples or on the vault of the head. They are not relieved by the usual pain medications and do not cause insomnia.

Sinusitis

Generally, pain from the paranasal sinuses manifests on the forehead from the frontal sinuses, on the cheeks from the maxillary sinuses, around the eyes from the ethmoid sinuses, and behind the eyes or on the vault of the head from the sphenoid sinuses. Pain is aggravated by bending forward, stooping, walking, and jumping. The pain of frontal sinusitis might be absent on awakening but begins in the midmorning and may subside in the late evening. Tenderness is present over the appropriate sinus, and pus might be visible in the nose, or the nasal mucosa might be edematous, particularly over the middle turbinate.

Intracranial Neoplasms

The pain from intracranial neoplasms is minimal at first, then becomes constant, severe, deep-seated, and increasingly difficult to control with analgesics. It is increased by stooping and straining (i.e., any maneuver that increases intracranial pressure or shifts the intracranial contents). Later, neurologic signs develop depending on the position of the tumor. Posterior fossa neoplasms cause occipital pain. Neoplasms of the frontal lobes are silent for long periods of time and then cause frontal pain.

Complete neurologic examination is mandatory. The optic discs must be examined to check for papilledema. Routine radiologic studies of the skull might show evidence of increased intracranial pressure, localized intracranial calcifications, shifting of a calcified pineal gland, or prominent vascular markings. Ancillary studies, such as computed tomography and angiography, are necessary for definitive diagnosis.

Viral Infections

Headache is a common component of all viral illnesses. Severe, acute headache, accentuated by straining and coughing, photophobia, fever, and increasing drowsiness, might indicate viral encephalopathy. A lumbar puncture is diagnostic. The cerebrospinal fluid pressure is raised and a mild to moderate number of lymphocytes are present per high-power field.

Bacterial Infections

Acute headache, accompanied by fever, nuchal rigidity, and photophobia, indicates an acute bacterial meningitis, which is easily determined by lumbar puncture. Meningitis, however, might be more indolent and be the cause of chronic headache.

Miscellaneous Factors

Ocular headaches are caused by conditions such as glaucoma, muscle imbalance, and errors of refraction. They present as pain in the forehead, vault of the head, or around the eyes.

SPECIFIC SYNDROMES

Horton's Syndrome

Horton's syndrome (cluster headaches, histamine cephalgia) is a controversial entity. Typically, the patient complains of episodes of severe, unilateral, periorbital and frontal headache, reddening of the eyes with lacrimation, and ipsilateral rhinorrhea. Episodes last for a few hours, occur in clusters over the span of a few days, and then cease for varying periods only to recur later. Treatment is mainly symptomatic because no uniformly successful maneuvers are available for handling this problem. Antihistamines, tranquillizers, mood elevators, and sympathomimetic drugs have all been tried with varying success.

Sphenopalatine Neuralgia

Sphenopalatine neuralgia (Sluder's neuralgia) is also a controversial entity. Symptoms are similar to those of cluster headaches but are more persistent and are usually unilateral. Theoretically, Sluder's neuralgia is caused by malfunction or irritation of the sphenopalatine ganglion. The nasal septum is frequently deviated to the ipsilateral side with spurs or ridges touching the middle turbinate. The diagnosis is confirmed by anesthetizing (with 4% cocaine or 4% lidocaine topically) the sphenopalatine ganglion duing an episode. The pain should be abruptly aborted. If this test is successful and if the nasal septum is grossly deviated, a septoplasty might be useful. Occasionally, excision of the sphenopalatine ganglion is successful.

Tic Douloureux

Tic douloureux is episodic, unilateral, severe, stabbing pain in one or two divisions of the fifth cranial nerve. The second division (cheek area) is the most frequently involved, and the first division is comparatively rarely affected. Tic douloureux begins in young adults (30 to 40 years old) and might persist for a lifetime if left unchecked. Pain is extremely severe, sharp, and stabbing and lasts for 30 seconds to 1 minute. The pain recurs in innumerable clusters over the space of a few days and then subsides, only to recur a few weeks, months, or years later. The features of tic douloureux are as follows:

A. Classic features
   1. Paroxysmal
   2. Provocable
   3. Trigeminal distribution only
   4. Unilateral in any single paroxysm
   5. No neurologic deficit

B. Less typical features
   1. Continuous or long-standing burning or aching
   2. Not provocable
   3. Radiates to neck or scalp
   4. Remains unilateral
   5. Spontaneous hyperesthesia

Characteristically, there are trigger areas on the face. These are points at which pressure might excite an acute attack during the active periods. Other possible precipitating factors, particularly during the clusters, are cold air, chewing, talking, and laughing. During the attacks, patients become extremely irritable, may refrain from washing, eating, and talking, and men will not shave.

The cause of tic douloureux is still controversial. Evidence suggests, however, the presence of a herpes-like virus in the gasserian ganglion of these patients, and more recently the concept of a vascular loop pressing on the ganglion has been promoted.

Diagnosis of tic douloureux is based on the history and a thorough physical examination that fails to reveal any other cause for facial pain. Radiologic studies of the skull and paranasal sinuses must be performed.

TREATMENT. The pain of tic douloureux does not respond to most analgesics. Therapeutic measures can be classified as medical or surgical.

MEDICAL THERAPY. A number of agents give useful, but usually temporary, relief (e.g., spraying of trichloroethylene on the cheek or diphenhydramine hydrochloride [Benadryl] taken orally). The most successful medication has been carbamazepine (Tegretol), beginning with 200 mg twice daily and gradually increasing the dose until an effective maintenance dose is achieved, which is usually around 800 mg/day.

SURGICAL THERAPY. Surgery is recommended only if medical treatment fails to adequately control symptoms and if the frequency of the episodes warrant. The following maneuvers have been used: section of the infraorbital nerve at its exit from the infraorbital canal; section of the rootlets of the gasserian ganglion (intracranial); injection of alcohol into the gasserian ganglion (extracranial); destruction of the gasserian ganglion by radiofrequency waves (extracranial); and elevation of vascular loops from the gasserian ganglion (intracranial).

Even surgery is not always successful. To a number of patients, the postoperative numbness of the cheek is almost as disturbing as the pain of tic douloureux.

Glossopharyngeal Neuralgia

Glossopharyngeal neuralgia is similar to tic douloureux, except that the symptoms are in the oropharynx. Episodes of severe, sharp, stabbing pain occur that last from 30 seconds to 1 minute and involve the area of the tonsil and hypopharynx. No demonstrable neurologic deficits develop. Examination should include digital palpation of the oral cavity, examination of the nasopharynx, hypopharynx, and larynx and a complete neurologic examination. Occasionally, the inferior end of an elongated styloid process is palpable and can be seen on a roentgenogram. Presumably, the glossopharyngeal nerve becomes stretched and irritated as it lies on the lateral aspect of the elongated styloid process.

Radiologic studies of the skull and mandible and computed tomography of the posterior cranial fossa should be obtained.

TREATMENT. Carbamazepine (Tegretol) should be tried, beginning with 200 mg twice daily and gradually increasing the dose to a maximum of 1200 mg/day. Resection of an elongated styloid process has occasionally been successful. Alternatively, and only if absolutely necessary, the rootlets of the ninth cranial nerve can be sectioned via a craniotomy.

Carotidynia

Carotidynia is still a controversial entity. Many physicians object to this term as a diagnosis. The patient complains of pain in the neck, which frequently radiates to the ear. Pain is often dull, persistent, and aggravated by extending the neck; however, the pain might also be episodic and sharper. The only positive physical finding is tenderness of the carotid artery and its major branches, which is elicited by careful palpation. Even the arteries of the face might be tender. No definitive satisfactory treatment is available for carotidynia. Corticosteroids, such as oral prednisone, may relieve the symptoms.

HEADACHE AND PAIN OF VASCULAR ORIGIN

Temporal Arteritis

Temporal arteritis is characterized by constant, throbbing pain in the temple, forehead, and into the scalp. The patient, however, might not give a clear-cut history and complains of a persistent headache that is not particularly localized. Other symptoms may occur such as temporary ipsilateral blindness, temporary ptosis, temporary hemiparesis, pain in the face, and even pain in the throat. Significant tortuosity, thickening, and tenderness of the superficial temporal artery develops on one side but without demonstrable neurologic deficits. Diagnosis is made by biopsy of the temporal artery. Histologically, there is thickening of the intima and adventitia and infiltration with giant cells.

Treatment is with analgesics and corticosteroids. Patients with temporal arteritis have an increased risk of cerebrovascular accidents.

Migraine

Migraine typically presents as episodic, severe, throbbing, unilateral headache that is accompanied by photophobia, scotoma, conjunctival injection, and, occasionally, symptoms of spasm of the cerebral vessels. Migraine is usually a problem of young adults, but children can also be affected. In children the symptoms are occasionally related to the abdomen with nausea, vomiting, and abdominal pain (abdominal migraine). With increasing age, the episodes become less frequent and milder. Typically, patients lie very still with eyes closed in a darkened room and the head turned way from any source of light. They will not move for fear of exacerbating the pain. Episodes may last from one to a few days and then remit spontaneously. Migraine is considered to be a vascular phenomenon. The initial event is presumed to be spasm of the intracranial vessels. Spasm is followed by vasodilation, which causes pain. Some evidence supports this theory.

The treatment of migraine is based on the theory of vascular spasm and dilatation and consists of taking small doses of vascular spasmodics (e.g., ergotamine tartrate [1 mg] and caffeine [100 mg] [Cafergot]) until the attack is aborted. One tablet of Cafergot is taken every half hour until symptoms abate or to a maximum of six tablets per episode. Overdosage with ergotamine causes peripheral arterial spasm. Prevention has been tried with drugs such as methysergide, but the possibility of side-effects is great. Generally, patients prone to migraine do better in less stressful situations.

FACIAL PAIN

The separation of facial pain from headache is artificial and is frequently impossible. Most of the important syndromes of facial pain have already been discussed in the previous sections of this chapter. The investigation of facial pain, however, requires certain mandatory steps. Some of these are routinely performed in patients with headache. These steps are as follows:

1. A complete neurologic evaluation.
2. A thorough, detailed examination of the head and neck, including nasopharyngoscopy.
3. Remember that pain in the face might originate from the infratemporal fossa or nasopharynx, and these areas must be investigated. Computed tomography has the advantage of showing soft tissues and is the only useful modality for assessing the infratemporal fossa.
4. Comprehensive radiologic studies of the paranasal sinuses, skull, and foramina at the base of the skull, including tomography.
5. Contrast angiography and other contrast studies of the cranial contents, as indicated.
6. Blood tests—routine CBC, white

blood cell count and differential, erythrocyte sedimentation rate, sickle cell screening, where applicable, VDRL, and antinuclear antibodies.

7. Lumbar puncture, if indicated.
8. Skin tests, if indicated by other examinations (e.g., for tuberculosis).
9. Biopsy if a mass lesion is identified.

Pain in the face is a common symptom. Most patients, however, complain of vague symptoms of heaviness in the cheek or forehead or a sense of tightness in the temporoparietal area. There are no positive clinical findings, and the problem is usually resolved by taking aspirin. These are primarily tension-type symptoms, but disease of the paranasal sinuses should be ruled out by physical examination and roentgenograms.

Facial pain might be part of a vascular syndrome (see the section on carotidynia in this chapter). Tenderness along the facial artery where it crosses the mandible usually occurs, and even the labial arteries might be tender. Multiple sclerosis occasionally presents with facial pain that is indistinguishable from tic douloureux.

Herpetic Neuralgia

Herpes zoster trigeminalis is a fairly common problem that usually involves the first division of the trigeminal nerve. Initially, severe pain occurs on one side of the forehead and around the ipsilateral eye. Pain is followed by vesicular eruptions in the distribution of the supraorbital and supratrochlear nerves, conjunctivitis, and lacrimation.

Treatment of the acute phase is symptomatic. The lesions are kept dry and clean by powdering with sterile talc. The disorder remits spontaneously but may leave an aftermath of postherpetic neuralgia, severe burning pain that sometimes persist for years. Postherpetic neuralgia is more frequent and more painful in the elderly. The treatment of postherpetic pain is unsatisfactory because there is little response to the safer analgesics, and peripheral nerve blocks are not generally successful.

Anesthesia Dolorosa

Anesthesia dolorosa is the phenomenon of burning pain in a denervated area. It is fairly common in the tongue following major surgical procedures in which the lingual nerves have been cut. There is no adequate treatment for anesthesia dolorosa.

Temporomandiblar Joint Syndrome

Dysfunction of the temporomandibular joint causes pain. The patient, however, complains of pain in the ear, a sensation of fullness in the ear, pain on mastication, and pain along the mandible. Pain might radiate to the temple, into the throat, and cause severe, recurrent headache. Neither hearing loss nor otorrhea develop. The temporomandibular joint is, therefore, a possible source of otalgia if the ear is negative on examination.

The most frequent problem of the joint is malalignment caused by malocclusion of the teeth; other problems are rheumatoid arthritis, stretching of the joint capsule during extensive dental work, and endotracheal intubation. Frequently, there is a history of bruxism. The pain is usually caused by spasm of the muscles of mastication: the masseter, temporalis, and pterygoid muscles.

Examination might reveal tenderness on pressure over the temporomandibular joint, which is best elicited on opening and closing of the mouth. Tenderness develops over the masseter and temporalis muscles and in the pterygoid muscles. The pterygoid muscles are palpated by placing a finger on the lingual surface of the angle of the mandible just anterior to the tonsil. The ears are normal. Treatment of dysfunction of the temporomandibular joint is directed to the causative factors. Malocclusion is corrected by fixing the teeth. Symptomatic relief is provided by a heating pad and analgesics. Occasionally, intermaxillary fixation is necessary. To prevent bruxism the patient wears an acrylic plate at night.

BIBLIOGRAPHY

Alling, C.C., III, and Mahan, P.E. (eds.): Facial Pain. 2nd Ed. Philadelphia, Lea & Febiger, 1977.

Costen, J.B.: Neuralgias and ear symptoms. J.A.M.A., 107:252, 1936.

Wolff's Headache and Other Facial Pain. 4th ed. Edited by D.J. Dalessio. New York, Oxford University Press, 1980.

Graham, J.R.: Treatment of Migraine. Boston, Little, Brown, and Co., 1955.

Jannetta, P.J.: Structural mechanisms of trigeminal neuralgia. J. Neurosurg., 26:159, 1967.

Kunkle, E.C., Pfeiffer, J.B., Wilhoit, W.M., and Hamrick, L.W.: Recurrent brief headache in cluster pattern. Trans. Am. Neurol. Assoc., 77:240, 1952.

Nair, K.K.: Carotid vasclar pain—a simple treatment. Laryngoscope, 91:605–608, 1981.

Reichert, F.L.: The neuralgias of the head and face. Am. J. Med. Sci., 187:362, 1934.

Sluder, G.: The role of the sphenopalatine (or Meckel's) ganglion in nasal headaches. N.Y. Med. J., 87:989, 1908.

Chapter 22

COMMON SURGICAL
PROCEDURES IN
OTOLARYNGOLOGY

THE EAR

Myringotomy

General anesthesia is required for children, local anesthesia for adults, and anesthesia is not necessary for infants.

INSTRUMENTS. The required instruments are a speculum, myringotomy knife (Figure 22.1), and a good headlight or operating microscope. An otoscope with off-center magnification can also be used.

INCISION. For drainage, the incision should be horizontal across the inferior half of the tympanic membrane. This type of incision usually gapes spontaneously. To insert a ventilating tube, a radial incision is made in the anteroinferior quadrant.

"Myringotomy and Tubes"

A myringotomy is performed as described above. The middle ear is then cleared by suction, and a plastic ventilating tube is placed through the incision, as shown in Figure 22.1. Many designs of ventilating tubes are available.

Exploratory Tympanotomy

This procedure is designed to expose the contents of the middle ear. Incisions are made in the skin of the bony external auditory canal to create a flap based at the annulus of the tympanic membrane. This "tympanomeatal" flap is elevated in continuity with the tympanic membrane, thereby exposing the posterior half of the tympanum (Figure 22.2). Bone is curetted from the posterosuperior bony annulus for wider exposure. The following structures are identified: annulus, chorda tympani, the handle and neck of the malleus, long process of the incus, incudostapedial joint, head of the stapes, stapedius tendon, crura and footplate of the stapes, oval window niche, horizontal part of the facial nerve, promontory, round window niche, and the hypotympanum.

Stapedectomy

A stapedectomy is a procedure that substitutes a prosthesis for a nonfunctioning stapes which is causing a conductive hearing loss. The procedure is used most frequently to treat otosclerosis and congenital anomalies. An exploratory tympanotomy is performed, and the ossicles are carefully examined and palpated to establish a diagnosis. The head, neck, and crura of the stapes are removed. A small hole is then carefully made in the footplate

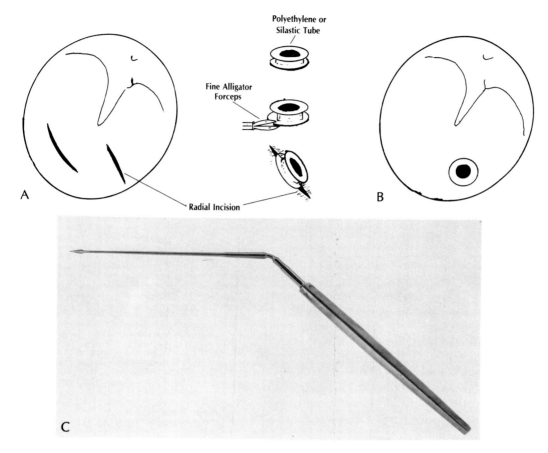

Fig. 22.1.   *A.* Myringotomy. A transverse or radial incision is made in the inferior half of the tympanic membrane. The middle ear is cleared by aspiration. *B.* Placing a ventilating tube (grommet). The ventilating tube is held by a flange. *C.* Myringotomy knife. The knife is angled to offset the surgeon's hands from the line of vision.

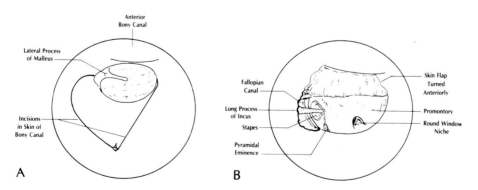

Fig. 22.2.   *A.* Exploratory tympanotomy (surgeon's view). Superior and inferior incisions outline the tympanomeatal flap, which is then elevated and reflected anteriorly. *B.* Removal of bone from the posterosuperior bony annulus, which exposes the long process of the incus and the stapes, stapedius tendon and round window niche.

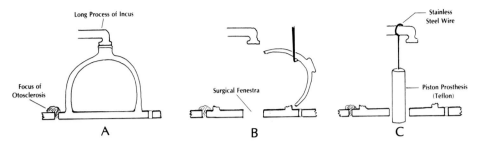

Fig. 22.3. Stapedectomy. *A.* The stapes is fixed by a focus of otosclerosis. *B.* The suprastructure of the stapes has been removed and an opening made in the footplate. *C.* The prosthesis (Teflon and stainless steel wire) has been introduced into the opening in the footplate, and the wire has been tightened around the long process of the incus.

of the stapes. A piston-like prosthesis made either of Teflon and stainless steel wire or stainless steel alone is introduced through the hole, and the wire is tightened around the long process of the incus (Figure 22.3). Gelfoam or fat is packed around the piston to prevent leakage of perilymph. Alternatively, the entire footplate can be removed and replaced by a prosthesis consisting of a plug of fat and stainless steel wire. Thick footplates require drilling.

Mastoidectomy

A mastoidectomy is an exenteration of the mastoid process for removal of infected tissue and to provide adequate drainage. There are basically two types of mastoidectomies: simple and radical. Presently, most mastoidectomies are performed via a postauricular incision. The alternative is an endaural (anterior) incision.

SIMPLE MASTOIDECTOMY. In a simple mastoidectomy the lateral cortex of the mastoid process is removed and all the mastoid cells are carefully exenterated using drills and curettes. The walls of the mastoid process, including the posterior wall of the external auditory canal, are kept intact. The aditus ad antrum is widened, and the epitympanum is cleaned (Figure 22.4). Neither the skin of the external auditory canal nor the tympanic membrane are disturbed. The ossicles are left in place, and the incision is closed over a drain.

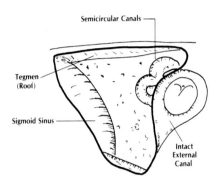

Fig. 22.4. Simple mastoidectomy. All the mastoid cells have been exenterated. The plate over the sigmoid sinus has been cleaned.

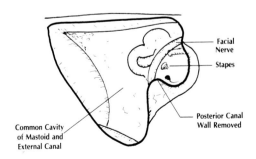

Fig. 22.5. Radical mastoidectomy. The mastoid process has been cleared of all its cells. Most of the posterior wall of the external auditory canal has been removed to create a common chamber between the mastoid and external canal.

RADICAL MASTOIDECTOMY. A radical mastoidectomy is designed to remove all disease and to provide for continued drainage of the mastoid process. In a radical mastoidectomy all cell walls are removed to create a single large cavity. The posterior wall of the external auditory canal is then removed so that the mastoid cavity and the external canal are joined into a common chamber. In addition, the malleus, incus, and tympanic membrane are removed. Only the stapes is left in place (Figure 22.5). The skin of the posterior external canal is preserved as a laterally based flap, which is positioned to line the mastoid bowl (Körner's flap).

MODIFIED RADICAL MASTOIDECTOMY. This is the same procedure as a radical mastoidectomy, except that the ossicles and tympanic membrane are kept intact or a tympanoplasty is performed.

Tympanoplasty

A tympanoplasty is a procedure for reconstruction of the tympanic membrane and sound conducting apparatus. Tympanoplasty was first described independently, but simultaneously, by two German otolaryngologists, Fritz Zoellner and Horst Wullstein.

AIMS OF TYMPANOPLASTY. The surgical aims of tympanoplasty are reconstruction of the sound-conducting mechanism and provision for phase difference between the oval and round windows. The creation of an air-containing buffer around the round window prevents sound waves from striking the oval and round windows simultaneously. The fluid mechanics of the inner ear require this difference in phases at the two windows for effective function.

Certain conditions are necessary for successful tympanoplasty:

1. The eustachian tube must be functioning normally, so that the middle ear will continue to be well aerated postoperatively.
2. The cochlear function should be ad-

equate to warrant surgery. Function can be measured by bone conduction.
3. All diseased tissue must be removed prior to tympanoplasty. Surgery should be performed only on ears that are likely to be stable after the eradication of all inflammatory disease.
4. The tympanoplasty should not jeopardize the patient by hiding cholesteatoma.
5. In type I and II tympanoplasties the ears should be dry before surgery.

TYPES OF TYMPANOPLASTY. There are five or six different types of tympanoplasties (Figure 22.6).

TYPE I. Indications: simple (dry) perforation of the tympanic membrane with an intact ossicular chain. Procedure: the perforation is freshened by excising its edges, and a tissue graft of temporalis fascia, perichondrium, or other soft tissue is used to close the perforation. The graft is placed either medial or lateral to the tympanic membranes and is held in place by pieces of Gelfoam (Figure 22.7).

TYPE II. Indications: dry perforation of the tympanic membrane and erosion of the handle of the malleus, but the incus is intact. Procedure: the edges of the perforation are excised, and a tissue graft of fascia, perichondrium, or other soft tissue is placed to close the perforation. Loss of the handle of the malleus necessitates placing the graft against the long process of the incus.

TYPE III. Indications: perforation of the tympanic membrane. The long process of the incus is eroded, but the head and crura of the stapes are present. The stapes is mobile. Procedure: the edges of the perforation are excised. The tissue graft used to close the perforation is depressed to make contact with the head of the stapes (Figure 22.8) and kept in place by packing.

TYPE IV. Indications: perforation of the tympanic membrane with the incus and head and crura of the stapes missing (usu-

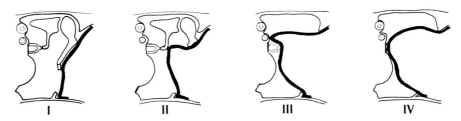

Fig. 22.6. Diagrammatic representation of some of the types of tympanoplasty. The heavy black lines are the fascial grafts.

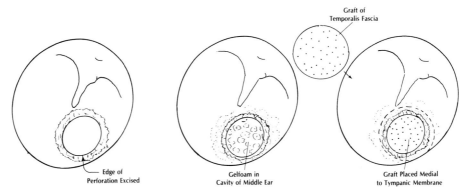

Fig. 22.7. Tympanoplasty Type I. The edges of the perforation are excised, and the squamous epithelium is pushed back from the edges to stimulate forward growth. The middle ear is filled with Gelfoam, and the free fascial graft is placed medial to the tympanic membrane.

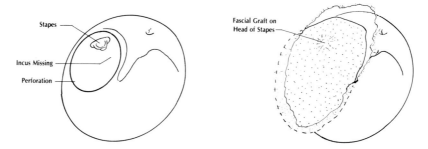

Fig. 22.8. Tympanoplasty Type III. The large posterior perforation has been sealed by a graft that is depressed onto the head of the stapes.

ally found with cholesteatoma). The footplate of the stapes is present and mobile. Procedure: a tissue graft replaces the tympanic membrane. The graft is placed in direct contact with the footplate of the stapes and promontory to separate the round and oval windows and create an air-containing chamber, the cavum minor, which extends from the orifice of the eustachian tube to the round window niche. The graft is held in place with packing.

TYPE V. Indications: clean middle ear, perforation of the tympanic membrane, erosion of the malleus and incus, and fixed stapedial footplate. Procedure: A small window (fenestra) is created in the wall of the horizontal semicircular canal. A tissue graft is placed to seal the middle ear and the fenestra, thereby providing a soft, mobile area that can transmit sound to the perilymph.

TYPE VI. Indications: missing ossicles and ankylosis of the stapedial footplate. Procedure: this is a different technique for handling the situation that was described for Type V. In Type VI the footplate is removed, and the oval window is filled with a plug of fat. The temporalis fascia graft is then laid onto the fat graft.

Surgery for Acoustic Neuroma

Depending on its size, an acoustic neuroma can be removed by one of three approaches: via the middle cranial fossa, transmastoid-translabyrinthine, or via an occipital craniotomy.

VIA THE MIDDLE CRANIAL FOSSA. This approach is reserved for small tumors that are confined to the internal auditory canal. The squamous temporal bone is removed, the dura of the middle cranial fossa is elevated, and the position of the internal auditory canal is determined by identifying the greater superficial petrosal nerve and tracing back to the geniculate ganglion and seventh cranial nerve. The roof of the internal canal is drilled away. The dura is opened, the facial nerve is identified and protected, and the tumor is excised.

TRANSMASTOID-TRANSLABYRIN-THINE. This surgical procedure is more successful for small to moderate-sized tumors that have a maximum diameter of 4 cm. The basis of this maneuver is first to perform a mastoidectomy and identify the facial nerve to the level of the geniculate ganglion. The semicircular canals are drilled out, and the dura of the internal auditory canal is exposed widely. The dura is opened, and the facial nerve is identified and preserved. The tumor is separated from the facial nerve, but the vestibular nerves are removed with the tumor.

OCCIPITAL CRANIOTOMY. This approach can be used for tumors of all sizes but is almost always necessary for large neoplasms. An occipital craniotomy is performed, the lateral lobe of the cerebellum is retracted, and the cerebellopontine angle is exposed. Tumors are totally excised or reduced in size by intracapsular decompression.

SURGERY OF THE NOSE AND SINUSES

Anesthesia

Two requirements are basic in surgery of the nose: adequate anesthesia and efficient hemostasis. Cocaine, applied topically (usually as a 4% solution), has the advantage of providing both anesthesia and hemostasis, but has the disadvantage of occasional severe reactions. Lidocaine (usually as 4% solution) mixed with a topical vasoconstrictor, such as 0.5 to 1.0% phenylephrine, also provides adequate anesthesia and effective vasoconstriction. Alternatively, anesthesia and vasoconstriction can be achieved by infiltrating the mucosa with a mixture of 1% lidocaine and 1:100,000 epinephrine solutions. Under general anesthesia, vasoconstriction is achieved by topical application of a solution of 1% phenylephrine.

Topical solutions are applied on pledgets of cotton or ribbon gauze. Infiltration anesthesia requires 1.0 to 1.5 in. long 25-gauge needles.

SEPTOPLASTY (SUBMUCOUS RESECTION). Indication: for repositioning of a grossly deviated nasal septum. Topical and local anesthesia are satisfactory, but there is no contraindication to general anesthesia. Procedure: on one side of the nasal septum a curvilinear vertical incision is made at the mucocutaneous junction and is carried into the floor of the nose (Figure 22.9). The mucoperichondrium of this side is carefully elevated from the skeleton of the septum. The septal cartilage is incised 5 mm from its caudal end, and through this incision the mucoperichondrium is elevated from the other side of the septal skeleton. The septal skeleton is refash-

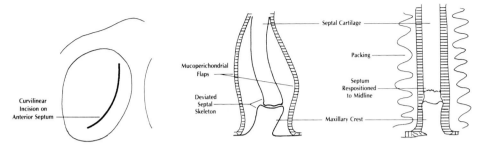

Fig. 22.9. Septoplasty. The standard incision is shown. The skeleton of the septum is exposed by elevation of mucoperichondrial flaps. The repositioned septum is kept in place by packing.

ioned by paring, cross-hatching, excision, and fracturing until the framework assumes the desired alignment in the midline. The mucoperichondrial flaps are allowed to fall back into position and are kept in place there by packing, which is removed in 24 hours.

NASAL POLYPECTOMY. Polypectomy can be performed with topical, local, or general anesthesia. If carefully applied, local anesthesia is preferred because it provides better hemostasis. Indications: nasal polyps of moderate to large size. Procedure: adequate lighting with a headlight is absolutely necessary. The patient is seated, and anesthesia is applied. Polyps are removed with snares (Figure 22.10) or punch forceps. A snare with a loop of stainless steel wire is passed into the nose.

The loop is carefully threaded around the polyp, gently manipulated to the base of the polyp, and tightened, thereby cutting the polyp off at its base. The polyp is extracted with suction or forceps. The amount of bleeding is variable and is controlled by packing with gauze impregnated with petroleum jelly.

ANTRAL LAVAGE. Antral lavage is the process of washing out the maxillary sinus. Two approaches are now in use: via the inferior meatus or by way of the natural ostium in the middle meatus (Figure 22.11). The patient is seated, and the area to be entered is anesthetized with pledgets of cotton soaked in topical anesthetic. Infiltrating the inferior meatus with a 1% xylocaine solution is helpful. A sharp-pointed cannula is then passed through the bone of the inferior meatus into the lumen of the maxillary sinus. Alternatively, after anesthetizing the area, a ta-

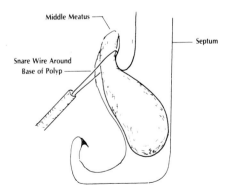

Fig. 22.10. Nasal polypectomy. A snare is passed around the polyp and tightened, thereby severing the polyp at its base.

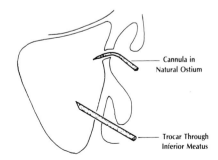

Fig. 22.11. Antral lavage. The two most popular techniques are shown. Irrigating solution is pumped into the sinus, via the cannula, and passes out through the natural ostium.

pered needle is passed deep to the middle turbinate into the ostium of the sinus.

The sinus is lavaged through the cannula with a normal saline solution, which exits through the natural ostium. Lavage is continued until the returning fluid is clear.

CALDWELL-LUC APPROACH. Caldwell (1893) and Luc (1897) simultaneously, but independently, described the sublabial anterior approach to the maxillary sinus. It is now the most frequently used approach for surgery on this sinus. Indications: any condition, such as chronic sinusitis, neoplasms, and cysts, that requires exposure of the cavity of the maxillary sinus. Procedure: a 4 cm long incision is made sublabially in the buccogingival sulcus down to and through the periosteum. The soft tissues of the cheek are elevated until they are just inferior to the infraorbital foramen. An opening about 2 cm in diameter is made in the anterior wall of the maxilla immediately above the canine fossa (Figure 22.12). The cavity of the sinus is inspected and the opening enlarged, if necessary. All diseased tissue is removed, and a new opening for drainage (nasoantral window) is fashioned through the medial wall of the sinus into the inferior meatus.

NASOANTRAL WINDOW. This is the creation of an opening in the inferior meatus for communication between the cavity of the maxillary sinus and the nasal passage. Indications: for drainage and possibly for biopsy of the maxillary sinus. Procedure: topical, local infiltration anesthesia, or general anesthesia can be used. The inferior turbinate is forcibly elevated and might even be fractured to expose the inferior meatus. Beginning about 2 cm from the edge of the pyriform aperture, an inferiorly based mucoperiosteal flap, 2 cm wide, is elevated from the bone and layered on the floor of the nose. The bone of the inferior meatus is then punctured with a special trochar. The small opening is widened with punch forceps to 2 to 3 cm in diameter. The flap of mucosa is repositioned into the floor of the opening to prevent contracture of the window.

ETHMOIDECTOMY. Ethmoidectomy is a procedure for exenteration of the ethmoid cells to convert the sinus into a single large chamber, which, in turn, is opened widely to the nasal cavity.

There are two approaches to the ethmoid sinus: intranasally and externally. Both are best performed under general anesthesia.

INTRANASAL ETHMOIDECTOMY. First vasoconstriction is accomplished by topical preparations. The middle turbinate is fractured medially, and, beginning at the bulla ethmoidalis, the ethmoid cells are exenterated with curettes and punch forceps. The thin intercellular walls are bro-

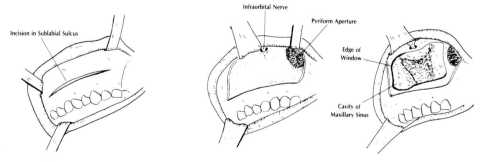

Fig. 22.12. The Caldwell-Luc approach to the maxillary sinus. The incision is in the buccogingival sulcus. The periosteum and soft tissues of the cheek are elevated. Bone 2 cm in diameter is removed from the anterior wall of the maxillary sinus.

ken down to the limits of the solid walls of the sinus, taking care not to penetrate the roof of the sinus into the anterior cranial fossa.

EXTERNAL ETHMOIDECTOMY. A curvilinear incision is made down to and through the periosteum midway between the medial canthus and the bridge of the nose. The periosteum is elevated, and the lacrimal sac is displaced laterally out of the lacrimal fossa. Continuing posteriorly, the periosteum is elevated from the medial wall of the orbit, which is the lamina papyracea of the ethmoid sinus, and the anterior ethmoid artery is clipped or coagulated. The ethmoid sinus is opened through the lamina papyracea, and all cells are exenterated (Figure 22.13). The sphenoid sinus is opened and drained, if necessary. The middle turbinate is usually totally or partially amputated. The external approach provides better exposure and control, and usually results in a more thorough exenteration of the sinus.

SURGERY OF THE FRONTAL SINUS. TREPHINATION. Trephination is a procedure in which an opening is created in the floor of the frontal sinus for drainage; this is usually done for the treatment of acute frontal sinusitis. An incision, 2 cm long, is made parallel and inferior to the medial end of the eyebrow. Soft tissues are divided, and the periosteum on the undersurface of the floor of the frontal sinus is elevated. Using a gouge or drill, an open-

ing 1 cm in diameter is made in the bony floor, and the sinus is entered. Samples are taken for cultures, and the cavity of the sinus is cleaned. A polyethylene or silicone tube-drain is passed into the sinus and sutured into place, and the incision is loosely approximated.

The sinus is irrigated daily until irrigation solution passes into the nose, which indicates patency of the nasofrontal duct.

FRONTAL SINUSECTOMY. Sinusectomy of the frontal sinus is the technique of eradication of all diseased tissue from the sinus, which usually entails removal of the entire mucosa.

There are many approaches to radical surgery on the frontal sinus. The most popular of these are the Lynch-Killian inferior approach and the more modern osteoplastic frontal sinusectomy.

THE LYNCH-KILLIAN OPERATION. Indication: chronic frontal sinusitis. Procedure: a 4 cm curvilinear incision is made the same as for an external ethmoidectomy but extended more laterally to give a wider exposure of the floor of the frontal sinus. After elevation of all soft tissue, the entire floor of the frontal sinus is removed, and the mucosal lining of the sinus is stripped away. The nasofrontal duct is widened by removal of bone and exenteration of the anterior ethmoid cells. A silicone tube is placed as a stent in the nasofrontal duct, and the external incision is closed. The stent is left in place for 6 weeks.

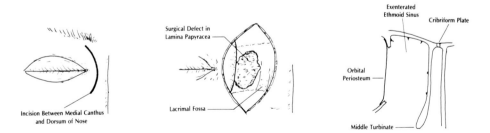

Fig. 22.13. External ethmoidectomy. The objective is to exenterate the ethmoid cells under direct vision. The incision that is shown can be lengthened in either direction. Note that the middle turbinate is preserved as long as possible because it protects the cribriform plate.

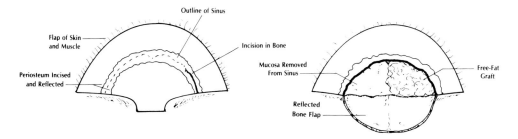

Fig. 22.14. *A.* Frontal sinusectomy via an anterior osteoplastic flap. Soft tissues have been elevated and the frontal sinus outlined. A saw-cut follows the line of the sinus. *B.* The flap of the anterior wall of the sinus is turned downward and the mucosa is stripped from the sinus. The cavity of the sinus is then filled with fat.

OSTEOPLASTIC FRONTAL SINUSECTOMY. In an osteoplastic frontal sinusectomy the anterior bony wall of the frontal sinus and its external periosteum are turned forward like a trapdoor and hinged inferiorly. This provides wide exposure of the cavity of the sinus. Indications: chronic frontal sinusitis, neoplasms, and fracture of the posterior wall of the frontal sinus. Procedure: first, a template of the frontal sinus is made from a Caldwell position roentgenogram. The template is made from x-ray film or from thin metal and is sterilized. The incision can be either a coronal incision just inside the hairline or, alternatively, the incision can be just above the eyebrow. The soft tissues are elevated from the periosteum, which is left on the bone. The template is then used to outline the superior edge of the frontal sinuses. The periosteum and bone are incised along this line, and the anterior wall of the sinus is turned downward as a flap that is hinged inferiorly (Figure 22.14). The mucous membrane is completely removed, and the bared bone is then drilled to provide a fresh bleeding surface. Fat is taken from the left side of the lower abdomen and packed into the sinus as a free graft. The bone flap is then repositioned and the periosteum sutured. The skin flap is replaced and sutured.

TRANSSPHENOIDAL HYPOPHYSECTOMY. The pituitary gland sits in the sella turcica, which is in the roof of the sphenoid sinus. The pituitary gland, therefore, can be easily approached via the sphenoid sinus. The sphenoid sinus is opened by way of an external ethmoidectomy or via the nasal septum because the septum articulates posteriorly with the anterior wall of the sphenoid sinus. The transseptal route is more frequently used at the present time. Either a sublabial incision or an incision in the caudal end of the septum gives access to the base of the septum. Septal mucosal flaps are elevated on each side, and the septal cartilage and bone are resected only if necessary. The mucosal flaps are kept apart by a special speculum. The sphenoid sinus is entered, the bulge of the sella is identified, and bone is removed to expose the dura over the pituitary gland. The dura is opened, and the gland or neoplasms are handled as indicated. The dural defect is plugged with a piece of fascia and fat and the mucosal flaps repositioned and kept in place with packing.

TONSILLECTOMY. Indications (see Chapter 16).

ANESTHESIA. General anesthesia is necessary for children, and either general or local anesthesia can be used for adults. With general anesthesia, an endotracheal tube is used, and the patient is placed in supine position. The mouth is opened with

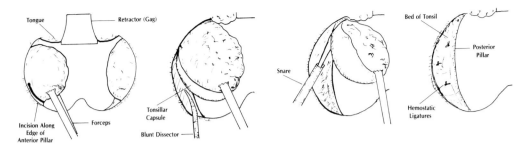

Fig. 22.15. Tonsillectomy. Viewed from the surgeon's position sitting at the head of the table looking toward the feet. The mouth gag keeps the tongue and anesthetic tube forward. Throughout the procedure, the tonsil is pulled inferiorly and medially. Hemostasis is achieved by cautery and ligatures.

a Davis gag, which is designed to keep the tongue and endotracheal tube out of the way. The surgeon usually sits at the head of the table looking toward the patient's feet.

PROCEDURE. The tonsil is grasped at its superior pole and pulled medially away from the soft palate. An incision is made in the mucosa along the anterior faucial pillar and is brought across the superior aspect of the tonsil (Figure 22.15). The mucosa is elevated from the superior pole of the tonsil and the shiny, white, smooth capsule of the tonsil is identified. The pharyngeal muscle is gently separated from the capsule along the length of the tonsil using blunt and sharp dissection as necessary. When only a small pedicle remains inferiorly, a snare is passed around the tonsil and pedicle, and the pedicle is crushed and cut. The other tonsil is removed in the same way. Meticulous hemostasis is achieved by packing, ligation, and cautery because postoperative bleeding is the major complication of tonsillectomy.

With local anesthesia, the patient is placed in a semisitting position, and the surgeon stands directly in front of the patient. The tonsillar fossa is anesthetized with a large volume of diluted anesthetic (0.5% xylocaine with 1:200,000 epinephrine). The tonsil is removed by the same technique as described above.

ADENOIDECTOMY. Adenoidectomy

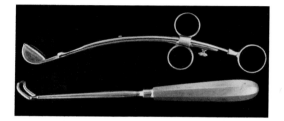

Fig. 22.16. A Le Force adenotome and adenoid curette. These are the most popular instruments used in adenoidectomy.

can be performed only with the patient under general anesthesia. The patient is placed in the supine position as for a tonsillectomy. The mouth is opened with a Davis gag. The hard palate is palpated for posterior notching, and if there is evidence of a submucous cleft of the soft palate, an adenoidectomy is not done. To perform an adenoidectomy, the nasopharynx is first palpated and the size of the adenoid mass is assessed. Using an adenotome and curettes, the central segment and lateral bands of the adenoid are removed (Figure 22.16). Adequacy of surgery is monitored by finger palpation. Smaller tags of tissue are removed with punch forceps. Alternatively, rubber catheters that are passed through the nose are used as retractors of the soft palate, and an angled mirror is used to view the adenoid mass. Bleeding, however, quickly obscures the view. Hemostasis is achieved with packs left in place for 10 to 15 minutes or longer, if necessary. Bleeding from the lower part of the surgical site can be cauterized.

COMPOSITE RESECTION (COMMANDO OPERATION) (Figure 22.17). This is a major surgical procedure that is performed for cancer of the oral cavity, oropharynx, or tonsil. It consists of partial or total excision of half of the mandible and adjacent tissue, sometimes including part of the tongue, and a radical neck dissection in continuity. A number of incisions can be used. The simplest is an apron flap of the skin of the neck with an incision that extends from the lower lip to the supraclavicular area, then loops posteriorly and upward to the mastoid process. The flap includes the platysma and is elevated to the level of the buccoalveolar sulcus, where the mouth is entered. The primary tumor is excised with adequate margins, and the mandible is sectioned in the appropriate places. A radical neck dissection is performed, taking care not to divide the tissue between the primary site and the neck. The mucosal margins are closed primarily, and the skin flap is closed in two

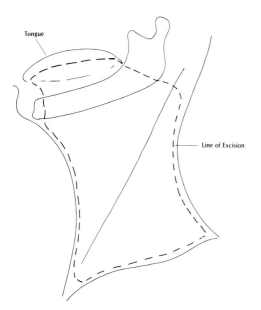

Fig. 22.17. Diagram of the large block of tissue removed with a composite resection.

layers over latex rubber drains or suction drains. A tracheostomy should be performed.

SURGERY OF THE LARYNX AND TRACHEA

Laryngectomy

Laryngectomy is usually performed for extirpation of a cancer. Laryngectomy may be either partial or total.

PARTIAL LARYNGECTOMY. Partial laryngectomy can be either in the horizontal plane (supraglottic laryngectomy) or in the vertical plane (frontolateral and vertical hemilaryngectomy).

SUPRAGLOTTIC LARYNGECTOMY. Supraglottic laryngectomy consists of excision of the superior half of the larynx, with the removal of all structures above the level of the vocal cords. A supraglottic laryngectomy is usually performed in continuity with a radical neck dissection.

Horizontal incisions can be used for easier access. The skin and platysma are elevated to expose the larynx, and the pharynx is opened at the level of the vallecula. The perichondrium is elevated from the thyroid cartilage and preserved. Horizontal incisions are made in the thyroid cartilage at the level of the vocal cords, and the portion of the larynx above the level of the vocal cord is removed by sharp dissection, taking care to preserve the arytenoid eminences, which ensures continued mobility of the vocal cords. A radical neck dissection is performed in continuity with the primary excision. The perichondrium of the thyroid cartilage is sutured to the base of the tongue to close the pharyngeal deficit. A myotomy of the cricopharyngeus muscle and a tracheostomy are performed.

THYROTOMY (LARYNGOFISSURE). This is a procedure that gives access to the interior of the larynx. Basically, it consists of a vertical section of the thyroid cartilage in the midline and separation of the vocal cords at the anterior commissure. The lam-

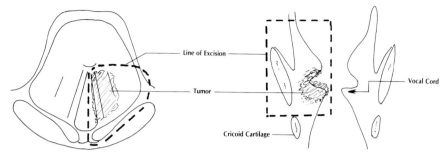

Fig. 22.18. Vertical hemilaryngectomy. The block of tissue removed is delineated by the broken line and includes a lamina of the thyroid cartilage.

inae of the thyroid cartilage are retracted laterally to expose the interior of the larynx.

CORDECTOMY. For early malignancies of the vocal cord, a cordectomy is successful. This consists of first performing a thyrotomy, then excising the vocal cord on the affected side with an adequate margin of normal tissue. Postoperatively, a band of scar tissue reforms a pseudocord. The voice is permanently hoarse.

VERTICAL HEMILARYNGECTOMY (Figure 22.18). If the neoplasm involves more than the cord but is still confined to one side of the larynx, a vertical hemilaryngectomy is performed. This procedure entails removal of the vocal cord, ventricular band, and the ipsilateral lamina of the thyroid

cartilage. The defect is lined with a split-thickness skin graft.

TOTAL LARYNGECTOMY (Figure 22.19). Indications. for extensive neoplasms of the larynx. Procedure: a "U"-shaped incision is made from the angles of the jaws to the lower neck. The flap is elevated and fascia incised over the larynx. The constrictor muscles are seperated from the larynx, and the superior laryngeal vessels and nerves are ligated. The pharynx is entered through the pyriform sinus, and the mucosa is incised along the medial walls of the pyriform sinuses into the vallecula on each side. The hyoid bone is usually removed with the specimen but can be left in place. Next, the trachea is divided obliquely at the second tracheal ring and separated from the esophagus as far

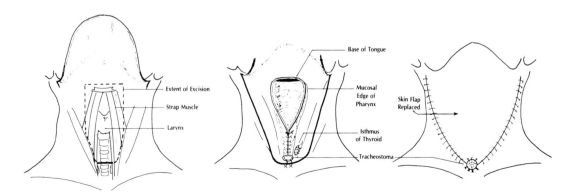

Fig. 22.19. Total laryngectomy. The "U"-shaped flap of skin and platysma are elevated. The strap muscles and isthmus of the thyroid gland are divided. The larynx is removed by severing the pharyngeal muscles and the trachea.

as the cricoid lamina, where the mucosa is incised. The larynx is freed by joining mucosal incisions. The lowest part of the skin incision is fashioned to accommodate the new tracheostoma, which is created by suturing the tracheal stump to the skin edges. A special tube is placed in the tracheostoma for a few days or weeks, as necessary. Postoperatively, the patient may learn esophageal speech or might use an electric "voice box." A more recently described technique for vocal rehabilitation is the placement of a hollow plastic button between the lumina of the trachea and esophagus, which directs air into the pharynx.

Radical Neck Dissection

Radical neck dissection was designed by Crile in 1907. Conceptually, it consists of an en bloc clearing of the neck, with removal of the lymph node-containing tissues and an adequate margin of normal tissue. Usually, only one side is done at a time. The following structures are removed: the sternocleidomastoid muscle, internal jugular vein and associated lymph nodes, the fat pad of the posterior cervical triangle and accessory nerve, the peripheral branches of the cervical plexus, the submandibular salivary gland, and digastric muscles. Occasionally, the ipsilateral lobe of the thyroid gland and the ipsilateral strap muscles are removed. The carotid artery, vagus nerve, brachial plexus and phrenic nerve, hypoglossal and lingual nerves, and the thoracic duct are left in situ.

Many incisions have been described for radical neck dissection, but the best utility incision is the "U"-shaped apron flap incision previously described in this chapter in the section on composite resection (Figure 22.20). The incision is carried through the platysma, and the flap of skin and platysma are elevated superiorly and held in place by sutures. The following sequence is the one I usually employ. First, the clavicular head of the sternocleidomastoid muscle is detached. The internal jugular vein is identified and doubly ligated. The phrenic nerve, vagus nerve, and common carotid artery are identified and cleared of soft tissue. Next, the supraclavicular fat pad is sectioned along the lines of the clavicle and the anterior edge of the trapezius muscle. The fat pad, sternocleidomastoid muscle, and the internal jugular veins are swept upward and dissected away from the carotid artery and the vagus and phrenic nerves. The branches of the cervical plexus are severed, and the hypoglossal nerve is identified and preserved. The submandibular salivary gland is removed from its bed in continuity with the block of tissue. The facial artery is usually divided during this maneuver. The upper end of the sternocleidomastoid muscle and the posterior belly of the digastric muscle are severed, and the upper end of the jugular vein is ligated (Figure 22.21). The specimen is removed, hemostasis is completed, and the flap is resutured into position over drains. A pressure dressing might be used.

ENDOSCOPIC PROCEDURES

Direct Laryngoscopy

Direct laryngoscopy is the technique of examining the larynx directly with a lar-

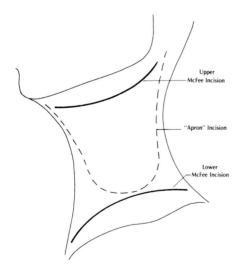

Fig. 22.20. Useful incisions for radical surgery on the neck. All have stood the test of time.

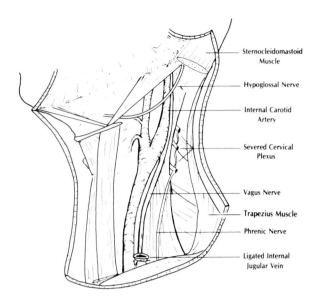

Sternocleidomastoid Muscle

Hypoglossal Nerve

Internal Carotid Artery

Severed Cervical Plexus

Vagus Nerve

Trapezius Muscle

Phrenic Nerve

Ligated Internal Jugular Vein

Fig. 22.21.   Radical neck dissection. The neck has been cleared of all lymph node-bearing tissue. More recently, the sternocleidomastoid muscle is being left in place.

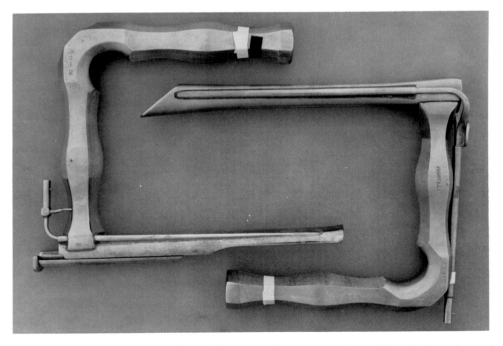

Fig. 22.22.   Diagnostic laryngoscopes. The straight tubular design and efficient bright light allows better direct vision of the endolarynx. One instrument has a removable panel that allows removal of the laryngoscope after an endotracheal tube or bronchoscope has ben emplaced.

yngoscope. There are many designs of laryngoscopes. Anesthesiologists use laryngoscopes with a flat-curved, open tongue blade. Otolaryngologists use laryngoscopes that are straight and tubular, usually with distal lighting (Figure 22.22). Direct laryngoscopy requires adequate anesthesia but can be performed without anesthesia in infants. For young children and adults, general anesthesia is necessary. Alternatively, adults can be examined endoscopically with topical and local anesthesia.

TECHNIQUE. After adequate anesthesia is obtained, the patient is placed in the supine position with his head slightly extended. The examiner stands or sits at the head of the table (Figure 22.23). The patient's teeth are protected with special guards or with a gauze sponge. The lar-

yngoscope is introduced just to one side of the midline. In sequence, the following structures are identified: the dorsum of the tongue, the soft palate and uvula, the posterior pharyngeal wall, and the epiglottis. The tip of the instrument is passed under the epiglottis to expose the larynx. The first structures that are seen are the arytenoid eminences posteriorly; as the tip of the instrument is rotated anteriorly, the aryepiglottic folds, ventricular bands, and vocal cords are identified and inspected. The beak of the laryngoscope is introduced into the ventricle, and the ventricular band is displaced laterally to expose the superior surface of a vocal cord and the ventricle. This maneuver is repeated on the opposite side. The beak of the instrument is then advanced to just below the level of one of the vocal cords, and the

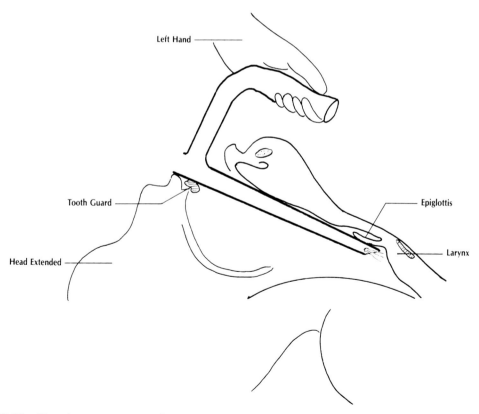

Fig. 22.23. Direct laryngoscopy. Note the protection of the upper teeth. The line of force is upward in the direction of the chin and not pivoted on the upper teeth.

vocal cord is displaced laterally to expose the undersurface of the cord and the subglottic area. Both sides are examined. If an endotracheal tube is in place, the laryngoscope is used to displace this anteriorly to expose the posterior commissure, which is inspected. The laryngoscope is then withdrawn from the larynx and passed into the pyriform sinuses. These are carefully and widely opened and inspected. All manipulation must be gentle, deliberate, and careful. Trauma causes swelling, which might obstruct the glottis.

Bronchoscopy

Two types of bronchoscopes are presently in use: rigid and flexible (Figure 22.24). The rigid instruments are metal tubes of different sizes, usually with distal lighting. Flexible instruments are fiberoptic bundles with flexible tips and channels for suction and for small biopsy forceps. Flexible bronchoscopes can be passed through an endotracheal tube. Bronchoscopy can be performed with the patient under either general or local anesthesia.

TECHNIQUE. The bronchoscope is passed into the larynx either directly or through a slotted laryngoscope, and the larynx is examined. The instrument is then passed into the subglottic area. The following structures are seen sequentially: the subglottic space, trachea (identified by its anterior, white, incomplete rings of cartilage and soft posterior wall), and the sharp carina at the lower end of the trachea with the openings of the right and left mainstem bronchi on either side. The right mainstem bronchus is almost in line with the trachea. The left mainstem bronchus is at an obtuse angle (Figure 22.25).

RIGHT BRONCHIAL TREE. The entrance to the superior lobe bronchus is on the right lateral wall of the mainstem bronchus. The entrance to the middle lobe bronchus is on the anterior wall, and the lower lobe bronchi are directly in line with the mainstem. Secondary bronchi can be examined directly with the flexible bronchoscope, but with the rigid instrument an oblique-viewing telescopic system is necessary.

LEFT BRONCHIAL TREE. The left mainstem bronchus is at a 120° angle to the trachea. The entrance to the superior lobe and lingula are on the left lateral wall and are not easily seen. The lower lobe bronchus is directly in line, and the segmental bronchi are easily seen.

Rigid bronchoscopes are best for manipulation, such as for the removal of foreign bodies and the biopsy of major segmental neoplasms. Telescopic systems are designed to examine secondary bronchi. Flexible bronchoscopes are easier to use with local and topical anesthesia and can be manipulated into the secondary segments.

Esophagoscopy

Like bronchoscopy, esophagoscopy is performed with rigid or flexible esophagosopes (Figure 22.26). Rigid esophagoscopes are made in different lengths and widths for use in different age groups of patients. To date, only one size of flexible esophagogastroscope is made for adults. Anesthesia can be either general or local and both are satisfactory.

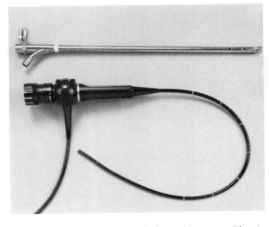

Fig. 22.24. Rigid and flexible bronchoscopes. The tip of the flexible scope can be bent in two directions.

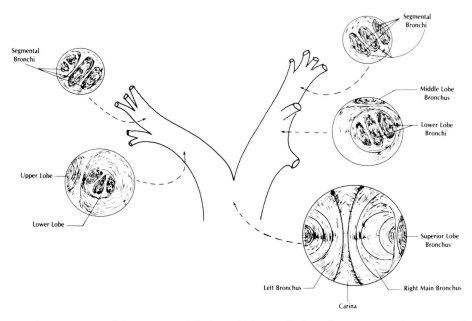

Fig. 22.25. Surgeon's view of the anatomy of the bronchial tree. The bronchi are examined systematically.

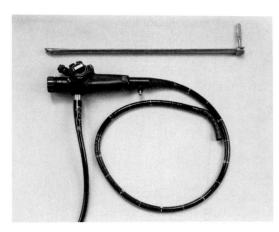

Fig. 22.26. Rigid and flexible esophagosopes. The flexible instrument is more popular for examining both the esophagus and stomach.

TECHNIQUE. When a rigid instrument is used, the patient is placed in the supine position. When the flexible esophagoscope is employed, th patient is placed on his side.

The upper teeth are protected with a guard or sponge when the rigid instrument is used. The lighted instrument is passed under direct vision into the right side of the mouth. It is gently manipulated past the right tonsil into the hypopharynx. The posterior pharyngeal wall is seen, and the instrument is then raised slightly forward, and the arytenoid eminences are identified. With these two structures as landmarks, the tip of the instrument is passed posterior and slightly to the right of the arytenoid eminences, first into the pyriform sinus, from which it slips easily into the region of the esophageal inlet. The cricopharyngeal sphincter may contract or dilate spontaneously under local anesthesia. Under general anesthesia, the cricopharyngeal sphincter is usually relaxed and dilated. The instrument is then passed gently through the cricopharyngeal sphincter into the cervical esophagus. The lumen is kept in the center of the field of vision at all times. The following are identified sequentially: the pulsation of the aorta on the left lateral wall, the bulge of the left mainstem bronchus on the anterior wall, and the pulsation of the left atrium

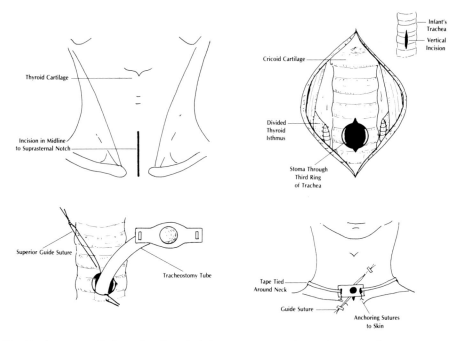

Fig. 22.27. Tracheostomy. Horizontal and vertical skin incisions may be used. A vertical incision is preferable in emergencies. In the adult a disc of the anterior tracheal wall is removed. In infants only a vertical slit is made in the trachea. No excision is made.

on the anterolateral wall. As the esophagus enters the stomach, the mucosa is thrown into vertically running longitudinal folds (rugae). The rigid instrument can be passed into the stomach for a short distance. The flexible instrument, however, is designed for concurrent examination of the stomach. Biopsies are taken through both instruments, as indicated.

Tracheostomy (Tracheotomy)

Tracheostomy is the technique of making an opening in the anterior wall of the trachea, through which a cannula is inserted. In infants and young children only a slit is made in the trachea (tracheotomy). In adults a small disc of the anterior tracheal wall is removed (tracheostomy).

PROCEDURE (Figure 22.27). General or local anesthesia can be used. Tracheostomy is easier and much safer if the airway is secured by endotracheal intubation. The patient is placed in the supine position with his head and neck extended to the maximum. The shoulders are elevated with a roll or inflatable pillow. The front of the neck and upper chest are scrubbed, and sterile drapes are applied. The lower midline of the front of the neck, from the cricoid cartilage to the sternal notch, is infiltrated with a solution of 1% lidocaine and 1:100,000 epinephrine. Either a vertical midline incision, 5 cm long in the adult, or a horizontal incision can be used. The subcutaneous tissues are divided and the strap muscles identified. The strap muscles are separated in the midline and retracted laterally. This exposes the isthmus of the thyroid gland, which overlies the third and fourth tracheal rings. The isthmus is cleaned, divided between hemostats, and the cut ends are suture-ligated. The trachea should now be visible from the cricoid cartilage to the fourth tracheal ring.

An opening is made in the trachea, centered on the third cartilaginous ring, and, in the adult, a disc of anterior tracheal wall, slightly smaller than the size of the tube to be used, is resected. In the infant and young child only a short vertical slit is made. In the child the tracheostoma must not involve the first tracheal ring. Free-standing guide sutures are placed on the edges of the tracheal opening. Hemostasis must now be meticulously accomplished. The endotracheal tube is slowly withdrawn and the tracheostomy tube inserted into the lumen of the trachea. The tracheostomy tube is anchored to the neck by sutures and further secured by tape around the neck. The incision might be left open or loosely and only partially closed.

In the adult, when the use of a ventilator is necessary, a cuffed tracheostomy tube is used. Otherwise, a regular metal or plastic tube is adequate.

Humidification and regular suctioning are necessary after tracheostomy to prevent crusting and obstruction of the tube.

BIBLIOGRAPHY

Montgomery, W.W.: Surgery of the Upper Respiratory System. Philadelphia, Lea & Febiger, 1971.
Ritter, F.N.: The Paranasal Sinuses. Anatomy and Surgical Technique. St. Louis, C.V. Mosby, 1973.
Shambaugh, G.E. and Glasscock, M.: Surgery of the Ear. Third Edition. Philadelphia, W.B. Saunders, 1980.

INDEX

Page numbers in *italics* indicate figures. Page numbers followed by "t" indicate tables.